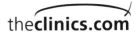

PSYCHIATRIC CLINICS
OF NORTH AMERICA

The Sleep–Psychiatry Interface

GUEST EDITOR
Karl Doghramji, MD

December 2006 • Volume 29 • Number 4

SAUNDERS

An Imprint of Elsevier, Inc.
PHILADELPHIA   LONDON   TORONTO   MONTREAL   SYDNEY   TOKYO

W.B. SAUNDERS COMPANY
A Division of Elsevier Inc.

1600 John F. Kennedy Boulevard · Suite 1800 · Philadelphia, PA 19103-2899

http://www.theclinics.com

PSYCHIATRIC CLINICS OF NORTH AMERICA	**Volume 29, Number 4**
December 2006	**ISSN 0193-953X**
Editor: Sarah E. Barth	**ISBN 1-4160-3821-3**

Psychiatric Clinics of North America (ISSN 0193-953X) is published quarterly by Elsevier Inc., 360 Park Avenue South, New York, NY 10010-1710. Months of issue are March, June, September, and December. Business and Editorial Offices: 1600 John F. Kennedy Blvd., Suite 1800, Philadelphia, PA 19103-2899. Customer Service Office: 6277 Sea Harbor Drive, Orlando, FL 32887-4800 Periodicals postage paid at New York, NY and additional mailing offices. Subscription prices are $194.00 per year (US individuals), $329.00 per year (US institutions), $97.00 per year (US students/residents), $232.00 per year (Canadian individuals), $400.00 per year (Canadian Institutions), $270.00 per year (foreign individuals), $400.00 per year (foreign institutions), and $135.00 per year (international & Canadian students/residents). Foreign air speed delivery is included in all *Clinics'* subscription prices. All prices are subject to change without notice. **POSTMASTER:** Send address changes to *Psychiatric Clinics of North America*, Elsevier Periodicals Customer Service, 6277 Sea Harbor Drive, Orlando, FL 32887-4800. Customer Service: 1-800-654-2452 (US). From outside of the US, call 1-407-345-4000.

Psychiatric Clinics of North America is covered in *Index Medicus, Current Contents/Social and Behavioral Sciences, Social Science Citation Index, Embase/Excerpta Medica,* and PsycINFO.

Printed in the United States of America.

The Sleep–Psychiatry Interface

GUEST EDITOR

KARL DOGHRAMJI, MD, Professor of Psychiatry, Department of Psychiatry and Human Behavior, Jefferson Medical College; and Director, Sleep Disorders Center, Thomas Jefferson University, Philadelphia, Pennsylvania

CONTRIBUTORS

SONIA ANCOLI-ISRAEL, PhD, Professor of Psychiatry, Department of Psychiatry, University of California San Diego School of Medicine, San Diego, California

PHILIP M. BECKER, MD, Clinical Professor, Department of Psychiatry, University of Texas Southwestern Medical Center at Dallas, Dallas, Texas; and Medical Director, Sleep Medicine Institute, Presbyterian Hospital, Dallas, Texas

RUTH M. BENCA, MD, PhD, Professor, Department of Psychiatry, University of Wisconsin-Madison, Madison, Wisconsin

KATHLEEN L. BENSON, PhD, Barnstable, Massachusetts; Formerly, Department of Psychiatry and Behavioral Sciences, Stanford University School of Medicine, Stanford, California; and Veterans Administration Palo Alto Healthcare System, Palo Alto, California

JED E. BLACK, MD, Assistant Professor, Department of Psychiatry and Behavioral Sciences; and Director, Stanford Sleep Disorders Center, Stanford University, Stanford, California

STEPHEN N. BROOKS, MD, Assistant Clinical Professor, Department of Psychiatry and Behavioral Sciences and Stanford Sleep Disorders Center, Stanford University, Stanford, California

JANA R. COOKE, MD, Clinical Instructor, Division of Pulmonary and Critical Care Medicine, University of California San Diego School of Medicine, San Diego, California

DENISE TROY CURRY, MD, Sleep Medicine and Research Center, St. John's Mercy Medical Center and St. Luke's Hospital, Chesterfield, Missouri

RHODY D. EISENSTEIN, MD, Sleep Medicine and Research Center, St. John's Mercy Medical Center and St. Luke's Hospital, Chesterfield, Missouri

MILTON K. ERMAN, MD, Voluntary Clinical Professor, Department of Psychiatry, University of California San Diego School of Medicine, San Diego, California; and President, Pacific Sleep Medicine, San Diego, California

CHRISTOPHER D. FAHEY, MD, Postgraduate Fellow of Sleep Medicine, Department of Neurology, Northwestern University Feinberg School of Medicine, Chicago, Illinois

PAUL GLOVINSKY, PhD, Adjunct Assistant Professor, Department of Psychology, Cognitive Neuroscience Doctoral Program, The City College of the City University of New York, New York; and Clinical Director, Capital Region Sleep/Wake Disorders Center, Saint Peter's Hospital, Albany, New York

MARINA GOLDMAN, MD, Research Fellow, Department of Psychiatry and Human Behavior, Treatment Research Center, University of Pennsylvania, Philadelphia, Pennsylvania

ANDREW D. KRYSTAL, MD, MS, Associate Professor with Tenure in Psychiatry and Behavioral Sciences; Director, Insomnia and Sleep Research Program; Director, Treatment-Resistant Depression Research Program; and Director, Quantitative EEG Laboratory, Duke University School of Medicine, Durham, North Carolina

SCOTT M. LEIBOWITZ, MD, Medical Director, The Sleep Disorders Center of CDS, Atlanta, Georgia

DIMITRI MARKOV, MD, Instructor, Department of Psychiatry and Human Behavior, Jefferson Sleep Disorders Center, Thomas Jefferson University, Philadelphia, Pennsylvania

THOMAS A. MELLMAN, MD, Professor and Vice Chair, Department of Psychiatry, Howard University, Washington, District of Columbia

LISA J. MELTZER, PhD, Assistant Professor of Clinical Psychology in Pediatrics, Division of Pulmonary Medicine, The Children's Hospital of Philadelphia and University of Pennsylvania School of Medicine, Philadelphia, Pennsylvania

JODI A. MINDELL, PhD, Professor of Psychology, Saint Joseph's University, Philadelphia, Pennsylvania; and Associate Director, The Sleep Center at The Children's Hospital of Philadelphia, Philadelphia, Pennsylvania

BRIAN J. MURRAY, MD, FRCP(C), D, ABSM, Assistant Professor, Division of Neurology, Department of Medicine, University of Toronto, Toronto, Ontario, Canada; Sunnybrook Health Sciences Centre, Toronto, Ontario, Canada; and Women's College Hospital, Toronto, Ontario, Canada

MICHAEL J. PETERSON, MD, PhD, Wyeth-HealthEmotions Research Fellow and Clinical Instructor, Department of Psychiatry, University of Wisconsin-Madison, Madison, Wisconsin

DAVID T. PLANTE, MD, Clinical Fellow in Psychiatry, Department of Psychiatry, Massachusetts General Hospital and McLean Hospital, Harvard Medical School, Boston, Massachusetts

CLAUDIO N. SOARES, MD, PhD, Associate Professor, Department of Psychiatry and Behavioural Neurosciences, McMaster University, Hamilton, Ontario, Canada; and Director, Women's Health Concerns Clinic, St. Joseph's Healthcare Hamilton, Hamilton, Ontario, Canada

ARTHUR J. SPIELMAN, PhD, Professor, Department of Psychology, Cognitive Neuroscience Doctoral Program, The City College of the City University of New York, New York; Associate Director, Center for Sleep Medicine, New York–Presbyterian Hospital, Weill Cornell Medical School, New York; and Center for Sleep Disorders Medicine and Research, New York Methodist Hospital, Brooklyn, New York

JAMES K. WALSH, PhD, Sleep Medicine and Research Center, St. John's Mercy Medical Center and St. Luke's Hospital, Chesterfield, Missouri

JOHN W. WINKELMAN, MD, PhD, Assistant Professor of Psychiatry, Divisions of Sleep Medicine and Psychiatry, Brigham & Women's Hospital, Harvard Medical School, Boston, Massachusetts; and Medical Director, Sleep Health Center Affiliated with Brigham & Women's Hospital, Brighton, Massachusetts

CHIEN-MING YANG, PhD, Associate Professor, Department of Psychology and Research Center for Mind, Brain and Learning, National Chengchi University, Taipei, Taiwan

PHYLLIS C. ZEE, MD, PhD, Professor of Neurology, Northwestern University Feinberg School of Medicine, Chicago, Illinois

The Sleep–Psychiatry Interface

> Sleep is a vital, highly organized process regulated by complex systems
> of neuronal networks and neurotransmitters. Sleep plays an important
> role in the regulation of central nervous system and body physiologic
> functions. Sleep architecture changes with age and is easily susceptible
> to external and internal disruption. Reduction or disruption of sleep can
> affect numerous functions varying from thermoregulation to learning
> and memory during the waking state.

> When patients report problems sleeping, a psychiatrist must determine
> their significance based on frequency, duration, and daytime impair-
> ment. Because up to 50% of adults report sleep problems in any year,
> it is necessary to define when insomnia becomes long-standing, severe,
> and a complication to daytime function. Psychiatrists must determine if
> a sleep disturbance reduces mood, motor performance, or cognitive
> function. If insomnia syndrome is present, major depression, dysthy-
> mia, and anxiety disorders commonly are comorbid. To assist in eval-
> uating insomnia, psychiatrists are urged to use the 6 Ps + M of
> insomnia model to conceptualize the characteristics of the insomnia
> and coordinate therapeutic intervention.

> Views on the etiology and morbidities associated with insomnia are
> evolving and affect clinicians' approach to the pharmacologic manage-
> ment of insomnia. Currently, benzodiazepine receptor agonists (BzRAs)
> and a single melatonin receptor agonist are recognized as safe and effi-
> cacious hypnotics. Variability in BzRAs, pharmacokinetics, and manip-
> ulation of dose provide clinicians with options that meet the needs of
> most patients. Other drugs (eg, sedating antidepressants) also are

used commonly in clinical practice to treat insomnia, but evidence is lacking to support this most cases. Improvement in managing insomnia will result from systematic research with these drugs, with drugs in development, and with novel uses, such as cotherapy.

Many psychiatric patients have significant sleep disturbance. Insomnia should be addressed directly even when comorbid with a psychiatric disorder. Nonpharmacologic treatments are effective and especially well suited for long-term management of sleep problems. Although the techniques themselves are fairly straightforward, they work best when applied with the kind of clinical insight and experience that psychiatrists regularly draw on in their practices. This article briefly reviews the evaluation of insomnia, with the aim of eliciting clinical material sufficiently comprehensive to inform the choice of treatment, and provides a practical overview of the basic nondrug approaches to insomnia, emphasizing what the clinician and the patient may expect from their application.

Excessive daytime sleepiness or pathologic sleepiness is a complaint found in patients who experience somnolence at unwanted times that adversely affects their daytime function. Although psychiatric illness, chronic medical illness, or medication side effects may be causes for fatigue, insufficient sleep is the most common cause of excessive daytime sleepiness in the general population. When an individual complains of frank sleepiness, in addition to insufficient sleep, important considerations in these patients are disturbances in the normal homeostatic mechanisms that govern sleep and wakefulness. This article summarizes the clinical presentation, the differential diagnosis, commonly used diagnostic tools, and treatment options for patients complaining of excessive daytime sleepiness.

Sleep disorders, including restless legs syndrome and periodic limb movement disorder, sleep apnea syndrome, and narcolepsy, are prevalent medical conditions, likely to be seen by practicing psychiatrists. Awareness of these conditions and their presentations, pathophysiology, and treatment allows psychiatrists to treat these conditions where appropriate, to minimize complications and health consequences associated with delayed diagnosis, and to reduce the burden of disease that these conditions may place on patients already experiencing primary psychiatric disorders.

Parasomnias are undesirable behaviors that arise from sleep but are not fully under voluntary control. Parasomnias are grouped broadly according to whether they arise from non–rapid eye movement (NREM) or rapid eye movement (NREM) sleep. NREM parasomnias are disorders of arousal that occur along a continuum of behavioral, affective, and autonomic activation. REM-related parasomnias include REM sleep behavior disorder, sleep paralysis, and nightmare disorder. Parasomnias can often be managed successfully using behavioral and pharmacologic therapies.

Circadian rhythm sleep disorders are characterized by a desynchronization between the timing of the intrinsic circadian clock and the extrinsic light–dark and social/activity cycles resulting in symptoms of excessive sleepiness and insomnia. This article explores the six recognized circadian rhythm sleep disorders: delayed sleep phase syndrome, advanced sleep phase syndrome, non–24-hour sleep–wake syndrome, irregular sleep–wake pattern, shift work sleep syndrome, and time zone change syndrome. Additionally discussed are the therapeutic roles of synchronizing agents, such as light and melatonin.

Sleep disturbances are among the most common symptoms in patients who have acute episodes of mood disorders, and patients who have mood disorders exhibit higher rates of sleep disturbances than the general population, even during periods of remission. Insomnia and hypersomnia are associated with an increased risk for the development or recurrence of mood disorders and increased severity of psychiatric symptoms. Sleep electroencephalogram recordings have identified objective abnormalities associated with mood disorders, providing insight into the neurobiologic relationships between mood and sleep. Future studies will continue to investigate this association and potentially improve treatment of sleep and mood disorders.

In untreated schizophrenia, psychotic decompensation is associated with profound insomnia, one of the prodromal symptoms associated with psychotic relapse. First- and second-generation antipsychotic medication can ameliorate this insomnia, but side effects may include sedation or residual insomnia. Patients who are clinically stable and medicated may continue to experience disturbed sleep, including long sleep-onset latencies, poor sleep efficiency, slow wave sleep deficits, and short rapid eye movement latencies. Schizophrenia also can be associated with comorbid sleep disorders, which may be enhanced or induced by antipsychotic medication. Sleep disorders in schizophrenia should be treated vigorously because normalized sleep and its restorative processes may be essential for a positive clinical outcome.

Sleep disturbances commonly are associated with anxiety disorders, in particular generalized anxiety disorder, panic disorder, and posttraumatic stress disorder. Sleep loss may exacerbate and contribute to relapse of these conditions. Core features of panic disorder and post-traumatic stress disorder occur in relation to sleep (sleep panic attacks or re-experiencing nightmares). Investigation of sleep in anxiety disorders provides clues to mechanisms of arousal regulation relevant to insomnia and pathologic anxiety. Established treatments for anxiety disorders and insomnia have many overlapping components; however, optimal sequencing and integration of the approaches remain underinvestigated.

Pediatric sleep disorders are common, affecting approximately 25% to 40% of children and adolescents. Although there are several different types of sleep disorders that affect youth, each disorder can have a significant impact on daytime functioning and development, including learning, growth, behavior, and emotion regulation. Researchers are only beginning to uncover the interaction between sleep and psychiatric disorders in children and adolescents, including depression, attention-deficit/hyperactivity disorder, and autism. This article reviews normal sleep and sleep disorders in children and adolescents, the assessment of sleep in pediatric populations, common pediatric sleep disorders, and sleep in children who have common psychiatric disorders.

For many older adults, aging is associated with significant changes in sleep. There are a variety of potential causes, including primary sleep disorders, circadian rhythm disturbances, insomnia, depression, medical illness, and medications. As with younger adults, the diagnosis requires a thorough sleep history and an overnight sleep recording when appropriate. Treatment should address the primary sleep problem and can result in significant improvement in quality of life and daytime functioning in older adults.

Claudio N. Soares and Brian J. Murray

Sleep disorders are more prevalent in women than in men. Sex hormones modulate sleep-wake behaviors and mood and may contribute to heightened risk across the life cycle of women. Sleep disorders may have a unique expression in women, emerging throughout their reproductive life cycle. These conditions require careful treatment strategy to manage medical, hormonal, and behavioral contributing factors to poor sleep efficiency and impaired quality of life. This review focuses on clinical evidence for sleep disorders in women and discusses existing evidence of risk factors and treatment options for insomnia and sleep-disordered breathing in women.

Andrew D. Krystal

Understanding of the relationship between co-occurring sleep and psychiatric disorders has undergone a radical change. The longstanding perspective that sleep problems invariably are a symptom of a psychiatric disorder is giving way to understanding that complex bidirectional relationships may exist. This change has opened doors to new directions in research and led to changes in guidelines for clinical practice. This article discusses promising future directions for building on this foundation, including developing lines of research currently underway, studying mechanisms that underlie the relationships between sleep and psychiatric disorders; and developing treatment strategies that target these mechanisms to lead to better treatment of sleep disorders and psychiatric disorders.

PSYCHIATRIC CLINICS
OF NORTH AMERICA

PSYCHIATRIC CLINICS
OF NORTH AMERICA

Preface

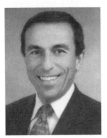

Karl Doghramji, MD

Guest Editor

Complaints regarding sleep and wakefulness are commonly voiced by patients suffering from a wide variety of psychiatric disorders. It is not surprising, therefore, that sleep and its disorders are of great interest to psychiatrists. One of the earliest theoreticians to focus on sleep was Sigmund Freud. In *The Interpretation of Dreams*, published in 1900, he advanced the notion that sleep and dreams are windows into the mysteries of the unconscious mind. Since then, dream analysis has played a central role in psychoanalytic technique. The search for a physiological basis for psychic phenomena led Hans Berger, a German psychiatrist, to record the first human electroencephalogram (EEG) in 1924. This was the technological foundation for the milestone discovery of rapid eye movement (REM) sleep by Aesrinsky and Kleitman in 1953. The subsequent surge in research into electrophysiological sleep, triggered by this discovery, further advanced the role of sleep as a probe into psychiatric phenomena. We now know, for example, that the sleep EEG of individuals suffering from major depression adopts characteristic and predictable patterns. Such findings have led to theoretical formulations regarding the pathophysiological underpinnings of affective illness.

The interface between sleep and psychiatric disease took on additional dimensions following observations that changes in sleep and wakefulness can independently predict psychiatric phenomena. Several longitudinal studies, spanning the course of up to 40 years, indicate that current and persistent complaints regarding sleep and wakefulness predict future vulnerability to psychiatric illness. A constellation of sleep EEG patterns in healthy individuals identifies vulnerability for depression and, in prior depressives, predicts future relapse; the correction of these EEG abnormalities in depressed individuals by certain antidepressants predicts subsequent antidepressant response.

0193-953X/06/$ – see front matter
doi:10.1016/j.psc.2006.10.001

Furthermore, certain behavioral manipulations of sleep have a positive impact on depressive symptoms, and the correction of sleep abnormalities with certain hypnotic agents in depressives receiving antidepressant treatment can impart benefit for depressive symptoms above and beyond the benefit derived from treatment with antidepressants alone. Disturbances of sleep and wakefulness can no longer be viewed, therefore, solely as symptoms of, and markers for, psychiatric disease. Rather, the results of decades of research, along with emerging data, support the additional viewpoint that they can be independent contributors to psychiatric phenomena, related to psychiatric illness in a bi-directional fashion.

That sleep disturbances can be primary is highlighted by the fact that the recently introduced International Classification of Sleep Disorders, Second Edition, lists more than 80 primary sleep disorders, many of which feature psychiatric symptoms. The understanding of these conditions is, therefore, of crucial importance to psychiatrists. The clinical evaluation and treatment of these disorders is the professional focus of thousands of sleep medicine physicians, many of them also psychiatrists. Sleep medicine is now an accepted medical subspecialty, and all diplomates of the American Board of Psychiatry and Neurology are eligible to complete training and become board certified in this field.

The goal of this issue of the *Psychiatric Clinics of North America* is to explore the multifaceted interface that exists between sleep and psychiatry, one that has been shaped by decades of research and clinical experience. We begin with a review of the neurophysiology of normal sleep and circadian rhythms. We then examine the sleep-related symptoms most commonly encountered by psychiatrists, insomnia and excessive sleepiness. We then elaborate upon commonly encountered sleep disorders that present with psychiatric symptoms, and specific psychiatric disorders that feature disturbances of sleep and wakefulness. We explore how sleep disturbances are affected by gender and age. Finally, we speculate as to how the future will define the multifaceted interface that exists between sleep and psychiatry.

I am indebted to the contributing authors of this issue. Many are luminaries in their individual areas of research and clinical work. Without them, an issue of this scope would have been impossible. I am also grateful to my family, Laurel Jeanne, Mark, and Leah, for their loving support.

Karl Doghramji, MD
Department of Psychiatry and Human Behavior
Jefferson Medical College
Sleep Disorders Center
Thomas Jefferson University
1015 Walnut Street, Suite 319
Philadelphia, PA 19107, USA

E-mail address: Karl.Doghramji@jefferson.edu

Normal Sleep and Circadian Rhythms: Neurobiologic Mechanisms Underlying Sleep and Wakefulness

Dimitri Markov, MD[a],*, Marina Goldman, MD[b]

[a]Department of Psychiatry and Human Behavior, Thomas Jefferson University, 1020 Sansom Street, Thompson Building, Suite 1652, Philadelphia, PA 19107-5004, USA
[b]Department of Psychiatry and Human Behavior, University of Pennsylvania, Philadelphia, Pennsylvania

T he cyclic repetition of sleep and wakefulness states is essential to the basic functioning of all higher animals, including humans. As understanding of the neurobiology of sleep increases, clinicians no longer view it as a passive state (ie, sleep as merely the absence of wakefulness). Sleep is an active neurobehavioral state that is maintained through a highly organized interaction of neurons and neural circuits in the central nervous system (CNS).

DEFINING SLEEP

Sleep physicians define human sleep on the basis of an individual's observed behavior and accompanying physiologic changes in the brain's electrical activity as the brain transitions between wakefulness and sleep. Behaviorally, human sleep is characterized by reclined position, closed eyes, decreased movement, and decreased responsivity to internal and external environment. The responsiveness to stimuli is not completely absent; a sleeper continues to process some sensory information during sleep, and meaningful stimuli are more likely to produce arousals than nonmeaningful ones. A sound of one's own name is more likely to arouse a sleeper than some other sound, and the cry of her infant is more likely to arouse a sleeping mother than a cry of another infant.

Constituents of Sleep

Sleep consists of two strikingly different states, rapid-eye-movement (REM) sleep and non-REM (NREM) sleep. NREM sleep can be subdivided further into four stages.

Polysomnography is the "gold standard" technique that simultaneously records the three physiologic measures that define the main stages of sleep and wakefulness. These measures include muscle tone, recorded through electromyogram (EMG); eye movements, recorded through electro-oculogram

*Corresponding author. E-mail address: dimitri.markov@jefferson.edu (D. Markov).

0193-953X/06/$ – see front matter
doi:10.1016/j.psc.2006.09.008

(EOG); and brain activity, recorded through electroencephalogram (EEG) [1]. The clinical polysomnogram, the purpose of which is to detect findings that are characteristic of certain sleep disorders, includes, in addition to these three variables, the following: monitors for airflow at the nose and mouth, respiratory effort strain gauges placed around the chest and abdomen, and noninvasive oxygen saturation monitors that function by introducing a beam of light through the skin. Other parameters include the electrocardiogram and EMG of the anterior tibialis muscles, which are intended to detect periodic leg movements. Finally, a patient's gross body movements are monitored continuously by audiovisual means.

The EEG pattern of drowsy wakefulness consists of low-voltage rhythmic alpha activity (8–13 cycles per second [Hz]). In stage 1 of NREM sleep, the low-voltage mixed frequency theta waves (4–8 Hz) replace alpha rhythm of wakefulness. Slow asynchronous eye movements are seen on the EOG in the beginning of stage 1 sleep and disappear in a few minutes. The muscle activity is highest during wakefulness and diminishes as sleep approaches. Individuals with behavioral characteristics of sleep and polysomnographic characteristics of stage 1 sleep may or may not perceive themselves as sleeping. Stage 1 is viewed as a "shallow" sleep, during which an individual can be easily aroused. With transition to stage 2, EEG patterns termed *sleep spindles* and *K complexes* appear on the EEG. Sleep spindles are 12- to 14-Hz synchronized EEG waveforms with duration of 1.5 seconds. Sleep spindle waves arise as a result of synchronization of groups of thalamic neurons by the GABAergic thalamic spindle pacemaker. The origin of K complexes is unknown. With the onset of stage 2, the arousal threshold increases, and a more intense stimulus is needed to arouse a sleeper. Stages 3 and 4 of NREM sleep are defined by synchronized high-amplitude (>75 µV) and slow (0.5–2 Hz) delta wave EEG pattern. Stages 3 and 4 collectively are referred as deep sleep, delta sleep, or slow-wave sleep. By definition, delta waves account for 20% to 50% of EEG activity during stage 3 and greater than 50% of EEG activity during stage 4 of sleep. Slow-wave sleep is associated with a higher arousal threshold than "lighter" stages of NREM sleep. No eye movements are detected on the EOG during stages 2, 3, and 4 of NREM sleep. The EMG tracks continued muscle tone decline as NREM sleep "deepens" from stages 1 to 4.

The cortical EEG pattern of REM sleep is characterized by low voltage and fast frequencies (alpha or 8–13 Hz). This EEG pattern is referred as *activated* or *desynchronized* and also is seen in the state of relaxed wakefulness (with eyes closed). *Activated* refers to an active mind (dreams) and the EEG pattern characteristic of wakefulness. Paradoxically, individuals in REM sleep, although activated, are behaviorally less responsive than during the wake state [2,3]. *Desynchronized* refers to the random-appearing wave pattern seen on the REM sleep EEG, which is contrasted with the *synchronized* uniform wave pattern seen on the NREM sleep EEG [2,3]. To be scored as REM sleep, a polysomnographic tracing must contain an *activated* EEG pattern and muscle atonia (EMG) and the presence of rapid eye movements (EOG). REM sleep can be subdivided further into two stages: *tonic* and *phasic*. The tonic stage is *continuous* and shows muscle atonia and desynchronized EEG as two main features. Superimposed on the tonic stage of REM are *intermittent* phasic events, which include bursts of rapid eye movements and irregularities of respiration and heart rate.

Sleep Architecture
Sleep typically begins with a "shallow" stage 1 of NREM sleep and "deepens" to NREM sleep stages 2, 3, and 4, which are followed by the first brief episode of REM sleep in approximately 90 minutes. After the first sleep cycle, NREM and REM sleep continue to alternate in a predictable fashion, each NREM-REM cycle lasting approximately 90 to 120 minutes [1]. In the course of the night, sleep cycles recur three to seven times. Stage 1 of NREM sleep, which lasts only a few minutes, serves as a transition from wakefulness to sleep and later during sleep serves as a transition between REM-NREM sleep cycles. Typically, stage 1 constitutes 2% to 5% of total sleep time. An increase in the amount or percentage of stage 1 sleep may be a sign of sleep disruption. The brief first period of stage 1 NREM sleep is followed by "deeper" stage 2, which lasts approximately 10 to 20 minutes. Stage 2 sleep normally constitutes 45% to 55% of the total sleep time. Stage 2 sleep progresses to stages 3 (lasting a few minutes) and 4 (lasting 40 minutes). Stage 3 constitutes 5% to 8% of the total sleep time, and stage 4 constitutes 10% to 15% of the total sleep time. Stages 3 and 4 of NREM sleep predominate during the first third of the night. The first REM period is brief and occurs approximately 90 minutes after sleep onset; subsequent REM cycles occur approximately 90 to 120 minutes apart. REM sleep episodes become longer as the night progresses, and the longest REM periods are found in the last third of the night [4,5]. NREM sleep accounts for 75% to 80% and REM sleep accounts for 20% to 25% of the total sleep time [1,3,6–8]. These proportions commonly vary with age (see later section on effects of age).

Physiologic Functions in Sleep
Autonomic nervous system during sleep
The parasympathetic drive is higher during all stages of sleep than in relaxed wakefulness. The sympathetic drive increases significantly during phasic REM, decreases slightly during tonic REM, and remains relatively unchanged during relaxed wakefulness and NREM sleep. The net effect is the dominance of the parasympathetic tone during NREM and tonic REM sleep, and the sympathetic dominance during phasic REM [9–11].

Body temperature regulation
The energy expenditure is lower during NREM sleep compared with wakefulness. The body temperature is maintained at a lower set-point in NREM than in wakefulness. During REM sleep, thermoregulatory responses of shivering and sweating are absent, and thermal regulation seems to cease (as in poikilothermic organisms) [9–11].

Control of respiration and cardiovascular function during sleep
The predominance of the parasympathetic tone and decreased energy expenditure during NREM sleep are responsible for decreased ventilation during this

stage. The respiration rate in NREM sleep is regular, and cardiovascular changes are consistent with decreased energy expenditure. In contrast, breathing patterns and heart rate during REM sleep are irregular [9–11]. The irregularities in cardiovascular parameters increase the risk of myocardial infarctions during REM sleep in vulnerable individuals. The changes in ventilation, respiration, and upper airway tone make REM sleep a vulnerable period for individuals with obstructive sleep apnea (Table 1).

Effects of Age

Age is likely the strongest factor that affects sleep continuity and the distribution of sleep stages through the night. The sleep pattern of newborn infants dramatically differs from that of adults. During the first year of life, infants sleep twice as much as adults and, in contrast to adults, enter sleep through REM. During the first year of life, REM sleep constitutes 50% of the total sleep time; the percentage occupied by REM sleep decreases to adult levels of 20% to 25% by age 3 years and remains at that level until old age. NREM-REM cycles, controlled by the *ultradian* process, are present at birth, but the 50- to 60-minute cycle periods in newborns are shorter than the approximately 90-minute periods in adults. Slow-wave sleep is not present at birth, but develops by age 2 to 6 months. The amount of slow-wave sleep steadily declines from maximal levels in the young to almost nonexistent amounts in the elderly [1,10,12]. In addition to loss of slow-wave sleep, sleep changes in the elderly

Table 1
Physiologic changes with stages of sleep

Parameter	NREM	REM
Heart	Decreases	Irregular with increases and decreases
Blood pressure	Unchanged and stable	Irregular with increases and decreases
Respiration	Decreased rate	Irregular rate in phasic stage
Ventilation	Decreased tidal volume; decreased hypoxic response	Decreased tidal volume in phasic stage; decreased hypoxic response
Upper airway muscle tone	Decreased	Further decreased
Temperature	Preserved thermoregulation	Increased temperature and poikilothermia
Pupils	Constricted	Constricted in tonic stage; dilated in phasic stage
Gastrointestinal	Failure of inhibition of acid secretion; prolonged acid clearance	Failure of inhibition of acid secretion
Nocturnal penile tumescence/clitoral enlargement	Infrequent	Frequent

Data From Refs. [9,35].

include sleep fragmentation, increased percentage of stage 1 sleep, and decreased ability to maintain continuous sleep at night and wakefulness during the day. Contrary to commonly held beliefs, the need to sleep does not decrease with the advancing age; what changes in the elderly is the ability to maintain sleep (Fig. 1) [10,12,13].

How Much Sleep Does One Need?
One needs a sufficient amount of sleep to feel alert and refreshed and to avoid falling asleep unintentionally during the waking hours. Most young adults average 7 to 8 hours of sleep nightly, but there is a significant individual and night-to-night variability in these figures. Genetics plays a role in determining sleep length, and voluntary sleep reduction plays a significant role in determining how much sleep an individual actually gets. Sleep restriction results in daytime sleepiness, and daytime sleepiness suggests that an individual's sleep needs have not been met [1].

REGULATION OF SLEEP AND WAKEFULNESS
Drives
Experimental studies in humans and animals led to the development of the *two-process model,* which accounts for regulation of sleep and wake time. According to the model, sleep is regulated by two basic processes: a *homeostatic process,* which depends on the amount of prior sleep and wakefulness, and a *circadian process,* which is driven by an endogenous circadian pacemaker, generating nearly 24-hour cycles of behavior. An *ultradian process* within sleep is believed to control the alternation between REM-NREM sleep every 90 to 120 minutes. It is hypothesized that the interaction of homeostatic and circadian processes is

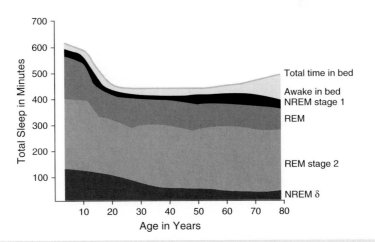

Fig. 1. Sleep and age. (*Data from* Williams RL, Karacan I, Hursch CJ. Electroencephalography (EEG) of human sleep: clinical applications. New York: Wiley & Sons; 1974.)

responsible for helping humans to maintain wakefulness during the day and consolidated sleep at night (Fig. 2).

Homeostatic Regulation of Sleep

Virtually all organisms have an absolute need to sleep. Humans cannot remain awake voluntarily for longer than 2 to 3 days, and rodents cannot survive without sleep for longer than few weeks [10,14]. The homeostatic factor represents an increase in the need for sleep (sleep pressure) with increasing duration of prior wakefulness. The presence of homeostatic factor is best shown through sleep deprivation studies. When a normal amount of sleep is reduced, the homeostatic drive is increased, leading to increased sleep pressure and sleepiness during the day and increased deep sleep at night. When normal sleep is preserved, the homeostatic factor represents a basic increase in sleep propensity during waking hours. The pull of this drive builds up during wakefulness and reaches its peak at sleep time. Its strength declines during sleep with the lowest point (nadir) on awakening in the morning.

It also is useful to differentiate sleepiness from tiredness or fatigue. A tired or fatigued individual does not have a propensity to fall asleep given an opportunity to do so. A sleepy individual is not only anergic, but also falls asleep given the opportunity to do so.

Circadian Rhythms

Humans have an endogenous circadian pacemaker with an intrinsic period of slightly more than 24 hours [15]. Virtually all living organisms exhibit metabolic, physiologic, and behavioral circadian (ie, about 24 hours) rhythms.

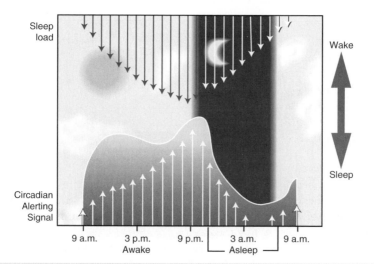

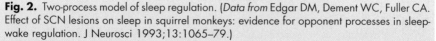

Fig. 2. Two-process model of sleep regulation. (*Data from* Edgar DM, Dement WC, Fuller CA. Effect of SCN lesions on sleep in squirrel monkeys: evidence for opponent processes in sleep-wake regulation. J Neurosci 1993;13:1065–79.)

The most obvious circadian rhythm is the human sleep-wake cycle. Examples of other circadian rhythms include the release of cortisol, thyroid-stimulating hormone, and melatonin. Most mammalian tissues and organs contain mechanisms capable of expressing their function in accordance with the circadian rhythm. The "master biologic clock," which regulates sleep-wake and all other circadian rhythms, resides in the suprachiasmatic nuclei (SCN) of the hypothalamus. SCN are bilaterally paired nuclei located slightly above the optic chiasm in the anterior hypothalamus.

Circadian clocks normally are synchronized to environmental cues *(zeitgebers)* by a process called *entrainment.* The process of entrainment of SCN cells is mediated through glutamate stimulating the *N*-methyl-D-aspartate receptor [16]. Light hitting the retina activates the release of glutamate through the retinohypothalamic tract projecting to the SCN [17]. In most mammals and humans, light-dark cycle is the most potent entraining stimulus. The modulation of the SCN by environmental cues and neurotransmitters/hormones is phase dependent. When light is given to a patient at night, it shifts the circadian clock back, whereas light exposure in early morning shifts the clock forward; melatonin is effective only in shifting the circadian clock when given at dawn or at dusk, but not during the daytime hours; cholinergic activation of the muscarinic receptors affects the clock only at night [18,19].

Circadian information from the SCN is transmitted to the rest of the body after input from the hypothalamus. Body organ responses (eg, sleep-wake cycle, core body temperature, the release of cortisol, thyroid-stimulating hormone, melatonin) to the circadian rhythm is controlled by the SCN and modulated by the hypothalamus. The release of melatonin from the pineal gland, signaled by the circadian rhythm, peaks at dawn and dusk. The SCN contains melatonin receptors, and the circadian clock can be reset by melatonin through a feedback mechanism [15,18,20]. In the absence of environmental cues (eg, under conditions of sensory deprivation), the endogenous rhythmicity of the circadian pacemaker persists independently of the light-dark cycle [18,21]. The genes of the SCN cells, through transcription-translation, are responsible for maintaining the 24-hour clock. Experimental mutation of these genes in animals produces prolonged or shortened circadian periods, whereas in humans such mutations result in abnormal circadian rhythms [18].

Neurotransmitters Involved in Sleep and Wakefulness

Adenosine had been identified as a possible mediator of the homeostatic sleep process. It is an endogenous sleep-producing substance [10,18,22–24]. A breakdown product of adenosine triphosphate (ATP), adenosine is believed to be a homeostatic sleep factor that mediates the transition from prolonged wakefulness to NREM sleep. Adenosine mediates this transition by inhibiting arousal-promoting neurons of the basal forebrain. Caffeine is believed to promote wakefulness by blocking adenosine receptors. ATP is an important energy reserve in neurons. Adenosine accumulates in certain areas of the brain when neurons consume energy in the form of ATP during prolonged wakefulness.

In animal studies, adenosine levels in the brain increased during sleep deprivation and returned to baseline during sleep [14,25,26]. Other substances hypothesized to be involved in promoting sleep and contributing to the homeostatic factor include proinflammatory cytokines (interleukin-1) [18,27] prostaglandin D_2, and growth hormone–releasing hormone [27].

Cholinergic neurons have a dual role: Some promote sleep, and others promote wakefulness. The serotoninergic, noradrenergic, and histaminergic wakefulness-promoting neurons have a discharge pattern nearly opposite that of the cholinergic sleep-promoting neurons. The discharge rate of serotoninergic, noradrenergic, and histaminergic neurons is fastest during wakefulness, decreases during NREM sleep, and virtually stops firing during REM sleep. Additionally, newly discovered peptides called *hypocretins* (also known as *orexins*) are thought to regulate wakefulness by interacting with histaminergic, aminergic, and cholinergic systems (Fig. 3).

Acetylcholine

Cholinergic neurons that originate in the laterodorsal and pedunculopontine tegmental nuclei (LDT/PPT) of the *midbrain reticular formation* reach the cortex by ascending through the thalamus and hypothalamus. These midbrain LDT and PPT areas contain two interspersed subsets of cholinergic neurons. One subset is responsible for the fast-frequency and low-voltage EEG pattern of "cortical activation," which appears in REM sleep and restful wakefulness. These are called *wake/REM-on* neurons [28]. The second subset is responsible for generations of REM sleep. These latter cholinergic neurons are called *REM-on* cells. The three physiologic components of REM sleep (muscle atonia, rapid

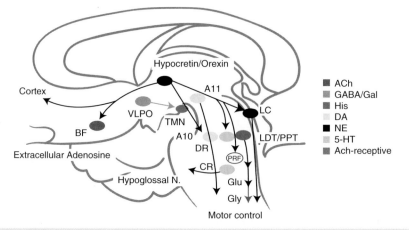

Fig. 3. Sleep: neurochemistry. BF, basal forebrain cholinergic nuclei; CR, caudal raphe; LDT/PPT, laterodorsal tegmental nuclei/pedunculopontine tegmental nuclei; PRF, pontine reticular formation; TMN, tuberomammillary nucleus; VLPO, ventrolateral preoptic nucleus. (*From* Mignot E, Taheri S, Nishino S. Sleeping with the hypothalamus: emerging therapeutic targets for sleep disorders. Nat Neurosci 2002;5:1072; with permission.)

eye movements, EEG activation/desynchronization) are controlled by different nulei located in the pontine reticular formation (PRF). The *REM-on* cholinergic neurons promote REM sleep by sending excitatory input to the PRF. This causes the rapid firing of the PRF, which produces the three cardinal physiologic components of REM sleep. The PRF is shut off during NREM sleep.

Cholinergic neurons that project from the *basal forebrain* to the cerebral cortex and limbic areas are part of the vigilance-waking system. The side effects produced by anticholinergic medications likely result owing to a disruption of the vigilance-wake producing cholinergic neurons and the wake/REM-on cholinergic neurons.

Serotonin and Norepinephrine

Serotoninergic neurons originate in the dorsal raphe nucleus and noradrenergic neurons originate in the locus caeruleus. Both sets of neurons act as suppressants of REM sleep (*REM off* cells) by inhibiting REM-promoting cholinergic neurons and by sending inhibitory input to the PRF. Serotonin and norepinephrine neurons promote cortical activation during wakefulness by rapid firing [29]. The noradrenergic wake-promoting system also was found to have an important role in the cognitive function of learning during the waking state. Activity of the noradrenergic system triggers an increase in the expression of genes associated with memory formation and learning [18]. The serotoninergic system was not found to have this close link to cognitive function.

During the NREM sleep period, at the beginning of the first sleep cycle, the serotoninergic and noradrenergic neurons significantly reduce their firing rate. This removes the inhibition from the *REM-on* cholinergic neurons; leading to the first REM sleep period approximately 90 minutes later.

Hypocretin

Hypocretins (also called orexins) are two neuropeptides (hypocretin 1 and hypocretin 2) with key roles in regulation of arousal and metabolism. They bind to their corresponding receptors (*Hcrtr1* and *Hcrtr2*) throughout the brain and spinal cord. These peptides are produced by hypothalamic neurons that surround the fornix bilaterally and in the dorsolateral hypothalamus. These hypothalamic regions are implicated in control of nutritional balance, blood pressure, and temperature regulation and endocrine secretion and arousal. Hypocretins likely play a role in all of these functions [30].

The hypocretin-producing neurons in the hypothalamus receive direct input from the SCN (the circadian rhythm clock) and project to the posterior hypothalamus (tuberomammillary nucleus [TMN]–histamine), basal forebrain (cholinergic vigilance-wake area), thalamus, locus caeruleus and dorsal raphe neuclus (norepinephrine and serotonin *REM off* cells), LDT, and PRF (cholinergic REM-on cells and muscle atonia) [30,31]. In accordance with circadian rhythm control of hypocretin levels (through SCN input), their concentration is highest during the waking period. Hypocretin levels also increase during a period of forced sleep deprivation. It is unclear whether this increase during sleep deprivation represents hypocretin opposing and attempting to override the sleep drive or producing a stress response to sleep deprivation. Hypocretin input to the brainstem REM-on cells controls the switch into REM by reducing the firing rate of the REM-on cells during the wake period [30].

Histamine
Antihistaminergic drugs that cross the blood-brain barrier are known to produce sedation. The neurotransmitter histamine plays a key role in maintenance of wakefulness. Histaminergic neurons originate from the TMN of the posterior hypothalamus and project diffusely throughout the brain. In the cortex, histamine facilitates cortical arousal. Histaminergic neurons fire most rapidly during cortical activation in the wake state and turn off during REM sleep [29,32].

Hypothalamus
The role of the hypothalamus as a key area of the brain involved in regulation of sleep and wakefulness was recognized after the pandemic of encephalitis lethargica swept the world in the early 1900s. Thought to be a viral infection of the brain, encephalitis lethargica induced severe sleep abnormalities in affected individuals. Most patients exhibited profound and prolonged sleepiness, whereas some had severe insomnia. Patients affected by sleepiness were discovered to have lesions in the *posterior hypothalamus*; patients affected by insomnia were found to have lesions in the *anterior hypothalamus* [23,33].

Since this clinical observation more than 70 years ago, numerous human and animal studies have elucidated further the role of the hypothalamus in the regulation of sleep. In accordance with these original observations, the ventrolateral preoptic nucleus in the anterior hypothalamus has been established as the key sleep-inducing region and the TMN of the posterior hypothalamus as one of the important wakefulness-promoting regions of the brain.

The anterior hypothalamus contains GABAergic cells. Activity of GABAergic cells in the ventrolateral preoptic nucleus region is implicated in production of NREM sleep, whereas the GABAergic cells in the area adjacent to the ventrolateral preoptic nucleus is thought to promote REM sleep by inhibiting the noradrenergic (locus caeruleus) and serotoninergic (dorsal raphe nucleus) REM-off nuclei of the brainstem [23]. The rapid firing of the anterior hypothalamus region during sleep leads to inhibition of the locus caeruleus and dorsal raphe nucleus in the brainstem. This in effect takes the "noradrenergic and serotoninergic breaks" off the hypothalamic sleep generator, reinforcing the sleep state [33].

The posterior hypothalamus/TMN receives histaminergic input and has hypocretin receptors (hctr2). Histamine and hypocretin produce activation of the TMN cells, which leads to sustained wakefulness [23]. At the same time, hypocretin activates the noradrenergic and seretoninergic cells in the brainstem, which send inhibitory signals to the anterior hypothalamus. This in effect takes the "GABAergic breaks" off the hypothalamic wakefulness generator, reinforcing the wake state.

From the point of view of evolutionary advantage, it may be important for most animals to be either in the fully awake or the fully asleep state and to spend little time in the transition state between sleep and wakefulness. The anterior and posterior regions of the hypothalamus work through a system of mutual inhibition in what has been referred to as a *flip-flop switch* (similar to a light switch) [33]. The hypothalamic *sleep switch* is quickly turned "on" and "off," with both positions being equally stable. It is hypothesized that the circadian, homeostatic, and ultradian drives are responsible for flipping the hypothalamic switch into the sleep and wake positions. The hypocretin tone, which also is influenced by the circadian and homeostatic drives, helps to stabilize the hypothalamic switch in the wake position and prevent intrusion of REM sleep into the waking state [23,33]. When the hypocretin tone is reduced, as in narcolepsy, this stability of the wake state is impaired resulting in abnormal shifts from wake to REM states (eg, cataplexy, sleep paralysis).

PHARMACEUTICALS AND RECREATIONAL DRUGS

All drugs that cross the blood-brain barrier may affect sleep. Selective serotonin reuptake inhibitors, tricyclic antidepressants, serotonin norepinephrine reuptake inhibitors, and monoamine oxidase inhibitors suppress REM sleep; acute withdrawal from these antidepressants is likely to produce a rebound increase in REM sleep. Barbiturates increase slow-wave sleep and suppress REM. Benzodiazepines suppress slow-wave sleep and do not affect REM. Psychostimulants, such as amphetamine and cocaine, increase sleep latency, fragment sleep, and suppress REM sleep [4,10,12].

SLEEPING AND DREAMING

Many theories attempt to explain the biologic function of sleep, without a clear winner. One such theory posits that sleep serves a restorative function for the brain and body. Normal sleep is subjectively associated with feeling refreshed on awakening. REM sleep is associated with increased CNS synthesis of proteins and is crucial for the CNS development of infants and young humans and animals. Growth hormone secretion is increased, while cortisol secretion is decreased during sleep. All these can be used to support the restorative theory of sleep [34]. Another theory of sleep function proposes that sleep has a central role in reinforcement and consolidation of memory. Sleep deprivation experiments have highlighted the important role of REM sleep in memory function [34]. Another theory suggests that sleep is important for thermoregulatory function. Experiments have shown that total sleep deprivation results in thermoregulatory abnormalities, NREM sleep maintains thermoregulatory function, and REM sleep is associated with impaired thermoregulatory responses (eg, shivering, sweating) [34].

Since the middle 1950s, when REM sleep was identified, sleep research has focused on understanding the physiology of dreams. Most dreams (about 80%) occur during REM sleep; the remainder occur during NREM sleep. REM sleep dreams are more complex, have more emotional valence, can be bizarre, and are easier to recall. NREM sleep dreams are more logical and realistic, but more difficult to recall possibly because awakening from NREM sleep leaves a person feeling more confused and disoriented than awakening from REM sleep. During REM sleep, neuronal signals originating from the brainstem are transmitted to the cerebral hemispheres and stimulate the cortical association areas to produce images that compose dreams [34].

SUMMARY

Sleep is a vital, highly organized process regulated by complex systems of neuronal networks and neurotransmitters. Sleep plays an important role in the regulation of CNS and body physiologic functions. Sleep architecture changes with age and is easily susceptible to external and internal disruption. Reduction or disruption of sleep can affect numerous functions varying from thermoregulation to learning and memory during the waking state.

References

[1] Sinton CM, McCarley RW. Neurophysiological mechanisms of sleep and wakefulness: a question of balance. Semin Neurol 2004;24:211–23.

[2] Doghramji K. The evaluation and management of sleep disorders. In: Stoudemire A, editor. Clinical psychiatry for medical students. Philadelphia: Lippincott; 1998. p. 783–818.

[3] Siegel JM. REM sleep. In: Kryger MH, Roth T, Dement WC, editors. Principles and practice of sleep medicine. Philadelphia: Saunders; 2005. p. 120–35.

[4] Carskadon MA, Dement WC. Normal human sleep: an overview. In: Kryger MH, Roth T, Dement WC, editors. Principles and practice of sleep medicine. Philadelphia: Saunders; 2005. p. 13–23.

[5] Markov D, Jaffe F, Doghramji K. Update on parasomnias: a review for psychiatric practice. Psychiatry 2006;3:69–76.

[6] Carskadon MA, Rechtschaffen A. Monitoring and staging human sleep. In: Kryger MH, Roth T, Dement WC, editors. Principles and practice of sleep medicine. Philadelphia: Saunders; 2005. p. 1359–77.

[7] Chokroverty S. An overview of sleep. In: Chokroverty S, editor. Sleep disorders medicine: basic science, technical considerations, and clinical aspects. Boston: Butterworth Heinemann; 1999. p. 7–20.

[8] Walczak T, Chokroverty S. Electroencephalography, electromyography, and electro-oculography: general principles and basic technology. In: Chokroverty S, editor. Sleep disorders medicine: basic science, technical considerations, and clinical aspects. Boston: Butterworth Heinemann; 1999. p. 175–203.

[9] Chokroverty S. Physiologic changes in sleep. In: Chokroverty S, editor. Sleep disorders medicine: basic science, technical considerations, and clinical aspects. Boston: Butterworth Heinemann; 1999. p. 95–126.

[10] Roth T, Roehrs T. Sleep organization and regulation. Neurology 2000;54(Suppl 1):S2–7.

[11] Parmeggiani PL. Physiology in sleep. In: Kryger MH, Roth T, Dement WC, editors. Principles and practice of sleep medicine. Philadelphia: Saunders; 2005. p. 185–91.

[12] Roth T. Characteristics and determinants of normal sleep. J Clin Psychiatry 2004;65(Suppl 16):8–11.

[13] Bliwise DL. Normal aging. In: Kryger MH, Roth T, Dement WC, editors. Principles and practice of sleep medicine. Philadelphia: Saunders; 2005. p. 24–38.

[14] Porkka-Heiskanen T, Strecker RE, Thakkar M, et al. Adenosine: a mediator of the sleep-inducing effects of prolonged wakefulness. Science 1997;276:1265–8.

[15] Czeisler CA, Duffy JF, Shanahan TL, et al. Stability, precision, and near-24-hour period of the human circadian pacemaker. Science 1999;284:2177–81.

[16] Hattar S, Liao HW, Takao M, et al. Melanopsin-containing retinal ganglion cells: architecture, projections, and intrinsic photosensitivity. Science 2002;295:1065–70.

[17] Berson DM, Dunn FA, Takao M. Phototransduction by retinal ganglion cells that set the circadian clock. Science 2002;295:1070–3.

[18] Pace-Schott EF, Hobson JA. The neurobiology of sleep: genetics, cellular physiology and subcortical networks. Nat Rev Neurosci 2002;3:591–605.

[19] Brzezinski A. Melatonin in humans. N Engl J Med 1997;336:186–95.

[20] Reiter RJ. Melatonin: clinical relevance. Best Pract Res Clin Endocrinol Metab 2003;17:273–85.

[21] Reppert SM, Weaver DR. Molecular analysis of mammalian circadian rhythms. Annu Rev Physiol 2001;63:647–76.

[22] Borbely AA, Achermann P. Sleep homeostasis and models of sleep regulation. J Biol Rhythms 1999;14:557–68.

[23] Mignot E, Taheri S, Nishino S. Sleeping with the hypothalamus: emerging therapeutic targets for sleep disorders. Nat Neurosci 2002;5(Suppl):1071–5.

[24] Borbely AA, Achermann P. Sleep homeostasis and models of sleep regulation. In: Kryger MH, Roth T, Dement WC, editors. Principles and practice of sleep medicine. Philadelphia: Saunders; 2005. p. 405–17.

[25] Boutrel B, Koob GF. What keeps us awake: the neuropharmacology of stimulants and wakefulness-promoting medications. Sleep 2004;27:1181–94.

[26] Porkka-Heiskanen T, Alanko L, Kalinchuk A, et al. Adenosine and sleep. Sleep Med Rev 2002;6:321–32.

[27] McGinty D, Szymusiak R. Sleep-promoting mechanisms in mammals. In: Kryger MH, Roth T, Dement WC, editors. Principles and practice of sleep medicine. Philadelphia: Saunders; 2005. p. 169–84.

[28] McCarley RW. Sleep neurophysiology: basic mechanisms underlying control of wakefulness and sleep. In: Chokroverty S, editor. Sleep disorders medicine: basic science, technical considerations, and clinical aspects. Boston: Butterworth Heinemann; 1999. p. 21–50.

[29] Jones BE. Basic mechanisms of sleep-wake states. In: Kryger MH, Roth T, Dement WC, editors. Principles and practice of sleep medicine. Philadelphia: Saunders; 2005. p. 136–53.

[30] Sutcliffe JG, de Lecea L. The hypocretins: setting the arousal threshold. Nat Rev Neurosci 2002;3:339–49.

[31] Peyron C, Tighe DK, van den Pol AN, et al. Neurons containing hypocretin (orexin) project to multiple neuronal systems. J Neurosci 1998;18:9996–10015.

[32] Siegel JM. The neurotransmitters of sleep. J Clin Psychiatry 2004;65(Suppl 16):4–7.

[33] Saper CB, Chou TC, Scammell TE. The sleep switch: hypothalamic control of sleep and wakefulness. Trends Neurosci 2001;24:726–31.

[34] Chokroverty S. An overview of normal sleep. In: Chokroverty S, Wayne AH, Walters AS, editors. Sleep and movement disorders. Philadelphia: Butterworth Heinemann; 2003. p. 23–43.

[35] Catesby JW, Hirshkowitz M. Assessment of sleep-related erections. In: Kryger MH, Roth T, Dement WC, editors. Principles and practice of sleep medicine. Philadelphia: Saunders; 2005. p. 1394–402.

Psychiatr Clin N Am 29 (2006) 855–870

PSYCHIATRIC CLINICS
OF NORTH AMERICA

ELSEVIER
SAUNDERS

Insomnia: Prevalence, Impact, Pathogenesis, Differential Diagnosis, and Evaluation

Philip M. Becker, MD[a,b,*]

[a]Department of Psychiatry, University of Texas Southwestern Medical Center at Dallas, Dallas, TX, USA
[b]Sleep Medicine Institute, Presbyterian Hospital Dallas, Dallas, TX, USA

R est is a basic biologic need. At a cellular level, periods of rest and activity can be identified. Increasing complexity of an organism results in more complex presentations of rest. In mammals, the most obvious times of rest are described as sleep and generally follow a rhythm defined by the light-dark cycle of day and night. Sleep is mediated through complex interaction of neural networks to regulate metabolism, catabolism, temperature, learning, and memory consolidation [1].

Humans are particularly susceptible to the disruption of the sleep-wake schedule that is called insomnia. Insomnia is a symptom that arises from multiple environmental, medical, and psychologic and mental disorders [2]. Insomnia can be transient, short-term, or chronic in its presentation. When patients have difficulty falling asleep, staying asleep, or waking early, they begin to dread the night and the daytime consequences of fatigue, mental clouding, and irritability. In a typical psychiatric practice, 50% to 80% of adult patients experience significant problems with falling or staying asleep during any year [3]. Research on sleep problems in the general population documents that between 10% and 18% of adults consider difficulty sleeping to be a serious, chronic problem and is seen more commonly in women and the elderly who fall in the lower quartile of socioeconomic status [4].

Although animal models for insomnia have been developed [5], none has provided sufficient representation of the human experience to elucidate common mechanisms or the most effective means of treatment of insomnia. The lack of representative animal models of insomnia results in the need for clinical human research of the biologic and psychologic processes of sleep. Research must define the normal perturbations in sleep versus long-term pathologic changes that have consequences for daily function.

*Sleep Medicine Associates of Texas, 5477 Glen Lakes Drive, #100, Dallas, TX 75231.
E-mail address: pbecker@sleepmed.com

0193-953X/06/$ – see front matter
doi:10.1016/j.psc.2006.08.001

The goal of this article is to review the frequency of sleep complaints in industrialized nations, the prevalence of the insomnia syndrome, the impact of insomnia on function, hypotheses regarding the pathogenesis of chronic insomnia, and how clinicians should evaluate the disorder and arrive at an appropriate differential diagnosis through the use of the "6 Ps + M" insomnia model.

PREVALENCE OF INSOMNIA: SYMPTOMS VERSUS SYNDROME

Sleep complaints are remarkably common in adults living in industrialized nations. When up to 50% of adults report problems of sleep during any year, it becomes important to distinguish between normal and abnormal perturbations of sleep. The frequency, duration, and impact of sleep disturbance must be explored with patients to determine if they have a symptom of insomnia or whether or not the insomnia syndrome is present, having an impact on physical and mental health.

The work of Ohayon and colleagues has proved valuable in distinguishing symptom from syndrome. In 2002, Ohayon reviewed various studies that used a systematic random dialing telephone survey as a means to assess sleep and sleep disorders. Questions about sleep symptoms, such as any problem falling asleep, staying asleep, or nonrestorative sleep, were posed to more than 24,000 adults. In any year, 30% to 48% of national samples reported some problem sleeping. When asked to report whether or not the sleep problem was often or always, 16% to 21% reported frequent disturbances of sleep. When asked if the problem was moderate or severe, 10% to 28% considered it to be so. To the question of dissatisfaction with either the quality or the quantity of sleep, 8% to 18% of the various national samples reported clinically significant reductions in sleep. When respondents were surveyed about their sleep and the consequences of lost sleep, 8% to 18% reported sleep disturbance that reduced daytime function. When diagnostic criteria were used for insomnia syndrome (discussed below), 6% of the respondents in multinational surveys indicated a disorder of insomnia that impaired daytime function [4]. The insomnia syndrome becomes chronic when it is present for a month or longer and is defined by whether or not it is primary or associated with comorbid disorders.

DEFINITION AND FEATURES OF INSOMNIA

The commonality of sleep complaints requires an operational definition of a disorder of insomnia to prevent nondisordered individuals from receiving a medical diagnosis or therapy that carries side effects. The Sleep Disorders Workgroup of the Diagnostic and Statistical Manual Committee of the American Psychiatric Association defines diagnostic criteria that require problems of sleep onset, maintenance, early awakening, or nonrestorative sleep on more than half of the days for at least 1 month that are associated with significant daytime dysfunction that impair performance of activities at home or work [6]. *The Diagnostic and Statistical Manual of Mental Disorders, Fourth Edition, Text*

Revision (*DSM-IV-TR*) segments chronic insomnia into primary insomnia or insomnia related to other conditions. The criteria for the diagnosis of primary insomnia are listed in Box 1. It is estimated that 10% to 15% of patients who have chronic insomnia are of primary origin. Insomnia that is comorbid with psychiatric disorders, medical disorders, circadian rhythm disorders, or substances or medications accounts for nearly 85% to 90% of chronic insomnia [4]. Table 1 summarizes the common comorbid conditions in relationship to the time of night when sleep is disturbed. A state-of-the-science conference held at the National Institutes of Health in 2005 described the circular rather than linear association among insomnia, psychiatric disorders, and medical illness, suggesting the term, "comorbid insomnia," to describe the association [7].

Primary insomnia subsumes several insomnia diagnoses in the *International Classification of Sleep Disorders* [8] including psychophysiologic insomnia, sleep-state misperception, idiopathic insomnia, and some cases of inadequate sleep hygiene. Psychophysiologic insomnia is a sleep disorder of somatized tension and learned sleep-preventing associations that results in a complaint of insomnia and associated decreased functioning during wakefulness.

Sleep-state misperception is characterized by complaints of insomnia accompanied by a marked discrepancy between subjective and objective estimates of sleep.

Idiopathic insomnia presents in childhood and has a lifelong course, presumably caused by an abnormality in the neurologic control of the sleep-wake system. Inadequate sleep hygiene results in sleep disturbance from behavioral practices that increase arousal or disrupt sleep organization (eg, working late at night, taking excessive day naps, or keeping irregular sleep hours). The

---

Box 1: Diagnostic criteria of primary insomnia

a. The predominant complaint is difficulty initiating or maintaining sleep or non-restorative sleep for at least 1 month.

b. The sleep disturbance (or associated daytime fatigue) causes clinically significant distress or impairment in social, occupational, or other important areas of functioning.

c. The sleep disturbance does not occur exclusively during the course of narcolepsy, breathing-related sleep disorder, circadian rhythm sleep disorder, or a parasomnia.

d. The disturbance does not occur exclusively during the course of another mental disorder (eg, major depressive disorder, generalized anxiety disorder, or delirium).

e. The disturbance is not caused by the direct physiologic effects of a substance (ie, drug abuse, medication) or a general medical condition.

From American Psychiatric Association. Diagnostic and statistical manual of mental disorders. 4th ed. text revision. Washington, DC: American Psychiatric Press; 2000; with permission.

Table 1
Causes of chronic insomnia based on time of presentation during the night[a]

Insomnia type	Causes
Sleep onset	Learned or conditioned activation (primary insomnia)
	Anxiety, including situational, panic disorder; generalized anxiety disorder; and obsessive compulsive disorder
	Mood disorders, including major depression, bipolar disorder I or II, and dysthymia
	Psychotic disorders during acute exacerbation
	Delayed sleep phase syndrome
	Restless legs syndrome
	Upper airway resistance syndrome (UARS) (and less commonly sleep apnea, either obstructive or central)
	Substances, such as caffeine, decongestants, and so forth
	Chronic pain, any type
	Cardiopulmonary disorders, in particular those exacerbated by the recumbent position
	Neuropathy
Sleep maintenance	Excessive time in bed
	Major depression dysthymia, or bipolar disorder in association with anxiety
	Sleep-disordered breathing: sleep apnea, UARS
	Periodic limb movements of sleep
	Chronic pain, in particularly arthritis of hips, shoulders, and neck and disc disease of the lumbosacral spine
	Respiratory disorders, in particular those exacerbated by the recumbent position
	Cardiovascular disease: heart failure, angina, atrial fibrillation, and others
	Neurologic disease: fatal familial insomnia, dementia, Parkinson's and other movement disorders, seizures, degenerative central nervous system disorders, peripheral nerve disease, and toxic exposure
Early awakening	Major depression
	Advance sleep phase syndrome
	Learned or conditioned activation (primary insomnia)
	Forced awakening for work or family responsibility

[a] Insomnia presentation may shift from onset to maintenance or early awakening in many of these disorders. The disorders that are listed in each category should be considered generally to present at a particular time of the night.

syndrome of insomnia (or insomnia disorder) must be distinguished from the manifestation of only some symptoms of insomnia.

In 2004, a workgroup of the American Academy of Sleep Medicine published criteria to be used in research trials for the insomnia syndrome [9]. It was an effort to systematize diagnosis of various disorders that cause insomnia. It recommended that in clinical trials, systematic data collection, such as sleep diaries or objective measures for sleep, be applied to patient complaints to determine inclusion and exclusion criteria for study eligibility. Research trials generally require a reported sleep-onset latency of 30 or more minutes to be eligible for enrollment. If the problem of sleep maintenance is to be studied, at least 30 minutes of wake after sleep onset may be required, with many recent trials using 60 or more minutes of wakefulness to establish eligibility for participation. Sleep efficiency (time asleep while in bed) must be less than 85%.

Although only 1 month of frequent insomnia is required in the *DSM-IV-TR* for characterization of sleep disturbance to be chronic, many patients experience sleep disturbance for several years. The duration of a sleep complaint often is reviewed in lectures to primary care physicians who are instructed to search for chronic insomnia while being aware of transient and short-term insomnia [10]. Transient insomnia presents and then passes after a few days, typically developing during a brief adjustment reaction, rotating shifts, or international travel. Transient insomnia does not come to the attention of physicians unless patients experience the transient insomnia in some consistent manner, resulting in the request for treatment of the predictable sleep disturbance. Transient insomnia likely represents the majority of the 30% to 48% of the adults in the Ohayon study [4] who reported disturbed sleep in any year. Short-term insomnia is characterized by 4 to 28 days of poor sleep and often proves stressful to patients. Short-term insomnia likely represents 10% to 20% of those reporting insomnia in any year. When the situation improves or a person's coping skills adapt to the stressful life event, the person again sleeps better. The most common precipitants for short-term insomnia include illness, job change, bereavement, dissolution of a relationship, or other significant life stressor [11]. As discussed later, individuals who are predisposed to short-term insomnia are at significantly increased risk for the development of chronic insomnia related to psychiatric disorders.

Although duration of the insomnia complaint is relevant to psychiatrists, selection of therapeutic intervention may be better based on the time of night that patients complain of sleep disturbance [12]. Subtypes of insomnia are demarcated along a continuum of sleep onset, sleep maintenance, and early awakening. Table 1 lists in descending order of likelihood the psychiatric, medical, and environmental disorders that disturb sleep at the beginning, middle, and end of the night. Approximately 40% of patients fall into each of these subtypes of insomnia, with some patients having onset, middle, or late insomnia. [13]. The challenge for therapy is that up to 50% of chronic insomnia patients during any year shift from onset to maintenance to early awakening and back.

There also are patients who have nonrestorative sleep who sleep 7 to 8 hours and yet experience significant daytime dysfunction. Ohayon used his systematic telephone survey to assess the prevalence of nonrestorative sleep in 25,000 individuals in seven European countries [14]. Overall prevalence of nonrestorative sleep was 10.8% with an impact more on women than men. Prevalence decreased with advancing age. Citizens of the United Kingdom (16.1%) and Germany (15.5%) had the highest prevalence and Spain (2.4%) showed the lowest prevalence of nonrestorative sleep. Several factors were associated positively with nonrestorative sleep: difficulty getting started in the morning, stressful life, presence of anxiety, bipolar or a depressive disorder, and having a physical disease. Respondents who had nonrestorative sleep reported greater daytime impairment than did those who had onset or maintenance insomnia. Partial or subsyndromal depression may be operative in that as many as 40% of patients who receive fluoxetine for depression report symptoms that are comparable to nonrestorative sleep [15].

IMPACT AND IMPAIRMENT FROM CHRONIC INSOMNIA

Chronic insomnia may result in impairments of physiologic and psychologic processes. The consequences of insomnia may or may not have relationship to sleep deprivation. When assessing a report from a patient who has chronic insomnia, the amount of sleep loss may not represent the principal reason for the daytime symptoms of the patient. In general, chronic insomnia patients sleep more than they recognize (referred to as sleep state misperception) [16]. Daytime impairment associated with insomnia includes reduction of attention and concentration, memory lapses, slowed reaction time, poor coordination, dysphoria, increased anxiety or worry about sleep, fatigue, tiredness, lethargy, and, occasionally, sleepiness. Cognitive disturbances of chronic insomnia increasingly are of interest to researchers [17]. The research is complicated by the definitions used to describe the sleep disturbance as insomnia symptoms versus syndrome and associated significance to other concurrent disorders. Studies of impairment have explored the psychiatric, medical, occupational, social, health economic, and cognitive impact of insomnia. Much of the work has been through epidemiologic studies that describe relationship but neither the direction nor cause of the relationship of the disorder to the sleep disturbance. As discussed later , disturbed sleep is a component of psychiatric disorders or medical disorders, yet insomnia symptoms may predict exacerbation of these disorders.

Psychiatric disorders, in particular anxiety and depressive disorders, include the symptoms of sleep disturbance in their definition [6]; yet, not all patients who have insomnia have a psychiatric disorder. Major depression, mania and hypomania, generalized anxiety, panic disorder, phobias, obsessive-compulsive disorder, alcohol abuse and dependence, and drug abuse are found either alone or in combination in 30% to 50% of all patients who have chronic insomnia [18–20]. Ford and Kamerow report that sleep-onset or maintenance insomnia of 2 weeks or longer were present in 10% of a large epidemiologic sample of the United States population. The insomnia group then was assessed for *DSM*-defined psychiatric disorders. In the insomnia group, major depression and dysthymia were present at a prevalence of 23% and anxiety disorders at a prevalence of 24% (weighted particularly by phobias) [21]. Ford and Kamerow report on the follow-up of subjects after 1 year and discovered a dramatic increase in the presentation of major depression if chronic insomnia lingers. There was a 40 times greater chance of converting from euthymia to major depression if euthymic patients who had insomnia symptoms continued to have insomnia in the intervening 1 year compared with the euthymic patients who were sleeping well at both time points [18]. Breslau and colleagues reported on more than 1000 adults who had a mean age of 31 years who were followed in a large metropolitan health maintenance organization population. The study showed that concurrrent insomnia increased the prevalence of multiple psychiatric disorders by a factor of 2 to 10 times. Breslau also found at a mean follow-up of 3.5 years that those complaining of insomnia at their first visit subsequently developed depressive disorders, anxiety disorders, and substance abuse disorders at a rate of 1.5 to 4 times higher than those who had no insomnia complaint [18].

Relevant to physicians, a study by Chang and colleagues shows that medical students who respond with insomnia under stress are at higher risk for developing depression years later. As part of a large health survey, male medical students were followed for 40 years. The cumulative risk of developing major depression was assessed. Of 887, 137 reported that during times of stress, such as semester examinations, sleep was poor. Over the first 17 years of follow-up, there was little difference between insomnia response and noninsomnia men in rates of depression. Twenty years into the project, the men who responded to stress with insomnia had a twofold increase in prevalence of major depression and 40 years later had a threefold greater prevalence of major depression. Chang and colleagues report that a significant predictor in 12 physicians who committed suicide was the insomnia response to medical school stress [19].

Medical illness also is associated with higher rates of insomnia. Katz and McHorney show that patients who have mild and severe insomnia have higher rates of medical and psychiatric comorbidities. The researchers used a self-administered patient assessment questionnaire in 3445 patients who had chronic medical and psychiatric conditions who participated in the Medical Outcomes Study [20,22]. Questions about sleep were posed to patients who had at least one of five physician-identified chronic conditions (hypertension, diabetes, congestive heart failure, myocardial infarction, or depression). Mild insomnia was defined as difficulty falling or staying asleep "some" or "a good bit" of the time during the preceding 4 weeks, whereas those who had severe insomnia had these difficulties "most" or "all" of the time. Table 2 presents the odds ratios corresponding to mild and severe insomnia in specific disorders. In recognition of the higher rates of insomnia in patients who have chronic medical illness, a study of a managed-care population shows that patients identified as having chronic insomnia showed increase use of health care services compared with subscribers who did not have insomnia [23]. Walsh calculates that chronic insomnia results in nearly $14 billion of direct expense to the United States health care system [24].

Insomnia also is associated with decrements in performance, although in a somewhat unpredictable manner. Epidemiologic study of chronic difficulties with sleep shows that workers who have the most significant insomnia have higher rates of absenteeism [25]. The National Sleep Foundation expresses concern that insomnia reduces driving performance and contributes to automobile

Table 2
Comparison of odds ratio of five chronic illnesses for mild and severe insomnia compared to patients who have no insomnia complaint

	Mild insomnia	Severe insomnia
Current depressive disorder	2.6	8.2
Congestive heart failure	1.6	2.5
Obstructive airway disease	1.6	1.5
Back problems	1.4	1.5
Hip impairment	2.2	2.7

Data from Katz DA, McHorney CA. Clinical correlates of insomnia in patients with chronic illness. Arch Intern Med 1998;158:1099–107.

accidents [26]. Although such epidemiologic data supports impairment from chronic insomnia, direct studies of patients who have primary insomnia demonstrate performance decrements of lesser concern. Patients who have chronic insomnia report that they sleep 1 to 3 hours less than age-appropriate norms, but as noted in a comprehensive review, objective measurement of daytime sleepiness through the multiple sleep latency test reveals no difference between patients and controls in their degree of daytime sleepiness [27]. Patients who have severe insomnia demonstrate impairment in reaction time but studies of attention, concentration, and short-term memory show variable evidence of performance decrement [28]. Schneider and colleagues show only mild decrements in alertness and selective attention in untreated patients who have primary insomnia, but the cognitive deficits were similar to patients who have narcolepsy and sleep apnea, disorders that result in recognized sleep disruption and increased daytime sleepiness [29]. Decrements in alertness and selective attention were noted in untreated patients who had psychophysiologic insomnia, narcolepsy, and sleep apnea. Narcoleptic and untreated patients who had obstructive sleep apnea had a lower threshold than controls or insomnia patients on the critical flicker fusion test. Self-rated tiredness or sleepiness was significantly more pronounced in the three groups of untreated patients than in control subjects. A study in older patients demonstrates that insomniac subjects who had relatively slow reaction times showed deficits in an electroencephalogram-derived measure of slow wave power in the 2- to 4-Hz bandwidth. These results suggest that performance deficits among some older insomniacs could be related to slow wave sleep deficiencies [30].

Bohnet and Arand reviewed in 1997 the nature of physiologic and cognitive hyperarousal and its relationship to primary insomnia [31]. Early studies of patients who had chronic insomnia were not able to document physiologic differences, but more recent studies demonstrate that patients who have primary insomnia on average take longer than control subjects to fall asleep on daytime nap study and have elevated body and brain metabolic rates and frontal cortical activation [32]. Bohnet and Arand opine that primary insomniacs suffer from a disorder of hyperarousal and that the elevated arousal produces the poor sleep and other symptoms reported by patients. They propose that treatment strategies be directed at reducing the heightened arousal [31]. To investigate the impact of cognitive and physiologic hyperarousal, Tang and Harvey took 54 healthy, good sleepers and completed assessment of subjective sleep reports and objective measurement of sleep-related movements (actigraphy) under three experimental conditions. Participants who were manipulated experimentally to experience anxious cognitive arousal or physiologic arousal during the presleep period reported longer sleep-onset latency and shorter total sleep time, and both groups exhibited a greater discrepancy between the self-reported and actigraphy-defined sleep, relative to participants who received no manipulation [33].

In summary, the symptom of chronic insomnia has impacts on physical and psychologic health, is associated with worsening of pscychiatric and medical disorders, and reduces occupational performance. Heightened cognitive and physical arousal may represent a common factor to be explored in future research.

EVALUATION OF THE COMPLAINT OF INSOMNIA—THE 6 PS + M OF INSOMNIA MODEL

There are many reviews of insomnia, its evaluation, and therapeutic strategies [13,34–41]. Each provides its own perspective on the process to manage insomnia, usually focusing on the chronic insomnia syndrome. To help organize a complex task, a model often proves helpful to psychiatrists when considering the differential diagnosis of a multifactorial syndrome, such as chronic insomnia. Psychiatrists can use the 6 P's + M of insomnia model to focus the process of evaluation with patients. In the next section, the model is applied to a patient.

Evaluation begins with establishing differential diagnosis. Historical review determines the significance of psychiatric, medical, circadian, and lifestyle factors to the sleep complaint. Seven or more days of sleep diary help establish the specifics of the sleep complaint and facilitate discussion with patients. If no recent medical work up has occurred, psychiatrists should consider a physical examination, particularly of the neurologic system, and laboratory testing for serum chemistry, B_{12} and folate deficiency, thyroid dysfunction, or other hormonal abnormalities. Questions about primary sleep disorders, in particular the nighttime symptoms of restless legs syndrome, sleep apnea, and delayed or advanced sleep phase syndrome, should be completed. Overnight polysomnographic testing is indicated in patients who report loud snoring or abnormal movements during sleep and particularly in those patients who report falling asleep when relaxed during the daytime.

The 6 Ps + M of insomnia model considers in a systematic manner the following categories: *p*redisposing, *p*recipitating, *p*erpetuating, *p*sychologic/psychiatric, *p*harmacologic/substances, *p*eriodicity/circadian plus *m*edical disorders (sleep, pain, and others). Table 3 outlines the 6 Ps + M of insomnia model.

The 6 Ps + M of insomnia are an expansion of the behavioral medicine conceptual model of chronic insomnia proposed by Spielman in 1987 [42]. Predisposed individuals are believed to develop insomnia because of heightened

Table 3
Evaluation of chronic insomnia by the '6 Ps + M of insomnia' model

Determine that the patient has a chronic syndrome of insomnia by diagnostic criteria of frequency, duration, and daytime dysfunction (see Table 1).	
Predisposition Examples:	Factors of genetics, parenting, relationships, and management skills that either worsen or allow weathering of stressful perturbations. genetics of short and long sleeping [44], early life trauma, limit setting of parents, social relationships, learning of adaptive coping mechanisms
Precipitants Examples:	Specific events that challenge or overwhelm coping mechanisms. job change or loss, separation, illness, death of a loved one, assault. Commonly experienced as a threat.
Perpetuation Examples:	Internal processes within the individual that reinforce maladaptive behaviors and misconceptions. spending excessive time in bed; trying to sleep; remaining in bed after becoming frustrated with being awake; working in bed; getting up to eat or work on the computer; worrying about sleep; unrealistic expectations: "I need 8 hours each night", "Losing sleep makes me a bad _____ (worker, mom, spouse, etc.)", "I won't be able to function without sleep"; and others.
Psychologic/ Psychiatric Disorders Examples:	Axis II disorders result in conflicts and disappointments with others, stressing adaptive coping mechanisms that are necessary for good sleep. Axis I disorders commonly exacerbate insomnia and insomnia also heralds developing mood or anxiety disorders. • Major depression and dysthymia are the most significant contributors to severe insomnia. Recurrence of episodic, serious insomnia point to mood disorder. • Mania-induced insomnia is recognized fairly easily, but hypomania and mixed states of mood may confuse the picture. • Panic attacks in the day, generalized anxiety, obsessive thoughts, and compulsive behaviors should be explored as reasons for nocturnal sleep disturbance. • Post-traumatic stress disorder results in heightened arousal and nightmares. • Acute exacerbation of psychotic disorders worsens insomnia, and sleep improves after therapy of the psychosis (occasionally obsessive concern for sleep lingers). • Abuse and dependence disorders of alcohol and recreational substances have variable effects on sleep and interact with axis I and II disorders that commonly disturb sleep.

Pharmacologic/ substances	Agents that have effects on central nervous system function can impact sleep. Certain individuals seem predisposed to these negative effects.
Examples:	caffeine, nicotine, decongestants, psychostimulants taken to late in the day, buproprion, monoamine oxidase inhibitors, diuretics, β-blockers, calcium channel blockers, SSRIs, and others. Alcohol sedates for 1 to 2 hours, then lightens sleep and increases wakefulness.
Periodicity	The human circadian clock has a periodicity of approximately 24 hours. Disorders of clock timing present as an insomnia complaint (noted in parentheses).
Examples:	advance sleep phase syndrome (sleep maintenance and early morning awakening insomnia), delayed sleep phase syndrome (sleep onset insomnia), shift work sleep disorder (onset and maintenance insomnia), irregular sleep-wake schedule (ill-defined bedtime and arising time), others
Medical disorders	Medical disorders that have an impact on sleep. These also include the traditional sleep disorders that contribute to insomnia.
Examples:	Primary sleep disorders: restless legs syndrome, periodic limb movement disorder, Obstructive or central sleep apnea, Narcolepsy Medical illnesses: chronic pain conditions, gastroesophageal reflux disease, respiratory disorders, congestive heart failure, angina, prostate disease, endocrinologic disorders, gynecologic disorders, Parkinson's disease, other movement disorders, and various neurologic conditions.

states of arousal, both psychologic and metabolic [32,43]. When these predisposed individuals are exposed to a precipitating event, psychologic and physiologic processes within individuals limit their ability to equilibrate to normal sleep [12]. Perpetuating processes generally are considered to be cognitive-behavioral factors that reinforce poor sleep [31]. Psychologic/psychiatric disorders expand on the 3 Ps of Spielman, focusing on the most common reasons for chronic insomnia. Pharmacology and substances represent ubiquitous agents in modern society that have the potential to alter sleep. Periodicity describes the circadian rhythms of the body and how shift work, circadian misalignment, and genetic factors contribute to insomnia. The addition of medical disorders recognizes how medical illnesses disturb sleep. The medical disorders include both primary sleep disorders, as outlined in Table 3.

APPLICATION OF THE 6 PS + M OF INSOMNIA MODEL TO A PATIENT

To apply the model, a representative case is offered. Ms. Smith is a 62-year-old single woman who has reported poor sleep dating back to her teens. She was educated through high school and held various clerical jobs until major depression and adult-onset diabetes mellitus resulted in disability. She never earned more than $18,000 annually. Her chief complaint was, "I can't fall asleep or stay asleep," leaving her tired and fatigued throughout the day. The 6 Ps + M of the model are explored with the patient.

Predisposition

To the question of what it was like to sleep in her family home, Ms. Smith reported that she had a regular bedtime, but the verbal fights of her parents sometimes interrupted sleep onset and maintenance. She felt unsafe. She remembered her mother sleeping in her bed when conflicts between her parents became more significant. Her mother had troubles sleeping and Ms. Smith considered her to be depressed, whereas her father drank excessively.

Precipitants

When did Ms. Smith start having more regular problems sleeping? "When I was in junior high school, I started having frequent troubles falling asleep." Did anything happen around that time that would have made it difficult to sleep? "My brother began to molest me at night." (This was only learned three sessions into treatment after rapport was established.) She reported stabilizing and managing through the regular routine of work and intermittent medication offered by her personal physician. She identified acute exacerbation of her chronic insomnia syndrome (a 60-minute delay into sleep and three awakenings of 30 to 60 minutes each at night) that presented during perimenopause and at approximately the same time that she was diagnosed with diabetes mellitus.

Perpetuation

Ms. Smith became increasingly more depressed as she struggled with her declining health, including complications from her diabetes mellitus. Soon after she began insulin, she was released from her job and she qualified for social security disability. Without the routine of work, she began to lie in bed for up to 16 hours per day, sometimes discovering that she "would lose track" of the television, suggesting that she would doze off. She kept the television on 24 hours per day. "The more I try to sleep, the more I think about my health, my money problems, and what is to become of me."

Psychologic/Psychiatric
Ms. Smith reported that she had chronic worries and concerns that dated back to her youngest years. Her first episode of major depression occurred in her early twenties after a relationship with a married male coworker ended badly. She identified recurrent episodes of moderate depression that manifested with hopelessness without suicidal ideation on diagnosis of diabetes mellitus. When asked about her friends, Ms. Smith reported that her only social contact was a woman whom she chatted with once or so per week when they met at the mailbox. "My biggest activities are going to see my doctors."

Pharmacologic/Substances
Ms. Smith avoided alcohol in view of the abuse problems of her father. She always had consumed coffee, drinking up to 6 cups per day as late as 9:00 PM. She smoked one-half pack of cigarettes per day. She denied the usage of recreational agents. Besides her insulin, she was on a statin, calcium channel blocker, selective serotonin reuptake inhibitor (SSRI), gabapentin, diazepam, and Cox-2 inhibitor. She had received a variety of sedative-hypnotic agents during her lifetime, although she noted that she had slept better when she was treated with imipramine (100 mg orally at bedtime), although xerostomia was significant.

Periodicity
Ms. Smith had not have a set bedtime or awakening time since her medical retirement. When asked to complete a sleep diary, she made a poor effort. As best that could be discerned, sleep onset occurred between 1:00 AM and 3:00 AM with intermittent wakefulness until she would get out of bed to make lunch at approximately 11:00 AM, suggesting a delayed sleep phase. Her longest time of sustained wakefulness began with watching *Jeopardy* in the later afternoon until moving to her bed to watch her evening television programs. She did not travel and never worked on rotating shifts.

Medical Disorders
Ms. Smith had only mild snoring without choking or obvious pauses in breathing (body mass index: 31) and she denied the complaints of restless legs. Her sheets and blankets often looked quite disturbed, but she did not know whether or not she had any abnormal movements during sleep. (After insufficient benefit from various therapeutic interventions, polysomnographic testing was completed and revealed mild obstructive sleep apnea/hypopnea at 12 per hour with periodic leg movements of sleep at 22 per hour but only 3 arousals per hour.) She showed a peripheral neuropathy that sometimes burned to such a significant degree that she found it difficult to fall asleep. She awoke

frequently because of nocturia. Because of osteoarthritis of the hips and knees, her awakenings at night intermittently were complicated by pain and stiffness.

SUMMARY

When patients report problems sleeping, a psychiatrist must determine its significance based on frequency, duration, and daytime impairment. Because up to 50% of adults, in particular older women, report problems of sleep in any year, it becomes necessary to define when insomnia becomes long-standing, severe, and a complication to daytime function. When sleep onset, sleep maintenance, early wake, or nonrestorative sleep are problems for 3 nights or more per week for 1 month or longer, a psychiatrist must determine whether or not the sleep disturbance reduces mood, motor performance, or cognitive function. If disturbed nocturnal sleep leads to daytime dysfunction for a month (and usually longer), as is the case in 6% of adults, the insomnia syndrome is present. In this chronic insomnia group, major depression (14% of all cases), dysthymia (9% of all cases), and anxiety disorders (24% of all cases) commonly are comorbid with the insomnia. Severity of insomnia increases as patients have more medical disorders. To assist in the evaluation of insomnia, psychiatrists are urged to use the 6 Ps + M of insomnia model to conceptualize the important characteristics of the insomnia and to coordinate therapeutic intervention.

References

[1] Jones BE. Basic mechanisms of sleep-wake states. In: Kryger MH, Roth T, Dement WC, editors. Principles and practice of sleep medicine. 4th ed. Philadelphia: Saunders; 2005. p. 136–53.
[2] Kupfer DJ, Reynolds CF. Management of insomnia. N Engl J Med 1997;336:341–6.
[3] Smith MT, Perlis ML, Park A, et al. Comparative meta-analysis of pharmacotherapy and behavior therapy for persistent insomnia. Am J Psychiatry 2002;150:5–11.
[4] Ohayon MM. Epidemiology of insomnia: what we know and what we still need to learn. Sleep Med Rev 2002;6:97–111.
[5] Shinomiya K, Shigemoto Y, Omichi J, et al. Effects of three hypnotics on the sleep-wakefulness cycle in sleep-disturbed rats. Psychopharmacology (Berl) 2004;173:203–9.
[6] American Psychiatric Association. Diagnostic and statistical manual of mental disorders. 4th ed. text revision. Washington, DC: American Psychiatric Press; 2000.
[7] National Institutes of Health. National Institutes of Health State of the Science Conference statement on Manifestations and Management of Chronic Insomnia in Adults, June 13–15, 2005. Sleep 2005;28:1049–57.
[8] American Academy of Sleep Medicine. International classification of sleep disorders. 2nd ed. Diagnostic and coding manual. Westchester (IL): American Academy of Sleep Medicine; 2005.
[9] Edinger JD, Bonnet MH, Bootzin RR, et al. American Academy of Sleep Medicine Work Group. Derivation of research diagnostic criteria for insomnia: report of an American Academy of Sleep Medicine Work Group. Sleep 2004;27:1567–96.
[10] Czeisler CA, Winkelman JW, Richardson GS, Phillipson EA, et al. Sleep disorders. In: Braunwald E, Fauci AS, Kasper DL, et al, editors. Harrison's principles of internal medicine. 15th ed. New York: McGraw Hill; 2001. p. 155–63.

[11] Vallieres A, Ivers H, Bastien CH, et al. Variability and predictability in sleep patterns of chronic insomniacs. J Sleep Res 2005;14:447–53.

[12] Becker PM. Pharmacologic and nonpharmacologic treatments of insomnia. Neurol Clin 2005;23:1149–63.

[13] Nowell PD, Buysse DJ, Reynolds CF 3rd, et al. Clinical factors contributing to the differential diagnosis of primary insomnia and insomnia related to mental disorders. Am J Psychiatry 1997;154:1412–6.

[14] Ohayon MM. Prevalence and correlates of nonrestorative sleep complaints. Arch Intern Med 2005;165:35–41.

[15] Nierenberg AA, Keefe BR, Leslie VC, et al. Residual symptoms in depressed patients who respond acutely to fluoxetine. J Clin Psychiatry 1999;60:221–5.

[16] Tang NK, Harvey AG. Time estimation ability and distorted perception of sleep in insomnia. Behav Sleep Med 2005;3:134–50.

[17] Morin CM. Cognitive-behavioral approaches to the treatment of insomnia. J Clin Psychiatry 2004;65(Suppl 16):33–40.

[18] Breslau N, Roth T, Rosenthal L, et al. Sleep disturbance and psychiatric disorders: a longitudinal epidemiological study of young adults. Biol Psychiatry 1996;39:411–8.

[19] Chang PP, Ford DE, Mead LA, et al. Insomnia in young men and subsequent depression. The Johns Hopkins Precursors Study. Am J Epidemiol 1997;146:105–14.

[20] Katz DA, McHorney CA. The relationship between insomnia and health-related quality of life in patients with chronic illness. J Fam Pract 2002;51:229–35.

[21] Ford DE, Kamerow DB. Epidemiologic study of sleep disturbances and psychiatric disorders. An opportunity for prevention? JAMA 1989;262:1479–84.

[22] Katz DA, McHorney CA. Clinical correlates of insomnia in patients with chronic illness. Arch Intern Med 1998;158:1099–107.

[23] Hatoum HT, Kong SX, Kania CM, et al. Insomnia, health-related quality of life and health-care resource consumption. A study of managed-care organization enrollees. Pharmacoeconomics 1998;14:629–37.

[24] Walsh JK. Clinical and socioeconomic correlates of insomnia [review]. J Clin Psychiatry 2004;65(Suppl 8):13–9.

[25] Leger D, Massuel MA, Metlaine A, SISYPHE Study Group. Professional correlates of insomnia. Sleep 2006;29:171–8.

[26] National Sleep Foundation. Report on highway safety. Washington (DC): National Sleep Foundation. January 17, 2005.

[27] Riedel BW, Lichstein KL. Insomnia and daytime functioning. Sleep Med Rev 2000;4:277–98.

[28] Hauri PJ. Cognitive deficits in insomnia patients. Acta Neurol Belg 1997;97:113–7.

[29] Schneider C, Fulda S, Schulz H. Daytime variation in performance and tiredness/sleepiness ratings in patients with insomnia, narcolepsy, sleep apnea and normal controls. J Sleep Res 2004;13:373–83.

[30] Crenshaw MC, Edinger JD. Slow-wave sleep and waking cognitive performance among older adults with and without insomnia complaints. Physiol Behav 1999;66:485–92.

[31] Smith MT, Perlis ML. Who is a candidate for cognitive-behavioral therapy for insomnia? Health Psychol 2006;25:15–9.

[32] Bonnet MH, Arand DL. Hyperarousal and insomnia. Sleep Med Rev 1997;1:97–108.

[33] Tang NK, Harvey AG. Effects of cognitive arousal and physiological arousal on sleep perception. Sleep 2004;27:69–78.

[34] McCall WV. Diagnosis and management of insomnia in older people [review]. J Am Geriatr Soc 2005;53(7 Suppl):S272–7.

[35] Krystal AD. The effect of insomnia definitions, terminology, and classifications on clinical practice. J Am Geriatr Soc 2005;53(7 Suppl):S258–63.

[36] Winkelman J, Pies R. Current patterns and future directions in the treatment of insomnia. Ann Clin Psychiatry 2005;17:31–40.

[37] Neubauer DN. Insomnia [review]. Prim Care 2005;32:375–88.

[38] Krahn LE. Psychiatric disorders associated with disturbed sleep. Semin Neurol 2005;25: 90–6.

[39] Sateia MJ, Nowell PD. Insomnia. Lancet 2004;364:1959–73.

[40] Benca RM, Ancoli-Israel S, Moldofsky H. Special considerations in insomnia diagnosis and management: depressed, elderly, and chronic pain populations. J Clin Psychiatry 2004; 65(Suppl 8):26–35.

[41] Schenck CH, Mahowald MW, Sack RL. Assessment and management of insomnia. JAMA 2003;289:2475–9.

[42] Spielman AJ, Caruso LS, Glovinsky PB. A behavioral perspective on insomnia treatment. Psychiatr Clin North Am 1987;10:541–53.

[43] Nofzinger EA, Buysse DJ, Germain A, et al. Functional neuroimaging evidence for hyper-arousal in insomnia. Am J Psychiatry 2004;161:2126–8.

[44] Xu Y, Padiath QS, Shapiro RE, et al. Functional consequences of a CKIdelta mutation causing familial advanced sleep phase syndrome. Nature 2005;434:640–4.

treatment decisions. Moreover, those few studies included in the meta-analyses had a median treatment duration of approximately only 1 week. Fortunately, since then, at least a few studies with longer treatment durations have been published.

In general, all currently approved BzRAs are absorbed rapidly, and thus, reduce sleep latency at recommended doses. The longer a drug's duration of action, the more sleep maintenance benefit is observed (ie, minimizing awakenings and WASO). The dose and elimination rate largely determine the duration of action, although delayed or ER properties also contribute for these formulations. Most BzRAs increase total sleep time, the net result of affecting sleep onset and sleep maintenance. The exception is zaleplon, which has a short duration of action and does not increase total sleep time reliably. This short duration of action, however, allows dosing for patients who may have only 4 to 5 hours left before they must rise in the morning or in treating patients who experience morning sedation with longer-acting agents. If zaleplon is administered with at least 5 hours of potential time in bed remaining, the residual sleepiness at wake time is a minimal risk [11].

Tolerance is not found in the majority of studies of a few weeks duration or longer. PSG studies of zolpidem and zaleplon reveal evidence of persistent efficacy over 5 weeks of nightly use [12,13]. In the few longer studies conducted to date, BzRAs seem to retain efficacy for at least several months. Oswald and colleagues report that patients described benefits for 5 to 6 months with BzRAs [14]. A large cohort study of primary insomniacs taking eszopiclone (3 mg nightly for 6 months) demonstrates persistent reduction in subjective sleep latency, fewer awakenings, decreased duration of awakenings, increased total sleep time, and improved quality of sleep compared with placebo [15]. After the double-blinded portion of the study, an open label 6-month extension of the study suggests sustained efficacy for up to 1 year and in fact revealed continued improvement compared with the patient's baseline [16].

Intermittent administration of hypnotics also has been investigated. Zolpidem (10 mg) was given for up to 12 weeks in a non-nightly regimen compared with placebo [17,18]. Patients reported improved sleep latency, frequency of awakenings, total sleep time, and sleep quality. On the nights hypnotics were not administered, rebound insomnia did not occur.

Effectiveness of BzRA hypnotics or any other sleep-promoting medication has not been evaluated systematically (effectiveness refers to systematic assessment of a therapy in the context of the usual clinical environment with clinically relevant endpoints, whereas efficacy refers to the observations in a controlled experimental study). Some relevant data have been collected, however, from clinical populations with surveys and from open-label studies. Ohayon and colleagues surveyed 532 patients, 66% of whom reported "a lot" of improvement in sleep quality and only 14% reported little or no improvement with prescription hypnotics [19]. In another survey, 74% to 84% of patients on triazolam, temazepam, or flurazepam reported satisfaction with their treatment and that they would take the medication again for the same purpose [20].

Few studies have been designed to examine the potential beneficial impact of hypnotics on daytime function and performance. A major barrier has been the failure to identify measurable deficits in waking function associated with untreated insomnia. Often it is difficult to tease out which daytime symptoms are secondary to insomnia and which are related to comorbid conditions. Nevertheless, it is reasonable to expect that insomnia treatment should lead to improvement in waking symptoms or consequences. Investigators recently have begun to focus on daytime outcome measures. During a study of 6-month treatment with eszopiclone, primary insomniacs reported improved daytime alertness, ability to function, and sense of well-being compared with placebo [14]. Multiple sleep latency testing measures of sleepiness improved in patients using hypnotics for insomnia who had comorbid rheumatoid arthritis [21] or periodic leg movements [22], and in a study of elderly insomniacs [23]. Further research into the waking state benefits of insomnia treatment is needed.

A related question deals with whether or not treatment of insomnia might improve one or more aspects of a comorbid medical or psychiatric illness. For example, in Walsh and coworkers' study of rheumatoid arthritis patients who had insomnia, duration of morning stiffness was reduced after 6 nights' treatment with triazolam as compared with placebo treatment (although other arthritis measures did not change) [21]. Recently, Fava and colleagues [24] reported that cotherapy with eszopiclone and fluoxetine was superior to fluoxetine and placebo in reducing ratings of depression on the Hamilton Depression Scale, even after removing the sleep-specific questions. Thus, it seems that assessing change in comorbid condition symptoms (eg, pain) represents a fertile insomnia research area.

Benzodiazepine receptor agonist safety and adverse reactions

Safety concerns for the BzRAs include the risk for dependence or abuse in susceptible individuals, impaired motor and cognitive function while blood levels are present (either at night or the next day), amnesia for events occurring when the drug is active, drug interactions, and toxicity. Importantly, the margin of safety (therapeutic index) is wide; that is, the ratio of effective dose to lethal dose is large and toxicity is rare. The most common side effects are headache, dizziness, and residual sleepiness; but symptoms generally are mild and infrequent.

The risk for residual sedation on the day after using hypnotic medication is determined by the dose and the rate of elimination. More slowly metabolized and eliminated medications (ie, those with intermediate or long half-lives) can exert their effects well into the next day, making drowsiness a potential problem (see Table 1). Short-acting hypnotics (eg, zolpidem and zaleplon) generally are free of residual effects in the morning. Residual sedation can affect performance on psychomotor tests and slow reaction time. It is reasonable to believe that driving and occupational impairment could result. However, it is problematic to extrapolate from the few studies performed on young, healthy volunteers using single doses of drug.

The impact of short- or long-term use of BzRAs on daytime cognition is unclear. Changes attributed to hypnotics, if any, probably are subtle [25] and the clinical significance is not clear [26]. Any meaningful study would have to investigate the impact of insomnia itself on cognition and that probably varies in primary insomniacs versus comorbid settings, and is compounded by the impact of multidrug regimens in many of these patients. Memory impairment can occur with BzRAs, but that is not specific to hypnotics and can be seen with alcohol or any sedating medications. Specifically, anterograde amnesia occurs (difficulty recalling events after the drug is ingested), the extent of which relates to the plasma concentration, with more memory difficulty occurring with higher plasma levels at the time of acquisition of information. Similarly, sleepiness itself can decrease recollection of events when they occur close to sleep onset.

The issue of falls and injury, particularly in the elderly, is a concern for many medications. Any sedating medication potentially could increase fall risk; but a large study of falls in Canada documents that the only medication groups that are independent predictors are narcotics, antidepressants, and anticonvulsants [27]. There are contradictory reports regarding fall and injury risk with BzRAs, and there is some suggestion that insomnia itself is a risk factor for falling, hip fracture, and so forth. Brassington and colleagues [28] find that reported sleep problems, but not use of psychotropic medication, are independent risk factors for falls in community-dwelling adults over 64 years of age. In another recent study, the risk for falls is significantly higher for insomnia without hypnotic use and for insomnia with hypnotic use, but not for hypnotics who did not have insomnia [29]. In other words, if the hypnotic relieves the insomnia, the hypnotic is not a risk factor for falling.

Although substance abusers show they self-administer BzRAs during the day and report a degree of "drug liking," there is no compelling data that BzRA hypnotic use by patients in a clinical situation leads to dependence. Most patients use hypnotic medications for 2 weeks or less [30,31]. Dose escalation is rare, even in patients using hypnotics for months or years [19], and patients generally do not administer hypnotics for purposes other than to promote sleep, such as daytime use. Experimental studies of self-administration indicate that when patients were allowed to self-medicate with triazolam, hypnotic use was stable and determined by symptom relief [32]. That is, insomnia severity, and in particular the perceived quality of sleep the previous night, determines the rate of hypnotic self-administration.

Rebound insomnia refers to a worsening beyond pretreatment measures when a drug is discontinued abruptly. When rebound occurs, it generally lasts only 1 night and can be minimized or prevented by using the lowest effective dose and then tapering before discontinuation [33]. Rebound is more likely after withdrawal of a short-acting or intermediate-acting drug, and the likelihood and severity of rebound is related to hypnotic dose but not necessarily the duration of use. Plasma concentrations slowly decline in the longer acting drugs and rebound is unlikely.

Melatonin Receptor Agonists

Background

Ramelteon, a MtRA, was approved by the FDA in July of 2005, for the treatment of insomnia characterized by difficulty with sleep onset; making it the first FDA-approved hypnotic that is not a BzRA and not a scheduled drug. Ramelteon is selective for the MT1 and MT2 melatonin receptor subtypes [34], which seem to be involved in the regulation of sleep and circadian rhythms. Ramelteon is absorbed (median t_{max} 0.5–1.5 hours) and eliminated (half-life 1–2.6 hours) rapidly but has an active metabolite, M-II, with a half-life of 2 to 5 hours.

Melatonin receptor agonist efficacy and effectiveness

The available details from early studies in primary insomniacs indicate that doses of 4 to 32 mg produce a modest but significant reduction in PSG sleep latency [35] that is maintained for up to 5 weeks (at doses of 8 to 16 mg) when administered nightly [36]. Similar improvements in subjective sleep latency are reported in elderly primary insomniacs treated with ramelteon (48 mg) for 5 weeks [37]. These studies have identified few if any differences in sleep latency over the 4- to 32-mg dose range and no increase in total sleep time beyond the reduction in sleep latency. Although in one study of ramelteon (16 and 64 mg) for transient insomnia, PSG sleep latency was reduced and total sleep time was increased essentially equally for both doses [38], reduction in patient-reported sleep latency is inconsistent.

It is possible that agonism of melatonin receptors promotes sleep onset without a detectable sedative effect, leading to an inconsistent perception of reduced time to sleep onset. This may be true particularly for patients having experience with traditional hypnotics. Ramelteon seems to have chronobiotic properties, producing a phase advance at doses as low as 4 mg [39], potentially explaining ramelteon's ability to promote sleep without appreciable sedation. Effectiveness in broad clinical populations is unstudied to date.

Melatonin receptor agonist safety

Safety trials have detected no potential for abuse relative to placebo and no withdrawal symptoms or rebound insomnia [40]. Ramelteon is found to increase prolactin levels in adult women and reduce testosterone levels in adult men. The clinical significance of these findings is not established nor have studies been conducted in adolescents. Ramelteon undergoes hepatic metabolism at cytochrome P450 1A2 (CYP1A2). Increases in serum concentration are seen even with mild liver disease, so caution is recommended for patients who have at least moderate liver disease. Fluvoxamine inhibits CYP1A2, dramatically increasing the serum concentration of ramelteon, and coadministration with potent CYP1A2 inhibitors should be avoided. Because of low abuse potential, ramelteon may have a role in the treatment of insomnia in individuals who have a history of chemical dependence; however, there are no published reports for that population.

Sedating Antidepressants Used as Hypnotics
Background

Although there are several FDA-approved drugs for insomnia, clinicians and their patients also have turned to many other drugs for the management of insomnia (Table 2). The reasons for this practice are multiple and include regulatory, third-party payer, economic, and clinical influences. Sedating antidepressants commonly are used off-label to treat insomnia.

Since the advent of amitriptyline in the United States in 1961, many antidepressants have been known to have sedating properties. Once considered an adverse effect sufficient for noncompliance by many patients, there is a significant trend to antidepressant medications being prescribed for insomnia management despite the relative absence of systematic research for this use. Several factors likely contribute to their use by physicians in spite of the absence of an established efficacious dose. Sedating antidepressants do not have a recommended limited duration of use on their package insert, in contrast to the BzRAs approved before 2004, leading to reduced scrutiny by regulators and third-party payers when prescribed for chronic treatment. The absence of this cautionary language in the inserts also is likely to contribute to the misperception that sedating antidepressants are safer than BzRAs and carry a lower risk for dependence. It will be interesting to observe whether or not prescribing behavior changes now that there are BzRA hypnotics (eszopiclone and

Table 2
Selected drugs used for insomnia without a Food and Drug Administration indication

Drug name	Drug type	Estimated dose[a]	Route of metabolism/ clearance	Elimination half-life
Trazodone	Antidepressant	50–150 mg	Hepatic/renal, fecal, biliary	3–6 h
Amitriptyline	Antidepressant	25–50 mg	Hepatic/renal	12–24 h
Doxepin	Antidepressant	25–150 mg	Hepatic/renal	10–30 h
Diphenhydramine	Antihistamine	50–100 mg	Hepatic:CYP450/ renal, fecal	6–8 h
Doxylamine	Antihistamine	6.25–25 mg	Unknown	6–12 h
Hydroxyzine	Antihistamine	25–50 mg	Hepatic/renal	7–25 h
Olanzepine	Antipsychotic	2.5–5 mg	Hepatic: glucuronidation, CYP1A2, 2D6/ renal and fecal	21–54 h
Quetiapine	Antipsychotic	25–50 mg	Hepatic: sulfoxidation, CYP3A4/renal and fecal	6–7 h
Melatonin	Hormone	1–10 mg	Hepatic/renal	30–60 minutes
Valerian	Plant extract	400–900 mg	Not established	Not established

[a]Therapeutic dose for insomnia is not established. Listed doses refer to those cited in the literature and used in clinical practice.

zolpidem ER and ramelteon) without a recommended limited duration of use in the label. Finally, insomnia frequently is interpreted solely as a manifestation of depression, and physicians may believe they are treating it only as a secondary condition.

Among the sedating antidepressants prescribed for the treatment of insomnia, trazodone, amitriptyline, and mirtazapine are used most commonly [2]. Although sedating antidepressants often are used for insomnia coexistent with a mood disorder, their use likely is not limited to that situation. As discussed previously, trazodone generally is prescribed at doses far below the range typically needed for the treatment of depression and often is prescribed in the absence of other antidepressant medications; both of which suggest use to treat insomnia in patients who are not depressed.

The neural mechanism mediating the sedating activity of these antidepressants is not identified, but the likelihood that one mechanism is common to all of these agents is low. Trazodone inhibits serotonin reuptake and antagonizes serotonin 2A and serotonin 2C receptors. Trazodone also blocks α_1-adrenergic receptors [41,42]. Amitriptyline inhibits the reuptake of serotonin and norepinephrine and blocks acetylcholine and histamine binding [43–45]. Mirtazapine antagonizes serotonin 2A, serotonin 2C, and serotonin 3 receptors; blocks α_1-adrenergic receptors; and is a strong histamine$_1$ antagonist [46,47]. The adrenergic, histaminergic, and cholinergic systems in the brainstem, midbrain, and basal forebrain all are implicated strongly in the promotion and maintenance of wakefulness; antagonistic activity in relevant portions of these systems easily could result in sedation. The serotonergic system plays a more controversial, less well established, and perhaps more complicated role in wakefulness.

Sedating antidepressants used as hypnotics: efficacy
The hypnotic efficacy of trazodone in insomniacs who are not depressed has been investigated twice (to the authors' knowledge). In the larger of the two studies, the effect of trazodone (50 mg) on subjective sleep measures was compared with zolpidem (10 mg) and placebo in a 2-week, placebo-controlled, parallel-group design. Trazodone and zolpidem shortened latency to sleep onset and increased total sleep time, with improvements with zolpidem greater than trazodone [48]. In an earlier study, PSG and subjective data were collected in nine individuals taking trazodone (150 mg a night for 3 weeks) with comparison made to measures taken before and after discontinuation of trazodone [49]. There was no improvement in sleep latency or total sleep time, but there was a reduction in stage 1 sleep and wakefulness and increased stage 3–4 sleep. Subjectively, there was an improvement in sleep quality. These findings suggest that trazodone may have some sleep-promoting effect in primary insomnia, at least short-term, but efficacy is not well established and the optimal dose remains undetermined. Amitriptyline and mirtazapine often are used as hypnotics for insomniacs who are not depressed, in the absence of published studies as to their efficacy in this group of patients.

Data also is limited for the sedating antidepressants used less commonly. Improved total sleep time was found in a trial of 15 primary insomniacs taking trimipramine (mean 166 mg ± 48 mg), but there was no parallel-placebo control, and PSG measures were made before an adequate period of washout from prior medications occurred [50]. Subjective sleep quality was improved by trimipramine (100 mg) when compared with placebo (taken nightly for 1 month) in a study by Hohagen and colleagues, but there were insignificant increases in total sleep time [51]. Doxepin (25–50 mg) produced increased total sleep time and improved subjective sleep quality [52].

Several studies have been performed investigating the efficacy of sedating antidepressants in depressed insomniacs, but small sample sizes and experimental design weaknesses limit the value of these studies. There was no consistent improvement in the continuity of sleep in subjects taking amitriptyline in two small studies that lacked placebo controls [53,54]. Subjective improvements in the latency to sleep onset and total sleep time were reported by six patients who had major depression when treated with mirtazapine for 2 weeks (15 mg increasing to 30 mg in the second week), again without a placebo control [55]. When a fixed dose of mirtazapine was compared with an escalating dose, similar subjective improvements in sleep latency and total sleep time were reported [47].

Sedating antidepressants used as hypnotics: safety and adverse reactions
The antidepressants as a class have more frequent and troublesome side effects in comparison to BzRAs. Tricyclic antidepressants in particular are known for their less than ideal side-effect profile, which has led in part to the greater reliance now placed on the selective serotonin reuptake inhibitors for the treatment of depression. The majority of safety data for the sedating antidepressants have been acquired from their use in mood or anxiety disorders at doses higher than those used for insomnia, and it is difficult to extrapolate the data to insomnia use. In trials of tricyclics used to treat primary insomnia, however, there are reports of leucopenia, thrombocytopenia, increased liver enzymes with doxepin [52]; dizziness, dry mouth, and nausea with trimipramine [56]; and daytime somnolence and weight gain with mirtazapine [56]. Given the pharmacokinetics of these drugs (mean half-lives of 9–30 hours for most drugs), residual sedation after bedtime administration is likely, although this has not been assessed directly.

Although trazodone is viewed by some as having a more favorable side-effect profile compared with the tricyclics, supportive data is lacking; moreover, the margin between lethal and safe dose is much smaller than that of the BzRAs. Troublesome side effects with trazodone include orthostatic hypotension, cardiac conduction abnormalities, and priapism [57].

At this time, there is insufficient data justifying the efficacious or safe use of sedating antidepressants for primary insomnia, and it cannot be recommended [57]. Their use for insomnia may have more to do with regulatory issues and perceived risks about the BzRAs that do not seem warranted based on available studies. Alternatively, individuals who have insomnia and coexistent depression may be a population for whom the sedating antidepressants are a reasonable choice, with the understanding that the side-effect profile of the BzRAs still seems more favorable than the profiles of any of the sedating antidepressants. Substance abusers are another patient group for whom sedating antidepressants may have a more favorable risk-to-benefit ratio, given the greater reinforcing effect of the BzRAs. As with any other treatment decision, the risks and benefits of a sleep medication regimen must be weighed and discussed with patients on an individual basis.

OTHER DRUGS AND SUBSTANCES USED AS HYPNOTICS
Prescriptive and Over-the-Counter Medications
In addition to off-label use of sedating antidepressants for insomnia, other prescription and OTC drugs use for this purpose include antihistamines (diphenhydramine and hydroxyzine), antipsychotics (quetiapine and olanzepine), muscle relaxants (cyclobenzaprine), and herbal supplements. Little is proved regarding their hypnotic efficacy, and safety concerns exist.

Diphenhydramine (at doses from 25 to 50 mg) has been evaluated in several brief and small trials lacking parallel placebo control, showing global improvement in general condition with treatment [58] and improvement in subjective sleep latency and sleep quality [59]. Histamine plays a role in maintenance of wakefulness. Tolerance to the sedative effect of diphenhydramine (25 to 50 mg two or three times per day) is, however, clearly shown to develop within 3 to 4 days [5,6].

The atypical antipsychotics, quetiapine and olanzepine, are active across a broad range of neurotransmitter systems, including H_1 receptors (antagonist); serotonin 2C (antagonist); and adrenergic, muscarinic, and dopaminergic circuits. Efficacy data for use in insomnia practically is nonexistent. Quetiapine and olanzapine at various dosages improved subjective measures of sleep in two small open-label studies of patients who had comorbid insomnia [60,61]. Although the sedative property of these medications (potentially mediated in part through histaminergic antagonism) makes them potentially useful; their broad activity across the CNS, resulting in several undesirable side effects, makes them less tolerable. Their troubling drug-drug/drug-enzyme interactions and concerns regarding increased risk for patients developing metabolic syndrome also are cautionary notes. Both of these antipsychotics reach peak plasma levels relatively slowly and have half-lives that make residual sedation likely. In the case of olanzepine, the duration of action is long (elimination half-life of 20–50 hours). In any event, their sleep-promoting effects are not assessed adequately for any form of insomnia.

Finally, patients who have chronic insomnia often resort to OTC remedies of questionable benefit. Most of these agents contain diphenhydramine and produce sedation through an antihistaminergic mechanism. Alcohol also is commonly chosen, however. There are significant concerns in that alcohol induces tolerance rapidly and exacerbates other sleep disorders (eg, restless leg syndrome and obstructive sleep apnea). After even acute administration of

sleep and dampens the circadian rhythm regulating sleep and wakefulness, which yields periods of extended wakefulness just as the poor sleeper anticipated.

Directly addressing dysfunctional thinking about sleep through education and targeted cognitive treatment has been associated with sleep improvement [52,53]. Such challenges to often long-held assumptions have become a cornerstone of nonpharmacologic treatment for insomnia.

Maladaptive Sleep Practices

Poor sleepers generally do not appreciate how important behaviors surrounding bedtime are in determining sleep quality. They rush home from an evening work shift and hope in vain to be sleeping an hour later. They exercise late at night in a bid to exhaust themselves, only to find that they are strangely energized at bedtime. Enjoyable and seemingly relaxing activities, such as phone calls to friends or video games, may prove so stimulating that sleep is deferred.

Behaviors meant to compensate for nocturnal wakefulness and improve daytime functioning ultimately may prove harmful to sleep. Coping strategies, such as keeping extended bedtimes, daytime napping, and weekend oversleeping, often bring short-term relief. In the long-term, however, they tend to reduce the sleep drive available to promote sleep at bedtime and disrupt the synchronization between the desired sleep/wake schedule and endogenous circadian rhythms. Box 1 lists common daily life practices that may interfere with sleep in these ways.

Emotional Arousal

Poor sleep is expected when individuals are under acute environmental stress or in emotional turmoil. As the autonomic nervous system and the hormonal system react to strong stresses or emotions, these physiologic processes may disrupt normal sleep mechanisms [42]. In addition to these direct physiologic effects, cognitive reactions to stressful and emotional situations, such as ruminative worrying, may interfere with sleep further.

Although transient insomnia resulting from acute stress is a nearly universal experience, some individuals are more vulnerable to sleep disruption than others [54]. Their insomnia tends to become chronic. Studies on personality traits in insomniacs have reported that individuals who tend to internalize conflicts through self-inhibition, denial, or suppression seem to be more susceptible to insomnia [55]. Other psychological factors, such as perfectionism, the need for control, excessive worrying, and depression, also have been found to be associated with insomnia [55–58].

Arousal at bedtime also can be a learned response. The repeated experience of poor sleep promotes an association between sleeplessness and presleep activities and the sleep setting. When these connections are established, the bedtime rituals and environment become contextual cues for arousal rather than for sleep [59].

Box 1: Sleep-related habits and daily life practices that may interfere with sleep

Practices that reduce homeostatic drive at bedtime

Daily life behaviors

- Insufficient activities during the day
- Lying down to get rest during the day

Sleep-related habits

- Napping, nodding, and dozing off during the day or evening
- In a trance, semiawake in the evening
- Spending too much time in bed
- Extra sleep on weekends

Practices that disrupt circadian regularity

Daily life behaviors

- Insufficient morning light exposure, leading to a phase delay in circadian rhythm
- Early morning light exposure, producing early morning awakening owing to a phase advance in circadian rhythm

Sleep-related habits

- Irregular sleep-wake schedule
- Sleeping-in in the morning during weekends

Practices that enhance the level of arousal

Daily life behaviors
- Excess caffeine consumption or caffeine later in the day
- Smoking in the evening
- Alcohol consumption in the evening
- Exercising in the late evening
- Late evening meal (may cause nocturnal acid reflux) or fluid (may cause frequent urination)
- Getting home late or insufficient time to wind down

Sleep-related habits
- Evening apprehension of sleep
- Preparations for bed are arousing
- No regular presleep ritual
- Distressing pillow talk
- Watching television, reading, engaging in other sleep-incompatible behaviors in bed before lights out, or falling asleep with television or radio left on
- Trying too hard to sleep
- Clock watching during the night
- Staying in bed during awakenings or lingering in bed awake in the morning
- Nonconducive sleep environment, such as bed-partner snoring, noises, direct morning sunlight, or pets in the bedroom

DEVELOPMENTAL MODEL OF INSOMNIA

Over the course of an evolving insomnia, the relative contribution of physiologic, psychological, and behavioral factors may vary. These factors also can be grouped temporally, into characteristics that *predispose* an individual to insomnia, events that *precipitate* the acute sleep disorder, and attitudes and practices that *perpetuate* the problem, transforming it into a chronic condition (Fig. 2) [60,61]. This conceptualization, which is known as the "3 P" model, is useful not only in enhancing understanding of the etiology of a particular insomnia case, but also in directing treatment efforts.

Common characteristics that predispose to insomnia include physiologic hyperarousal, manifested by such markers as an increased metabolic rate, an overactive hypothalamic-pituitary-adrenal axis, and elevated muscle tension. Cognitive hyperarousal, reflected in mind racing, chronic worrying, and a "hair trigger" startle response, is another common trait that increases the risk of developing insomnia. Another predisposing factor is the degree to which one's preferred timing of sleep (so called night types and morning types) deviates from societal norms.

Precipitating events usually are readily identified as the "cause" of insomnia. These triggers can be dire, as in grave illness, divorce, or job loss; full of excitement and apprehension, as with the birth of a child or a promotion at work; or relatively trivial, such as a switch of mattress. Often a triggering event resolves with the passage of time, and sleep regroups.

Insomnia may persist long after its precipitating event has resolved, however. In this situation, the contribution of perpetuating attitudes and practices has moved to the forefront. As discussed earlier, the poor sleeper through repeated experience of sleeplessness may have learned to associate the bedroom with anxiety or adopt temporarily beneficial but ultimately counterproductive

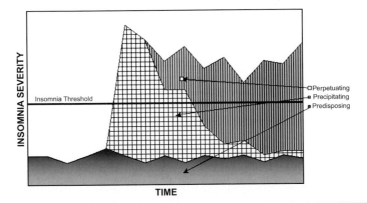

Fig. 2. The "3 P" model of insomnia, in this case illustrating the major contributions of *precipitating* and *perpetuating* factors and the minor contribution of *predisposing* factors. (*Adapted from* Spielman AJ, Caruso LS, Glovinsky PB. A behavioral perspective on insomnia treatment. Psychiatr Clin North Am 1987;10(4):541–53; with permission.)

practices, such as oversleeping or relying on caffeine to compensate for the effects of sleep loss. By the time an individual contending with chronic insomnia comes to clinical attention, these perpetuating factors often present the most opportune target for behavioral treatment.

This is not to say that the other two factors in the "3 P" model should be overlooked as targets of intervention. Predisposing characteristics generally are insufficient in themselves to yield chronic insomnia, but they can bring individuals so close to the threshold that only a slight perturbation is required to precipitate sleeplessness. If a trait such as physiologic hyperarousal has been identified in the course of evaluation, the clinician may wish to consider adding relaxation training or increased exercise to more specific treatments. Similarly, to the extent that precipitating events can be mitigated, sleep may respond in turn. If marital strife is seen as directly inducing sleep loss, conjoint counseling is likely bring improved sleep among its other benefits. Box 2 lists common factors contributing to insomnia grouped according to the "3 P" model and the three processes governing sleep and wakefulness.

EVALUATION

The heart of the clinical evaluation of insomnia is the interview. The clinical history should include the chief sleep complaints, daytime consequences, the circumstances of the onset and course of the insomnia, typical weekday and weekend sleep patterns, beliefs about sleep and the sleep problem and compensatory responses, probes for concurrent sleep disorders, general medical status, medication and substance use, the effects of prior treatments, family history, and assessments of psychological and social functioning.

The evaluation is facilitated by the use of a daily sleep log kept for 1 or 2 weeks (Fig. 3). The patient records various time-locked aspects of the sleep pattern, including retiring times, sleep-onset latencies, distribution and duration of sleep episodes, arising times, and daytime naps. Although bedtimes and rising times may be supplied by glancing at a clock, the other nocturnal parameters should be estimated in the morning as a "best guess," rather than fastidiously supplied by watching the clock all night. The patient supplies a subjective rating of sleep quality and, in the evening as the next bedtime is being marked down, a rating of fatigue during the day just passed. Events such as caffeine and alcohol intake, exercise, light exposure, and medication use also are logged. Although sleep logs are available in various formats, the authors favor a graphic log for its ability to convey quickly changes in sleep patterns from week to week.

Sleep logs provide the clinician with diagnostic clues and identify opportunities for therapeutic intervention. They also offer patients an opportunity to gain a wider perspective—countering their tendency to see sleep as totally random or to fixate on the worst or most recent nights at the expense of supplying a more comprehensive picture.

If the patient's history suggests the possibility of underlying physiologically based sleep disruption, such as a sleep-related breathing disorder or a sleep-

**Box 2: Common contributing factors associated
with the development of insomnia**

Predisposing factors

Homeostatic process

- Abnormality or weakness of the neurophysiologic system that generates sleep

Circadian process

- Extreme circadian type—"owls" predisposed to the late evening or "larks" inclined to the early morning as an individual trait
- Less flexible circadian system

Arousal system

- Anxiety-prone and depressive personality traits and tendencies toward neuroticism and somatization lead to a higher level of emotional and physiologic arousals
- Personality traits associated with sustained level of arousal, such as perfectionism and excessive need for control
- Heightened or more sensitive physiologic arousal system

Precipitating factors

Homeostatic process

- Lack of or decrease of daytime activities, such as retirement

Circadian process

- Change of sleep-wake schedule, such as jet lag or start of a night shift job

Arousal system

- Life stressors or events lead to emotional and physiologic distress

Perpetuating factors
Homeostatic process
- Increased resting in bed
- Discharge of the sleep drive by sleeping outside of the nocturnal sleep period, such as increased daytime naps or frequent dozing offs
- Reduced daytime activities

Circadian process
- Sleep-in during weekend to catch up on sleep
Arousal system
- Dysfunctional beliefs and attitudes about sleep that lead to increased emotional arousals and worries over sleep loss
- Conditioning between bedtime cues and arousal

Adapted from Spielman AJ, Caruso LS, Glovinsky PB. A behavioral perspective on insomnia treatment. Psychiatr Clin North Am 1987;10(4):541–53; with permission.

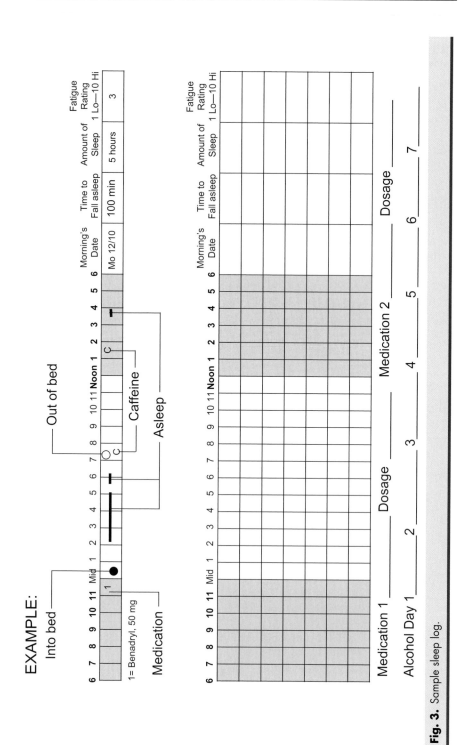

Fig. 3. Sample sleep log.

related movement disorder, referral to a sleep center for a nocturnal polysom-nographic recording is necessary to establish the diagnosis. Similarly, appropriate psychiatric or medical consultation should be recommended when comorbidities are judged to be pertinent to the sleep problem. In such cases, behavioral treatment of insomnia may proceed apace; often, concurrent treatment of predisposing and perpetuating factors yields the best treatment response.

COGNITIVE BEHAVIORAL INTERVENTIONS

Cognitive behavioral interventions for insomnia generally are well accepted and tolerated [62]. Nonetheless, there are some general issues of perception that the clinician would be wise to anticipate: From the patient's point of view, the entire gamut of cognitive behavioral treatment components often is reduced to the notion that a pill is not being swallowed. As opposed to the security of having a small bottle in the medicine cabinet, requiring just a few seconds and a glass of water to deploy, these treatments may require patients to carve out blocks of time, perform homework-like exercises, and deny themselves short-term relief. They may even dictate practices, such as leaving a warm bed in the middle of the night for a chair in the living room or setting an alarm clock to awaken oneself early in the morning after just having gotten to sleep that seem downright ridiculous.

As with other treatments in which conditions often get worse before they get better, it is important to impart an understanding to the patient of the rationale behind such seemingly onerous recommendations and the expected time course toward recovery. It is beneficial to declare at the outset that improvement is likely to take weeks rather than a few nights. It also is helpful to secure an early victory with regard to at least some part of the problem. Although the treatments present many challenges for patients in terms of adherence, they usually do produce a fairly quick and dramatic reduction in the time it takes to fall asleep. This benefit should not go unheralded.

Stimulus Control Instructions

One of the first behavioral treatments specifically developed to address the problem of insomnia is stimulus control instructions (SCI) [59]. SCI aims to break the maladaptive association between bedtime cues and conditioned arousal that accrues with the repeated experience of sleeplessness. SCI treatment consists of eliminating sleep-incompatible behaviors, such as eating, talking, and worrying in bed. Re-establishing the connection between going to sleep in bed and rapid sleep onset is accomplished by having patients get out of bed if not asleep after about 20 minutes; they spend time reading in a chair or engaged in a sedentary, distracting, but not overly engrossing activity, returning to bed when they feel sleepy (see Box 3 for detailed instructions). Initially, patients may spend a considerable amount of time out of bed following the 20-minute rule and experience some sleep loss. The ensuing partial sleep deprivation tends to foster rapid sleep onset. Over time, the repeated association of bedroom cues with rapid sleep onset is said to bring sleep under the

Box 3: Stimulus control instructions

1. Go to sleep only when you feel sleepy.
2. Do not use your bed or bedroom for anything except sleep (sexual activity is the only exception).
3. If you have not fallen asleep within approximately 20 minutes, get up and go into another room. Engage in relaxing activities, such as non–work-related light reading, and go back to bed when you feel sleepy or are ready for sleep.
4. If you cannot fall back to sleep, repeat step 3.
5. Set the alarm for the same time each morning.

Adapted from Bootzin RR. Stimulus control treatment for insomnia. Proc Am Psychol Assoc 1972;7:395–6.

"stimulus control" of the bedroom environment. Patients should be informed at the outset that some daytime deficits are to be expected at the initiation of treatment, and that the treatment requires a few weeks to show consistent effects.

The clinician is likely to hear several reservations regarding SCI treatment. First, the patient may argue that there is no chance of sleep occurring at all if the bed is abandoned. Second, patients may declare that they become wide awake when they allow themselves to read for a short while. Third, they may balk at sitting all alone in a cold, less hospitable room in the middle of the night. Finally, they may complain of daytime deficits after nights that have contained several stints away from bed.

Skeptical patients should be encouraged to consider that their experience with SCI treatment is properly compared with a night spent tossing and turning in bed and its daytime aftermath—the presenting complaint—rather than to some idealized sleep experience. An easy chair in the next room can be furnished with a cozy throw and a focused reading light—it can be comfortable as long as it is not too soporific. The clinician also might point out that a fair amount of sleep loss already is occurring, accompanied by frustration and helplessness. SCI treatment, by contrast, puts more "control" in the hands of the patient. Although it cannot make sleep appear on command, it does allow the patient to refuse the totally passive role heretofore assigned.

Sleep Restriction Therapy

Sleep restriction therapy (SRT) addresses the dilution of the homeostatic sleep drive and the dysregulation of the circadian sleep/wake cycle that is characteristic of chronic insomnia, often secondary to excessive time spent in bed as patients attempt to cope with sleep loss (Box 4).

As its name implies, SRT induces a mild-to-moderate sleep debt at the beginning of treatment, heightening sleep drive [61,63]. It corrals whatever sleep does accrue into a more consistent time slot and precludes compensatory daytime napping, enhancing the circadian sleep/wake cycle. As with SCI, it also

Box 4: Sleep restriction therapy

1. From information provided on a sleep log completed for at least 1 wk, set the initial time in bed equal to the reported average total sleep time. To avoid severe sleep deprivation, minimum time in bed is 5 h.

Version 1

2. Increase time in bed by 15–30 min when the average reported sleep efficiency (sleep efficiency = average sleep time/time in bed × 100%) for 5 days is ≥90% (≥85% in older individuals).

3. When sleep efficiency from 5 days documented on a sleep log is <85% (<80% in older individuals), decrease time in bed by 15 min.

4. When sleep efficiency from 5 days documented on a sleep log is 85–90% (80–85% in older individuals), keep time in bed the same.

Version 2

2. Following the original restriction, increase time in bed progressively by 15–30 min each week until the patient is spending 7 h in bed. Further changes are made based on daytime functioning, fatigue, and sleepiness.

Adapted from Spielman AJ, Caruso LS, Glovinsky PB. A behavioral perspective on insomnia treatment. Psychiatr Clin North Am 1987;10(4):541–53; with permission.

addresses the anticipatory anxiety that builds up with chronic sleeplessness by consistently producing more successful entries into sleep.

SRT treatment begins with a 1- to 2-week baseline sleep log. Average nightly total sleep time is estimated from this log, and initial bedtimes are set so that the time spent in bed is equal to this reported sleep duration. A patient who spends 8.5 hours in bed but typically gets only 5.5 hours of sleep would be instructed to spend 5.5 hours in bed at the start of treatment. The exact bedtime and rising time are negotiated with the patient, taking work and social obligations and when the bulk of nocturnal wakefulness is occurring into account. If difficulty with sleep initiation is paramount, the patient would be assigned a relatively late bedtime, whereas a patient who is plagued by early morning awakenings would be given a relatively early rising time. The initial time in bed is not set at less than about 5 hours, even when patients subjectively report just a few hours of sleep or none at all, to avoid extreme sleep loss over time.

In the authors' original formulation of SRT, subsequent time in bed was adjusted weekly based on reported subjective sleep efficiency (total sleep time/ time in bed × 100%) as gleaned from ongoing sleep logs according to the rules that are detailed in Box 4.

More recently, the authors have been employing an alternative SRT approach that progressively increases time in bed each week, after the initial restriction, so long as the patient's subjectively estimated wake time in bed is 45 minutes or more [64]. Fifteen-minute increments in time in bed are preferred to give the treatment time to work, but 30 minutes might be allowed if daytime sleepiness becomes too pronounced. This approach avoids the dispiriting effect of reducing bedtime again after the shock of the initial truncation has been assimilated.

Despite this modification, SRT can remain a formidable experience for the patient. The main objections to be addressed are usually daytime sleepiness and the perceived inanity of waking to an alarm clock when sleep is finally present; patients also are at a loss for things to do during their extra hours of wakefulness, and they may report that they are plenty sleepy earlier in the evening, but experience a "second wind" by the time their assigned bed-times roll around.

The clinician's challenge is to contrast the short-term discomfort produced by SRT treatment against the months or years that insomnia has been allowed to progress unabated and to impart sufficient understanding of the homeostatic and circadian processes regulating sleep to motivate patients to stick out the first weeks of treatment. The clinician needs to focus on the shorter sleep laten-cies that begin to appear on the logs, the increasing consistency of sleep, and the reduction in anticipatory anxiety that occurs when night-to-night variability sleep lessens. The clinician explains to the patient that over the long run, put-ting together a string of nights of sleep of relatively short duration but greater depth and consolidation is preferable to the haphazard pattern the patient began with.

Patients who experience a second wind should be counseled to become more physically active or intellectually engaged in the early evening. They are likely on the verge of sleep too early in the night and need to understand that, similar to a pilot gauging final approach, they should adjust their "altitude" relative to when they want to touch down. The later bedtimes to which they have been assigned according to SRT still should allow for a buffer period of several hours, containing less demanding activity, in which to unwind. Finally, the cli-nician should not lose the opportunity to point out that sleepiness in itself is often a sign of progress in cases of chronic insomnia. Contending as they do with hyperarousal seemingly around the clock, it is common for patients to welcome sleepiness as a sign that their sleep mechanisms are still viable. On such recognition, their goal becomes one of prodding sleepiness into making an appearance at the right time and place.

Relaxation Training

Insomnia is a problem that can be brought about, in individuals who are pre-disposed, not only by maladaptive behaviors, but also merely by thinking. Thoughts themselves might be inimical to sleep, such as concerns over how the bills are to be paid or worries about what a pending laboratory result might show. In addition, the way in which one thinks might be sufficient to waylay sleep, even when thought content is benign. Many patients complain of a "rac-ing mind" in which trifling observations or jingle snippets may be accelerated, as in a cyclotron, to highly energized (and energizing) states.

The interaction of sleep with waking behavior and thought can be put to good therapeutic effect—that is, sleep may be facilitated by activities that promote mental calm and physical relaxation. Many cognitive behavioral techniques that originally were developed to reduce tension and anxiety have been deployed successfully in the management of insomnia. Examples include progressive muscle relaxation, which reduces muscle tension by sequentially tensing and relaxing the main muscle groups [65,66]; autogenic training, which promotes somatic relaxation by inducing sensations of warmth and heaviness [66]; and guided imagery that shepherds potentially wayward cognitions toward a relaxing scene [67]. Biofeedback also has been used to help patients achieve behavioral and mental states more conducive to sleep [68,69].

Regardless of modality, relaxation training usually starts with an in-office demonstration (Box 5). This training session can be recorded to facilitate home practice; commercial tapes and disks also are available. The clinician should be prepared to "lower the bar," if necessary, over what constitutes a relaxed state because it is important to send the patient home flush with at least a modicum of success in this endeavor. Many insomnia patients display hyperarousal around the clock—just keeping their eyes closed and breathing paced for a few minutes without interjecting some comment or question may represent progress.

Patients should be instructed to practice the chosen technique at home once or twice per day. They should assess their subjective level of relaxation before and after each practice session with a simple rating scale to monitor their progress—it may take weeks for some individuals to develop the skill to relax. Some patients express great frustration over their inability to do so. Patients may be encouraged by the clinician noting that relaxation, in contrast to sleep, is a state that can be made to materialize on cue, whereas sleep usually scoffs at those who strive mightily to achieve it.

Patients initially should avoid using the procedure to try to induce sleep at night. The stakes are too high at bedtime; their interim goal should be to foster successful efforts at rest as opposed to sleep. "Rest" is a state often bypassed completely by insomniacs as they struggle to initiate or return to sleep. Even when attained, it may be defined as a failure to sleep, as opposed to a rewarding state in its own right. When restfulness is properly valued and even indulged in, it can serve as an effective staging ground for sleep in bed.

Cognitive Therapy

This article already has discussed how faulty beliefs and attitudes about sleep have been associated with insomnia, and how challenging it may be to break a vicious cycle of anxiety and arousal [48,50,52]. Common dysfunctional cognitions about sleep can be classified into five categories: (1) misconceptions concerning the causes of insomnia, (2) misattributions or amplifications of its consequences, (3) unrealistic sleep expectations, (4) diminished perceptions of control, and (5) mistaken beliefs about the predictability of sleep [48].

Misconceptions about sleep may be corrected with sleep hygiene. Cognitive restructuring also is used to address the sleep-disturbing cognitions directly;

> **Box 5: Relaxation training (progressive muscle relaxation, autogenic training, slow deep abdominal breathing, guided imagery)**
>
> 1. Explain the rationale for the specific technique.
> 2. The clinician demonstrates the technique for the patient during an office visit.
> 3. The patient practices the technique at home once or twice a day (for about 10 min) in between office visits.
> 4. The clinician's instructions and demonstration can be recorded, or commercial tapes can be used to facilitate the practice at home.
> 5. It may take a few weeks of practice before the patient develops the skill required.
> 6. The patient is told not to use the technique for sleep until a moderate level of skill in performing the technique is achieved.

such treatment replaces the thoughts with more realistic assessments and positive ideas [47,48]. With the help of the clinician, patients usually are able to identify several dysfunctional thoughts that may interfere with their sleep (Box 6). These thoughts and beliefs are held up to challenge and replaced by more realistic and adaptive notions. The patient is enlisted as a coinvestigator in this effort. A patient may declare that she is unable to function at work if she does not get 8 hours of sleep. She may be asked to rate job performance every day and to log these ratings along with her sleep data. The relationship between sleep quality and job performance is then examined to refute or at least modify her belief. The opportunity also might be taken to educate the patient in this scenario about how circadian rhythms and the arousal system can rally individuals to meet the day's challenges even when they have slept poorly the night before.

Sleep Hygiene Education

Sleep hygiene refers to the habits and practices of everyday living that affect sleep. The hour one chooses to sit down to dinner, how much and what one

> **Box 6: Cognitive therapy**
>
> 1. Discuss with patients their general beliefs regarding sleep and their sleep problems. Subjective rating scales on sleep beliefs, such as the Dysfunctional Beliefs and Attitudes Scale [48], can be used to help evaluate the patient's sleep cognitions.
> 2. Identify the counterproductive beliefs.
> 3. Enlist the patient as a coinvestigator to help gather data that would test and refute the dysfunctional beliefs.
> 4. Provide correct information to address the specific dysfunctional beliefs.

[80] Sasseville A, Paquet N, Sevigny J, et al. Blue blocker glasses impede the capacity of bright light to suppress melatonin production. J Pineal Res 2006;41:73–8.
[81] Campbell SS, Dawson D, Anderson MW. Alleviation of sleep maintenance insomnia with timed exposure to bright light. J Am Geriatr Soc 1993;41:829–36.
[82] Singer CM, Lewy AJ. Case report: use of the dim light melatonin onset in the treatment of ASPS with bright light. Sleep Res 1989;18:445.
[83] Edinger JD, Sampson WS. A primary care "friendly" cognitive behavioral insomnia therapy. Sleep 2003;26:177–82.
[84] Mimeault V, Morin CM. Self-help treatment for insomnia: bibliotherapy with and without professional guidance. J Consult Clin Psychol 1999;67:511–9.
[85] Hauri P, Linde S. No more sleepless night. New York: John Wiley & Sons; 1990.
[86] Jacobs G, Benson H. Say good night to insomnia: the six-week, drug-free program developed at Harvard Medical School. New York: Henry Holt & Company; 1998.
[87] Bastien CH, Morin CM, Ouellet MC, et al. Cognitive-behavioral therapy for insomnia: comparison of individual therapy, group therapy, and telephone consultation. J Consult Clin Psychol 2004;72:653–9.
[88] Verbeek I, Declerck G, Knuistingh NA, et al. Sleep information by telephone: callers indicate positive effects on sleep problems. Sleep Hypnosis 2002;4:47–51.
[89] Strom L, Pettersson R, Andersson G. Internet-based treatment for insomnia: a controlled evaluation. J Consult Clin Psychol 2004;72:113–20.
[90] Espie CA, Inglis SJ, Tessier S, et al. The clinical effectiveness of cognitive behaviour therapy for chronic insomnia: implementation and evaluation of a sleep clinic in general medical practice. Behav Res Ther 2001;39:45–60.

Excessive Daytime Sleepiness: Considerations for the Psychiatrist

Scott M. Leibowitz, MD[a],
Stephen N. Brooks, MD[b], Jed E. Black, MD[b],*

[a]Sleep Disorders Center of CDS, Atlanta, GA
[b]Department of Psychiatry and Behavioral Sciences and Stanford Sleep Disorders Center,
Stanford University, 401 Quarry Road, #3301, Stanford, CA 94305, USA

Fatigue and daytime sleepiness are common complaints in psychiatric patients. Patients who experience sleepiness (used synonymously with the term *somnolence* in this article) at unwanted times that adversely affects their daytime functioning are said to have pathologic sleepiness or excessive daytime sleepiness (EDS). Although psychiatric illness or medication side effects may be a cause of sleepiness, insufficient sleep is the most common cause of EDS in the general population. When an individual complains of frank sleepiness, other important etiologies to consider, in addition to insufficient sleep, are disturbances in the normal homeostatic mechanisms that govern sleep and wakefulness, which may manifest clinically as EDS. These syndromes may coexist with underlying psychiatric illness, complicating the diagnostic workup and treatment. Syndromes involving sleep fragmentation, circadian timing misalignment, or primary central nervous system (CNS) disorders are a frequent cause of EDS in the general population and should be considered in all patients complaining of EDS or fatigue. Lack of an understanding of these conditions not only leads to their being misdiagnosed or overlooked, but at times also results in gross mismanagement (eg, the use of antipsychotic medications in patients with narcolepsy-related hypnagogic hallucinations or the institution of antidepressant therapy in patients complaining of hypersomnolence who are misdiagnosed with depression).

A distinction should be noted between EDS and fatigue, although these descriptors frequently are used interchangeably in clinical practice. A patient with EDS often struggles to maintain wakefulness in monotonous situations, whereas a patient with the complaint of fatigue may have EDS, but may have no feeling of sleepiness and may be experiencing listlessness or lethargy, rather than a tendency to fall asleep. Although there is considerable overlap between these two complaints, and both complaints may indicate a significant problem, the former is a more specific symptom complex, usually indicating

---

*Corresponding author. E-mail address: jedblack@stanford.edu (J.E. Black).

0193-953X/06/$ – see front matter © 2006 Jed E. Black, Scott M. Leibowitz, and Stephen N. Brooks.
doi:10.1016/j.psc.2006.09.004   psych.theclinics.com

a specific physiologic state, whereas the latter is a nonspecific complaint that may represent numerous chronic or acute physiologic or psychological processes.

The American Academy of Sleep Medicine defines EDS in the International Classification of Sleep Disorders (ICSD) as "a complaint of difficulty in maintaining desired wakefulness or a complaint of excessive amount of sleep" [1]. The ICSD notes that excessive sleepiness (also referred to as *excessive somnolence*) is a subjective report of difficulty maintaining the alert awake state, usually accompanied by a rapid entrance into sleep when the individual is sedentary [1]. The severity criteria for sleepiness in the ICSD are based on frequency and degree of associated daytime impairment. This article summarizes the clinical presentation, differential diagnosis, commonly used diagnostic tools, and treatment options for patients complaining of EDS.

EPIDEMIOLOGY OF EXCESSIVE DAYTIME SLEEPINESS

Although a substantial portion of the general population experiences sleepiness, the reported prevalence figures for EDS vary widely. The largest and most comprehensive representative population survey [2] was performed across four Western European countries (United Kingdom, Germany, Spain, and Italy). Substantial EDS, defined as meeting three parameters of marked sleepiness during 3 or more days a week, was reported in 15% of this combined population. In the United States, smaller population surveys have been conducted. Polls suggest that 15% to 16% of the US population 18 years old and older may experience EDS that interferes with daily activities a few days a week or more [3,4] These polls did not differentiate between causes of EDS.

EVALUATION OF THE PATIENT WITH EXCESSIVE DAYTIME SLEEPINESS
Medical History

A detailed history and physical examination are crucial in evaluating the patient complaining of EDS. Important points of the sleep history that the clinician should document include, but are not limited to, total daily 24-hour sleep time, daily sleep patterns, number of nocturnal awakenings, prolonged sleep latencies, snoring, witnessed apneas, symptoms of restless legs syndrome, periodic limb movements of sleep (PLMS), and restless sleep. Medical conditions and alcohol or drug use can be significant contributors to EDS; if any of these are suspected, appropriate evaluation should ensue. Long-term use of any sedating medications should be noted.

Questionnaires and Inventories

Several questionnaires have been developed to help clinicians screen for and evaluate patients for sleepiness and its impact on daily living, including the Epworth Sleepiness Scale (ESS) [5], the Stanford Sleepiness Scale [6], and the Sleep-Wake Activity Inventory [7]. The ESS is the most commonly used questionnaire because of its ease of use and its small but statistically significant correlation with an objective test of sleepiness known as the multiple sleep latency test (MSLT) [8–10]. Although ESS scores are not entirely representative of true level of sleepiness, and the test is neither highly specific nor sensitive for the existence of pathologic sleepiness, the ESS serves as a useful screen for patients who are severely sleepy [11]. Given the test's ease of use and the high prevalence of sleepiness among the general population, the authors advocate administering the ESS to all adult patients in any clinical practice (Fig. 1).

To characterize a patient's sleep further, a sleep log can be helpful in establishing circadian tendencies and patterns of sleep. If the patient is unable to give a reliable history or nightly sleep times are in question, monitoring for several days with actigraphy (using a device that registers movement by the patient) may be useful in evaluating patterns of waking and sleep (Fig. 2).

Polysomnography

After a thorough history and physical examination have been performed, if a physical sleep problem is considered, the primary diagnostic tool is the nocturnal polysomnogram. The polysomnogram is used to evaluate sleep disturbances leading to sleep fragmentation, including sleep-related breathing disorders, periodic limb movement in sleep, rapid-eye-movement (REM) sleep behavior disorder, other sleep-related movement disorders and parasomnias, and, more rarely, nocturnal seizures. Polysomnographic techniques are described elsewhere in this issue.

Multiple Sleep Latency Test

The MSLT is useful in objectively quantifying the extent of sleepiness. The MSLT consists of four or five 20-minute polysomnographically monitored daytime nap opportunities separated by 2-hour intervals; for the nap opportunities, the patient is placed in a sleep laboratory bed in a dark room with instructions

Epworth Sleepiness Scale

How likely are you to doze off or fall asleep in the following situations, in contrast to feeling just tired? This refers to your usual way of life *in the past week, including today.* Use the following scale to choose the most appropriate number for each situation.

Situation	Chance of dozing			
	0 would never doze	1 Slight chance	2 Moderate chance	3 High chance
1. Sitting and reading	0	1	2	3
2. Watching TV	0	1	2	3
3. Sitting, inactive in a public place (e.g. a theatre or a meeting)	0	1	2	3
4. As a passenger in a car for an hour without a break	0	1	2	3
5. Lying down to rest in the afternoon when circumstances permit	0	1	2	3
6. Sitting and talking to someone	0	1	2	3
7. Sitting quietly after a lunch without alcohol	0	1	2	3
8. In a car, while stopped for a few minutes in the traffic	0	1	2	3

Total:

Fig. 1. Epworth Sleepiness Scale.

Daily Sleep Log

Today's Date >>				
1. How long (in min.) did you nap yesterday?				
2. What sleep medications did you take last night? (include dosage)				
3a. What time did you get in bed?				
3b. What time did you turn off the light intending to go to sleep?				
4. How long (in minutes) did it take you to fall asleep?				
5. What was your planned wake-up time this morning? (write "none" if you didn't have one)				
6. What time did you wake up for your final awakening (i.e. no more sleep occurred after this time) this morning?				
7. What time did you get out of bed?				
8. How many times did you wake up during the night?				
9. Estimate the total amount of time (in minutes) you were awake during the night after you fell asleep.				
10. How much time (in minutes) elapsed from the time you turned off the light out the time you finally get out of bed?				
11. How much sleep total (in minutes), did you get last night?				
12. Rate the quality of your sleep last night. 1 = very poor 10 = excellent				
13. Rate how sleepy, overall, you felt yesterday. 1 = not sleepy at all.....10 = extremely sleepy				
14. Rate how tired/fatigued, overall, you felt yesterday. 1 = not tired at all....10 = extremely tired				

Fig. 2. Daily sleep log.

to fall asleep. The primary assessments made by the MSLT are the rapidity of sleep onset, which correlates to degree of sleepiness, and the occurrence of REM sleep if sleep occurs during the nap opportunity. REM sleep episodes (a period of sleep during which dreams occur) at or close to sleep onset are known as sleep-onset REM periods.

Typical sleep latencies in a normal adult are 10 to 20 minutes; pathologic sleepiness is manifested by a latency of less than 5 to 8 minutes [12,13]. The MSLT should be performed only after the patient has received an adequate amount of nocturnal sleep (approximately 8 hours per night for a typical adult) for at least 2 weeks and immediately after a nocturnal polysomnogram to exclude other causes of EDS resulting from sleep fragmentation or insufficient sleep. If the polysomnogram is positive for other causes of EDS, these conditions should be treated adequately before an evaluation of EDS with MSLT is pursued.

Maintenance of Wakefulness Test

The maintenance of wakefulness test is another diagnostic test used in the sleep laboratory. Rather than evaluating the tendency to fall asleep, as the MSLT does, the maintenance of wakefulness test assesses the capacity to maintain wakefulness in a sedentary setting during the patient's regular waking hours.

This test often is used to evaluate the impact of treatment for sleep disorder–related EDS in heavy equipment operators and airline pilots [14,15].

SYNDROMES OF EXCESSIVE DAYTIME SLEEPINESS

Insufficient Sleep

Insufficient sleep is the most common cause of EDS in Western culture. Although the exact prevalence is unclear, in the 2002 Sleep in America Poll conducted by the National Sleep Foundation [3], 37% of adults reported sleeping less than 7 hours a night on weeknights, and 68% reported sleeping less than 8 hours. Although sleep requirements vary among individuals, the poll found that total weeknight sleep times averaged 6.9 hours compared with 7.5 hours on weekends. This discrepancy between weeknight and weekend sleep times implies ongoing voluntary sleep restriction during the week with sleep compensation on the weekends.

The number of hours of experimental sleep loss in normal volunteers is directly proportional to the degree of increased daytime sleepiness as assessed by the MSLT [16]. The effects of sleep deprivation may be cumulative [8], but this accumulated sleep debt may be countered by extending sleep time over several days [17]. Insufficient sleep may be due to lifestyle choices, job or school demands, shift work, or poor sleep hygiene.

Sixteen percent of the US workforce is engaged in shift work [18]. Research has suggested that despite subjectively experiencing adequate sleep, shift workers, in the absence of shift-work sleep disorder, sleep approximately 5 to 7 hours less per week compared with diurnal workers [19]. Studies consistently have shown that workers who regularly work night shifts experience more disrupted sleep and sleepiness during waking hours compared with day workers [20,21]. The tendency to feel sleepy or to doze may be as great for a worker during the night shift as for an individual with untreated narcolepsy [22].

Although insufficient sleep might be expected to lead to frank EDS, a constellation of other subjective complaints more commonly is seen, including tiredness, lack of energy, or fatigue. Decrements in attention, learning capacity, short-term memory, and psychomotor performance, with or without EDS, also may be present. Irritability, poor impulse control, or other forms of mood instability may exist alone or in combination with these features in individuals with insufficient sleep.

Circadian Influences

Circadian rhythms and their disorders are described in greater detail elsewhere in this issue. Circadian rhythm disorders are chronic conditions that occur when sleeping patterns are not synchronized with environmental cues for sleep and wakefulness. These disorders manifest when an individual cannot sleep at suitable times or desires to sleep at unsuitable times. Genetically determined individual variability in circadian phase results in some individuals' manifesting "night owl" sleep-wake behavior, whereas others are "morning larks." If an individual's circadian phase does not coincide with social or work demands, sleep time may be curtailed, and residual EDS may occur.

Fragmented Sleep

Several physical conditions may lead to fragmented sleep, predominantly in the form of microfragmentation and short awakenings. Sleep fragmentation appears on an electroencephalogram (EEG) recording as a cortical microarousal (1–3 seconds), brief arousal (3–15 seconds), or short awakening (15 seconds to 1–2 minutes)–activity typical of wakefulness, but followed immediately by a return to sleep. These episodes are not incorporated into memory and are not recalled on full awakening. In healthy individuals, the frequency of these events is generally less than 5 to 10 per hour. A much higher rate of sleep fragmenting activity may be caused by many sleep disorders that are associated with EDS, such as sleep-related breathing disorder (SRBD) (eg, obstructive sleep apnea, central sleep apnea, mixed apneas, upper airway resistance syndrome, and snoring) or a disturbance resulting from abnormal movements during sleep, most commonly in the form of PLMS. Additionally, the cause of sleep fragmentation is unclear in many cases. These sleep fragmenting events may lead to full awakenings from sleep at various times during the sleep period, but usually the individuals who have them are unaware of the sleep fragmentation when full awakenings do not occur–they simply know that they have compromised daytime functioning or disrupted sleep. Sleep fragmentation has been postulated to disrupt the normal restorative processes of sleep and has been shown to produce sleepiness and daytime performance deficits when induced by various subtle sensory stimuli in normal subjects in a manner that simulates the frequency of microfragmentation that occurs in common sleep disorders [23,24].

Fragmented sleep may not always lead to EDS, however, especially in children. Although children with an SRBD are generally sleepier than normal children, and their degree of sleepiness tends to increase with the severity of the SRBD [25], they also are more likely to display inattention, irritability, or hyperactive behavior as opposed to EDS [26–29]. In addition, more recent evidence strongly suggests that children with primary snoring, in the absence of obstructive sleep apnea, experience significant neurobehavioral deficits compared with children who do not snore, probably in part because of the sleep fragmentation that always accompanies regular snoring [30]. Findings paralleling those of SRBD in children manifesting attention-deficit and hyperactivity–like behaviors also have been reported in children with PLMS. A surprising percentage of children who have been diagnosed as having attention-deficit/hyperactivity disorder have been found to have PLMS, and many children with PLMS also have been found to have attention-deficit/hyperactivity disorder [31,32].

SLEEP-RELATED BREATHING DISORDERS

SRBDs are highly prevalent in the United States, with an estimated 20% of adults with mild to asymptomatic disease and at least 5% of adults with significant disease [33]. Prevalences of 10% to 25% have been reported for primary snoring in children 3 to 12 years old [34,35], and the prevalence of obstructive sleep apnea has been found to be 1% to 3% in the general pediatric population [36]. The clinician should suspect obstructive sleep apnea syndrome or some other form of SRBD in any patient complaining of EDS, loud or chronic snoring, or unrefreshing sleep. Despite popular belief, obstructive sleep apnea syndrome is not confined to obese individuals. Although its prevalence is greater in the obese white population, even greater prevalences are found in Asian and other populations [37,38]. Longitudinal data from the Wisconsin Sleep Cohort Study [39] showed that among patients with mild obstructive sleep apnea at baseline, a 10% increase in body weight is associated with a six-fold increase in the risk of developing moderate or severe obstructive sleep apnea.

Because sleep disruption commonly is reported by patients with obstructive sleep apnea, patients complaining of fitful, restless sleep, multiple nighttime awakenings, or sleep maintenance insomnia also should be evaluated for this disorder, regardless of body mass index. A more recent study found that one third of patients with SRBD have difficulty initiating or maintaining sleep [40]. Many variants of insomnia may manifest with similar symptoms, including those with a psychiatric etiology; SRBD should be considered in all of these patients, especially if comorbidities exist that might increase clinical suspicion.

Groups that have a higher risk of SRBD include men, postmenopausal women [41], and the elderly [42]. An analysis of data collected from the large multicenter Sleep Heart Health Study showed that the effect of male sex and body mass index on obstructive sleep apnea tends to diminish with advancing age [42] for unclear reasons, and the overall prevalence of obstructive sleep apnea plateaus after age 65 years [43]. In addition to patients who snore, patients with a history of cardiovascular disease [44], including hypertension [45], congestive heart failure [46], cardiac arrhythmias [47], coronary artery disease [48], and stroke [49], should be referred to a sleep center for screening to exclude the presence of obstructive sleep apnea.

Obstructive Sleep Apnea Syndrome

Obstructive sleep apnea syndrome is a condition in which cyclical or repetitive obstructive respiratory events occur during sleep, with microarousals occurring at the termination of a respiratory event [50,51]. In addition to the increased frequency of microarousals, alterations in the pattern of sleep stage activity, known as *sleep architecture*, commonly are observed in patients with obstructive sleep apnea. These changes are typified by reductions in the percentages of slow-wave sleep (stages 3 and 4—also known as delta or deep sleep) and REM sleep, with corresponding increases in lighter sleep. Sleep-related EEG alterations do not consistently correlate, however, with measures of sleepiness severity [52,53]. Patients with obstructive sleep apnea complain more often of tiredness, fatigue, or lack of energy than of frank sleepiness [54]. Obstructive sleep apnea is discussed in greater detail elsewhere in this issue.

Central Sleep Apnea Syndrome

In addition to obstructive sleep apnea syndrome, two other types of apneas have been described: central sleep apnea and mixed sleep apnea [55]. Central sleep apnea occurs when the drive to breathe during sleep is intermittently absent. Mixed sleep apnea begins as a central event, but changes to an obstructive event as respiratory effort begins during a period of airflow cessation. Although central apneas seem to be a unique physiologic event, mixed apneas seem to be most commonly the result of more severe obstructive sleep apnea that over time produces cyclical alterations in respiratory drive in combination with obstructive events; alternatively, sometimes these so-called mixed events are simply obstructive apneas in which respiratory effort is undetected at the beginning of the apnea. Both types of apnea are associated with arousals and fragmented sleep with resultant EDS; however, patients with pure central sleep apnea complain less frequently of EDS than do patients with obstructive sleep apnea [56,57]. Central sleep apnea may be seen in infants with immature central respiratory control systems, whereas in adults it may occur with cerebrovascular or neuromuscular disease, hypoventilation syndromes, or in association with congestive heart failure and Cheyne-Stokes breathing. It is notably present in patients with low cardiac output heart failure [58].

Upper Airway Resistance Syndrome

Upper airway resistance syndrome is an SRBD in which there is increased breathing effort during periods of increased upper airway resistance, but in the absence of hypopneas or apneas [53]. Patients with this disorder have frequent microarousals associated with increased respiratory effort, and many also have EDS. Snoring is often the first symptom reported by patients (or more commonly bed partners or roommates), who are later diagnosed has having obstructive sleep apnea or upper airway resistance syndrome. Snoring alone implies increased resistance of the upper airway during sleep, although the data are mixed on the actual influence of snoring without hypopnea or apnea on EDS and cardiovascular function.

PERIODIC LIMB MOVEMENT DISORDER

PLMS consist of brief repetitive flexion of the toes, feet, legs, thighs, or arms during sleep, lasting 0.5 to 5 seconds, recurring every 5 to 90 seconds, and manifesting a remarkably stable intermovement interval [59]. These cyclical stereotypic movements generally occur during the first one third to one half of the sleep period. Intermittently, cortical microarousals occur with movements. Periodic limb movement disorder is a condition in which PLMS are observed with polysomnography in a patient complaining of nonrestorative sleep or EDS. Cross-sectional studies suggest that periodic limb movement disorder occurs in approximately 3.9% to 5% of adults [60] and about 1.2% of children [61] in the absence of other sleep disorders. Clinically, patients with periodic limb movement disorder may present with EDS, although more often, it is the complaint of the bed partner of excessive movements, jerks, or kicking during sleep that brings it to the clinician's attention.

Some controversy exists regarding the impact of PLMS on sleep disturbance and subsequent daytime functioning in adults. When PLMS occur at rates of five or more per hour of sleep, with or without arousals, they may be associated with EDS, and periodic limb movement disorder may be diagnosed [62]. Several studies have shown no positive correlation of EDS, however, with the number of periodic limb movement arousal complexes per hour of sleep as measured by MSLT [63,64]. Given the conflicting research data, the significance of PLMS and associated arousals remains poorly understood, and clinical correlation is needed to understand the significance of each individual case.

RESTLESS LEGS SYNDROME
Restless legs syndrome is separate from but related to periodic limb movement disorder. It consists of an intensely uncomfortable or unpleasant feeling that occurs predominantly in the legs, but may involve the arms; it occurs more often in the evening and usually is relieved by moving or stretching. Periodic limb movement disorder is a condition of sleep that is confirmed by polysomnography, whereas restless legs syndrome occurs during waking hours and is, by definition, a subjective diagnosis based on the patient's report. Although 80% to 85% of all patients with restless legs syndrome have PLMS, only 18% of patients with periodic limb movement disorder experience symptoms of restless legs syndrome [65]. Although the mechanism of both disorders likely involves problems with dopamine production or use and possibly iron metabolism [66,67], they are distinct clinical disorders as classified by the ICSD. Although restless legs syndrome is predominantly a waking phenomenon, patients commonly report significantly interrupted sleep and sleep curtailment, often reporting only 4 hours of sleep a night because of these uncomfortable sensations [68]. Restless legs syndrome is discussed in greater detail elsewhere in this issue.

PRIMARY DISORDERS OF EXCESSIVE DAYTIME SLEEPINESS
Many disorders are regarded as primary disorders of EDS. This section considers narcolepsy, idiopathic hypersomnia, recurrent hypersomnia, and post-traumatic hypersomnia. Similar to patients with the disorders discussed in the previous sections, patients with CNS-mediated EDS syndromes commonly are misdiagnosed as having a mood disorder and are treated inappropriately with antidepressant therapy.

Narcolepsy
Narcolepsy is the best known and most studied of the primary disorders of EDS. Epidemiologic studies have shown that narcolepsy has a prevalence of approximately 1 in 2000 worldwide, but the prevalence varies substantially between races [69,70]. Narcolepsy is characterized by excessive daytime sleepiness with an increased propensity to fall asleep throughout the day. When in sedentary situations, patients need to exert an extra effort to avoid nodding

or dozing. This tendency toward sleep often manifests as an irresistible or un-controllable urge to sleep, described as "sleep attacks." Contrary to popular be-lief, "sleep attacks" are not sudden lapses into sleep, but rather episodes of profound sleepiness similar to the sleepiness experienced by individuals with marked sleep deprivation or other severe sleep disorders. ESS scores of 15 or greater are common in untreated patients [71,72]. In addition to frank sleepiness, the EDS of narcolepsy, as in other sleep disorders, can cause related symptoms, including poor memory, reduced concentration or attention, and irritability.

Because narcolepsy likely represents a disorder of sleep-state boundary con-trol, patients with narcolepsy often present with other symptoms in addition to EDS, including cataplexy, hypnagogic or hypnopompic hallucinations, and sleep paralysis, all of which manifest features that create the appearance of REM sleep phenomena intruding into wakefulness. Patients with narcolepsy also may report automatic behaviors, and 90% of patients complain of disrup-ted nocturnal sleep [73]. Symptom onset typically occurs during adolescence or young adulthood; however, narcolepsy has been seen to begin in early child-hood or in the fifth or sixth decade of life or later.

The impact of narcolepsy on the individual is dramatic; studies have shown that its effect on quality of life is equal to that of Parkinson's disease [74]. Di-agnosis of narcolepsy may be elusive because no symptom or sign of narco-lepsy is specific to it. Cataplexy unrelated to narcolepsy may occur, although rarely, as an isolated symptom or in conjunction with other conditions.

Cataplexy

Cataplexy is the partial or complete bilateral loss of voluntary muscle tone in response to strong emotion. The range of severity of cataplectic events is broad. Reduced muscle tone may be minimal, occurring in only a few muscle groups and causing minimal symptoms, such as bilateral ptosis, head drooping, slurred speech, and dropping things from the hand. At the other extreme, cataplexy can be so severe that total body paralysis occurs, resulting in complete collapse. Cataplectic events typically last a few seconds to 1 or 2 minutes and occasion-ally last longer [75]. During an event, the individual is usually alert and ori-ented despite an inability to respond. Any strong emotion is a potential trigger for cataplexy, although laughter and other positive emotions are a more common trigger than negative emotions [76]. Startling stimuli, stress, physical fatigue, and sleepiness also may be important triggers or factors that exacerbate cataplexy.

Depending on how cataplexy is defined, epidemiologic studies suggest that 60% to 100% of patients with narcolepsy experience cataplexy. Typically, pa-tients begin to experience cataplexy at the same time or within a few months of developing EDS, but in some cases cataplexy does not develop until years after the initial onset of EDS [65].

Hypnagogic or hypnopompic hallucinations

Hypnagogic hallucinations occur at the transition from wakefulness to sleep, and hypnopompic hallucinations occur at the transition from sleep to wakefulness. They may occur in many forms; they may be visual, tactile, auditory, or multisensory. They are usually brief, but occasionally continue for a few minutes. Hallucinations simultaneously may contain elements from dream sleep and consciousness and are often bizarre or disturbing to the dreamer. Patients who experience hypnagogic or hypnopompic hallucinations occasionally have been misdiagnosed as having a psychotic syndrome and inappropriately treated with antipsychotic medications. Antipsychotic drugs provide no benefit to these patients.

Sleep paralysis
Sleep paralysis is the inability to move during the transition from sleep to wakefulness or from wakefulness to sleep; these episodes may last a few seconds to a few minutes. This phenomenon, similar to hypnagogic and hypnopompic hallucinations, seems to be an intrusion of a component of REM sleep, specifically REM sleep atonia, into wakefulness. Episodes of sleep paralysis can be quite alarming to the individual experiencing them, especially when combined with a hypnagogic event. Often patients report the terrifying experience of the sensation of being unable to breathe. Although accessory respiratory muscle activity is absent during these episodes, diaphragmatic activity continues, and air exchange remains adequate, in the same way that air exchange continues during the atonia of REM sleep.

Fragmented nocturnal sleep
Fragmented nocturnal sleep is another common symptom of narcolepsy. Generally, individuals with narcolepsy have many more and longer nocturnal awakenings than others, a seemingly paradoxical finding [77]. Narcolepsy is a condition of disrupted continuity of wakefulness and sleep, however, with intrusion of each of these states into the other at various inappropriate times.

Automatic behaviors
Automatic behaviors are another symptom commonly reported in narcolepsy patients. These are "absent-minded" behaviors or speech that is often nonsensical and that the patient does not remember. Although hypnagogic hallucinations, sleep paralysis, and automatic behaviors are seen in healthy individuals and in patients with narcolepsy, these symptoms are far more common and occur with much greater frequency in patients with narcolepsy.

Diagnosis of narcolepsy
The diagnosis of narcolepsy depends on the clinical history, coupled with confirmatory diagnostic testing. The primary diagnostic tool used when narcolepsy is suspected is the MSLT. In patients with narcolepsy, the MSLT usually shows substantially reduced sleep latency and sleep-onset REM periods. In normal control subjects with adequate, nonfragmented nocturnal sleep, REM sleep does not occur during daytime naps, and the first REM period during nocturnal sleep usually does not occur until at least 90 minutes after sleep onset. Average MSLT sleep latency for untreated narcolepsy with cataplexy is approximately 2 to 3 minutes [61]; however, substantial variability across

patients and within patients can be seen. Sleep-onset REM periods are not specific for narcolepsy. Sleep deprivation, REM-suppressant medication rebound, altered sleep schedule, obstructive sleep apnea, and delayed sleep phase syndrome are a few circumstances in which sleep-onset REM periods commonly are seen on the MSLT. The occurrence of two or more of these events during the MSLT in a patient with objective marked sleepiness and in the absence of another explanation for their occurrence suggests narcolepsy, however.

When cataplexy accompanies EDS, a straightforward diagnosis of narcolepsy can be made. In these cases, nocturnal polysomnography is not an essential diagnostic tool, although it remains an important part of the evaluation process. It is used primarily to exclude other conditions that occur in narcolepsy at a higher rate than normal (obstructive sleep apnea, periodic limb movement disorder, and REM sleep behavior disorder) that could add to the sleepiness or nocturnal sleep disruption and daytime sleepiness the patient may be experiencing [78].

In addition to the MSLT, numerous adjunctive tests exist that may help to confirm the diagnosis of narcolepsy in a patient with a confusing clinical presentation. Hypocretin, an excitatory, wake-promoting neurotransmitter produced in the hypothalamus, is found to be low or undetectable in the cerebrospinal fluid of many, but not all, patients with narcolepsy [79,80]. A low cerebrospinal fluid level of hypocretin is not specific for narcolepsy, but when used to assess a patient for narcolepsy, cerebrospinal fluid hypocretin is a more specific test than the MSLT and may be more sensitive.

A strong but incomplete correlation exists between narcolepsy (with cataplexy) and the HLA subtype DQB1*0602. This subtype is common in the general population (approximately 20% in the US population), however, and is neither specific nor sensitive for narcolepsy [60]. HLA testing should be reserved for cases in which there is a high degree of clinical suspicion of narcolepsy, but cataplexy is not present.

Idiopathic hypersomnia

Idiopathic hypersomnia (previously called *idiopathic CNS hypersomnia*) is another important primary disorder of EDS that should be considered in a patient complaining of sleepiness. This diagnosis historically has been given to individuals who complain of EDS when other disorders that cause hypersomnolence have not been found or clearly characterized. There are numerous documented cases of patients having been misdiagnosed as having idiopathic hypersomnia when they had other disorders that cause EDS, such as narcolepsy without cataplexy, delayed sleep phase syndrome, and upper airway resistance syndrome [53].

True idiopathic hypersomnia is believed to be less common than narcolepsy, but estimating prevalence is difficult because there are no strict diagnostic criteria, and no specific biologic markers have been identified. The first symptoms tend to occur in late adolescence or early adulthood. No cause for idiopathic hypersomnia has been clearly identified, but viral illnesses, including those that may lead to Guillain-Barré syndrome, hepatitis, mononucleosis, and atypical viral pneumonia, may be a harbinger of the onset of EDS in a subset of patients. EDS may occur as part of the acute illness, but persist after the other symptoms subside. HLA-Cw2 and HLA-DR11 have been noted to occur with increased frequency in some rare familial cases [81]. Most patients with idiopathic hypersomnia have neither a family history nor an obvious associated viral illness, however. Autonomic nervous system dysfunction has been associated with some of these cases, including orthostatic hypotension, syncope, vascular headaches, and peripheral vascular complaints. Little is known about the pathophysiology of idiopathic hypersomnia, and no animal model is available for study. Neurochemical studies using cerebrospinal fluid have suggested that patients with idiopathic hypersomnia may have altered noradrenergic system function [82–84].

Clinically, the presentation of idiopathic hypersomnia varies among individuals. Idiopathic hypersomnia commonly is mistaken for narcolepsy. Because the predominant symptom in both disorders is EDS, and age at onset is similar for the two diseases, it is understandable that one may be mistaken for the other. With careful history taking and diagnostic testing, however, essential differences between the disorders become apparent. Patients with idiopathic hypersomnia present with EDS but without cataplexy or significant nocturnal sleep disruption [85]. The sleepiness they complain of typically interferes with normal daily activities, and occupational and social functioning may be severely affected by sleepiness. Nocturnal sleep tends to be long and unrefreshing, and patients usually are difficult to awaken in the morning. They may become irritable or abusive in response to others' efforts to rouse them. In some patients, this difficulty may be substantial and include confusion, disorientation, and poor motor coordination, a condition called "sleep drunkenness" [86]. These patients often take naps, which may be prolonged, but usually are unrefreshing. No amount of sleep ameliorates the EDS. "Microsleeps," with or without automatic behaviors, may occur throughout the day. This diagnosis is distinctly different from that of major depression because patients with idiopathic hypersomnia commonly lacks the generalized anhedonia usually associated with a major depressive episode and are much sleepier on objective testing than a patient with an atypical depression.

Polysomnographic studies of patients with idiopathic CNS hypersomnia usually reveal shortened initial sleep latency, increased total sleep time, and normal sleep architecture (in contrast to the studies of narcoleptic patients, which exhibit significant sleep fragmentation and altered sleep architecture). Mean sleep latency on the MSLT is usually reduced, often in the 8- to 10-minute range, but sometimes dramatically shorter. Also in contrast to narcolepsy, sleep-onset REM periods typically are not seen. As with narcolepsy, other disorders that produce EDS (eg, insufficient sleep, SRBDs, periodic limb movement disorder, other sleep fragmenting disorders, circadian rhythm disorders, and psychiatric illnesses) must be ruled out before the diagnosis of idiopathic hypersomnia is made.

Idiopathic CNS hypersomnia is often difficult to treat and responds poorly to medications. Lifestyle and behavioral modifications, including good sleep hygiene, are appropriate, but treatment with stimulant or wake-promoting medication, as with narcolepsy, is usually necessary.

RECURRENT HYPERSOMNIAS

Kleine-Levin Syndrome

Another group of disorders to consider in the differential diagnosis of a patient who presents with EDS, although rare, are recurrent hypersomnias. Kleine-Levin syndrome is a form of recurrent hypersomnia that occurs primarily in adolescents [87] with a male preponderance. It is characterized by episodes of EDS and frequently is accompanied by hyperphagia, aggressiveness, and hypersexuality. These episodes may last days to weeks and may be separated by asymptomatic periods lasting weeks or months. During symptomatic periods, affected individuals sleep 18 hours per day and are usually drowsy (often to the degree of stupor), confused, and irritable when they are awake. During these episodes, polysomnographic studies show long total sleep time with high sleep efficiency and decreased slow-wave sleep. MSLT studies show short sleep latencies and sleep-onset REM periods [88]. The etiology of this syndrome is obscure. Symptomatic cases of Kleine-Levin syndrome associated with structural brain lesions have been reported, but most cases are idiopathic. Single-photon emission computed tomography has shown hypoperfusion in the thalamus in one patient and in the nondominant frontal lobe in another [89]. Treatment with stimulant medication is usually only partially effective. The effects of treatment with lithium, valproic acid, and carbamazepine have been variable but generally unsatisfactory. In most cases, episodes become less frequent over time and eventually subside.

Menstrual-Related Hypersomnia

Another form of recurrent hypersomnia is menstrual-related periodic hypersomnia, in which EDS occurs during the several days preceding menstruation [90,91]. The prevalence of this syndrome has not been well characterized. Likewise, the etiology is unknown, but presumably the symptoms are related to hormonal changes. Some cases of menstrual-related hypersomnia have responded to the blocking of ovulation with estrogen and progesterone (birth control pills) [92].

Idiopathic Recurring Stupor

Another less commonly seen form of recurring hypersomnias is idiopathic recurring stupor. Numerous cases have been reported in which, in the absence of obvious cause, individuals are subject to stuporous episodes lasting hours to days. This syndrome affects predominantly middle-aged men. Individuals experience normal levels of alertness between episodes, and the episodes occur unpredictably. Elevated plasma and cerebrospinal fluid levels of endozepine-4, an endogenous ligand with affinity for the benzodiazepine recognition site at the γ-aminobutyric acid A receptor, have been found in several of these

Selected Sleep Disorders: Restless Legs Syndrome and Periodic Limb Movement Disorder, Sleep Apnea Syndrome, and Narcolepsy

Milton K. Erman, MD[a,b,*]

[a]Department of Psychiatry, School of Medicine, University of California San Diego, CA, USA
[b]Pacific Sleep Medicine, 10052 Mesa Ridge Court, Suite 101, San Diego, CA 92121, USA

Complaints of disturbed sleep are common in psychiatric patients and are associated with the diagnosis of specific disorders, such as mania and major depression. Despite this, clinicians often perceive sleep complaints to be a symptomatic reflection of the therapeutic response to treatment: If the treatment for depression is effective, sleep complaints should resolve. Most practicing psychiatrists have received little formal instruction about sleep disorders during their training in medical school and residency [1]. This leaves them incompletely prepared to recognize symptoms of sleep disorders, which often are subtle in their presentations, and the symptomatic complaints of which may overlap with various psychiatric syndromes.

The specific sleep disorders discussed in this article all are likely to be seen by practicing psychiatrists and may be misinterpreted by them as reflecting an element of a comorbid psychiatric syndrome. Additionally, the presence of these conditions may interfere with treatment efforts being provided for psychiatric conditions. For these reasons, awareness of these disorders and their presentations allows psychiatrists to function more effectively in clinical care.

Use of sleep studies to establish the diagnosis of several of these conditions is addressed later in this article. Polysomnography (PSG) techniques for establishing sleep stages have been reviewed elsewhere in this issue and include the electroencephalogram, electro-oculogram, and submental electromyogram. The typical clinical PSG also includes an electrocardiogram, respiratory effort (usually including measures of chest and abdominal effort), bilateral anterior tibialis electromyography, measurement of airflow (using a thermistor or a pressure transducer), and measurement of oxygen saturation (pulse oximetry). The studies must be performed in a temperature-controlled, sound-attenuated,

*Pacific Sleep Medicine, 10052 Mesa Ridge Court, Suite 101, San Diego, CA 92121, USA. E-mail address: merman@scripps.edu

0193-953X/06/$ – see front matter
doi:10.1016/j.psc.2006.09.007

and light-attenuated environment to ensure that the data obtained would not be disrupted by outside environmental factors. Guidelines for the use of PSG in the practice of sleep medicine have been established by a committee of the American Academy of Sleep Medicine [2]. Alternative methods for the diagnosis of various sleep disorders, including narcolepsy and sleep apnea, have been proposed, and are discussed in the sections pertaining to these diseases.

SLEEP APNEA

The term *apnea* refers to absence of ventilation and is derived from the Greek word *apnoia,* meaning "absence of respiration." As identified on PSG, two major categories of sleep apnea exist, obstructive and central. A third type, mixed, contains elements of the obstructive and central types [3]. Obstructive and central sleep apnea syndromes are defined on the basis of the relative preponderance of obstructive and mixed components for the former and central components for the latter (Figs. 1–3).

Sleep apnea syndrome has existed as an unrecognized disorder throughout history and was descibed by Dickens in the *Pickwick Papers* in 1836. His description of Joe, the "Fat Boy," led to use of the term *Pickwickian syndrome* by Burwell and colleagues to describe a disorder of excessive sleepiness, associated with carbon dioxide retention. Burwell's observations focused only on the daytime findings, likely delaying recognition of the specific nighttime findings of this disorder. Although apnea was described in the medical literature independently by two groups in 1965, it took until the 1970s for recognition of the significance of this disorder to begin to have an impact on medical diagnosis and treatment in the United States.

Obstructive sleep apnea (OSA) syndrome is the most common form of the two types of sleep apnea syndromes. It is best understood as a state-dependent disorder of breathing. Obstructive apneas occur because of obstruction in the upper airway, developing as a result of the combined effects of reduced muscle tone in sleep and the impact of negative upper airway pressure as a consequence of inspiratory effort. Typically, individuals with OSA exhibit no breathing abnormalities in the waking state, but are variably affected when they fall asleep.

Central sleep apnea syndrome is characterized by absent ventilation as a result of an absence of ventilatory effort. The classic pattern of crescendo-decrescendo breathing can be seen in patients with heart failure, neurologic lesions affecting the brainstem or other areas involved in regulation of respiration, and metabolic or toxic encephalopathies. This pattern may be present only in sleep or may be found during wakefulness as well. Central sleep apnea may follow other neurologic events, such as nocturnal seizures and strokes. True central sleep apnea is a rare and complicated disorder. Its evaluation and treatment are best left to specialists, and it is not discussed further in this chapter.

Diagnosis

The diagnosis of sleep apnea syndrome often may be strongly suggested based on history and physical examination, but the Practice Parameters of the

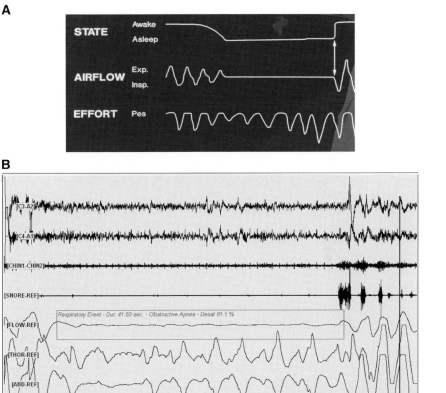

Fig. 1. OSA. (A) Breathing pattern in sleep. (B) PSG recording.

American Academy of Sleep Medicine still define PSG as the "reference or 'gold standard'" in the evaluation of sleep-disordered breathing. The issue of the use of portable monitoring devices in the investigation of suspected obstructive sleep apnea also has been reviewed by the American Academy of Sleep Medicine, with the general finding that none of these devices were believed to be suitable for use in an unattended setting [4].

Limitations of these devices as effective diagnostic instruments are based on the data that they obtain and the setting in which they are usually used. Limited recording devices, often using only four channels of physiologic data, typically provide no information on body position, arousals, or movement. More importantly, because they provide no formal electroencephalogram data, sleep states cannot be differentiated from awake states, and rapid-eye-movement (REM) sleep cannot be differentiated from non-REM sleep.

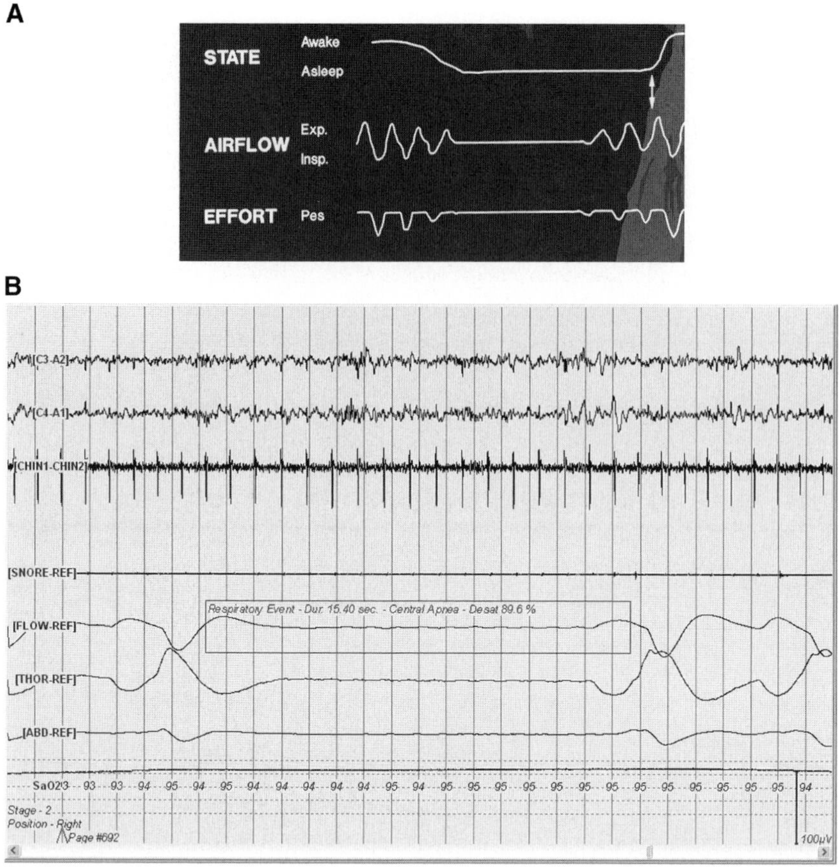

A

B

Fig. 2. Central sleep apnea. (A) Breathing pattern in sleep. (B) PSG recording.

The fact that these limited studies usually are performed in an unattended fashion in the patient's home often is considered desirable by the patient, in contrast to the need to come to the sleep laboratory for study. The patient's home is a poorly controlled, often chaotic, environment, however. Movement and activity by bed partners, family members, and pets may disrupt studies, as would the impact of noise and light in the sleep environment. When the studies are performed without a sleep technician present, no observations can be made about body position, movement, or the sleep environment. When continuous positive airway pressure (CPAP) titration has been performed, the presence of a sleep technician may be crucial with regard to mask fit and comfort during the first critical night of treatment, improving compliance and the probability of acceptance of CPAP treatment on a long-term basis.

The most common clinical signs of OSA are loud snoring, interrupted or absent breathing in sleep observed by a bed partner or family member, and

A

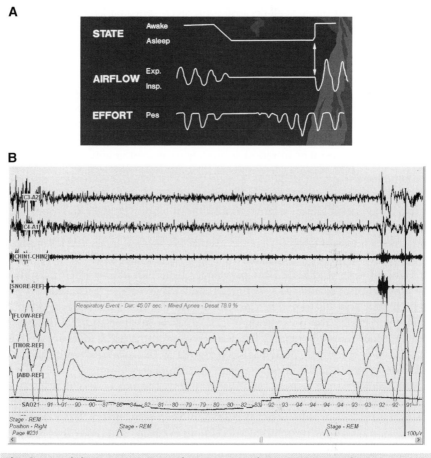

B

Fig. 3. Mixed sleep apnea. (A) Breathing pattern in sleep. (B) PSG recording.

excessive daytime sleepiness. The patient himself or herself is usually unaware of the existence of a problem, often boasting that they have no sleep problem—"I can fall asleep anywhere." Patients often deny the presence of these symptoms, and it is helpful to have a bed partner or family member present when symptoms suggesting sleep apnea are reviewed.

Some patients report awareness of awakening from sleep with a sensation of choking, at times associated with dreams of drowning or suffocating. Other common symptoms include a history of restless sleep, morning headache, morning sore throat, and daytime fatigue.

Specific abnormalities in the physical examination often are seen in patients with OSA. Many patients are obese and have a large neck or crowded upper airway, and a history of weight gain associated with increased severity of snoring or apnea often is reported. It should not be assumed that all patients, however, are morbidly obese or obese at all because some sleep apnea patients have a normal body habitus. Common structural abnormalities, such as narrow nasal passage, long soft palate, large tonsils, or a short (retrognathic or micrognathic) mandible contribute to airway obstruction.

OSA is associated with an increased risk of cognitive abnormalities and of affective disorders, such as depression [5]. Cognitive impairment associated with apnea may be misdiagnosed as dementia, with capacity for substantial improvement in cognition associated with effective treatment. Similarly, untreated apnea may exacerbate depression severity or limit response to therapy, with substantial improvement in mood seen after treatment is initiated [6].

Epidemiology

OSA is a common disorder. The Wisconsin Sleep Cohort Study [7], using restrictive methodologies in a large population of employed men and women 30 to 60 years old, reported a prevalence rate for OSA of approximately 15% in men and 5% in women based on an Apnea Hypopnea Index (AHI)—number of apneas or hypopneas, episodes of partial apnea, per hour of sleep—of 10 or higher. Other studies of OSA prevalence using laboratory PSG to estimate the prevalence of severe OSA, defined as an AHI greater than 15, report 7% to 14% in men and 2% to 7% in women. If mild disease is considered (AHI >5 events per hour), the prevalence is 17% to 26% in men and 9% to 28% in women older than 20 years. The presence of mild disease is relevant because an AHI of 5 events per hour has been shown to be associated with increased risks for hypertension and other health consequences.

Some patients may be unaware of or may deny the existence of snoring; confirmation of snoring may be particularly difficult for patients who sleep alone. Often, bed partners acknowledge that they have been driven from their bed and shared bedroom by their partner's loud snoring. Although they may be able to comment on snoring from the past, they can say little about the presence or absence of apneic pauses at the present time.

Another factor that may limit the reliability of information provided by a spouse or bed partner is hearing loss, a problem seen most frequently in older patients and their spouses. Some spouses may deny or may be unaware of the severity of their hearing loss, affecting their ability to provide accurate information about snoring and apneas.

Pathophysiology and Consequences

OSA involves repetitive obstructions of the airway in sleep, leading to oxyhemoglobin desaturation, inspiratory efforts against the occluded airway, and termination of the event by arousal from sleep. The daytime sleepiness and fatigue characteristic of OSA is likely a consequence of the fragmented sleep associated with this disorder, generated by the need for recurrent arousals to avoid suffocation and death.

Patients with OSA have an increased incidence of hypertension compared with individuals without OSA, and OSA seems to be an independent risk factor for the development of hypertension. OSA seems to be implicated in stroke and transient ischemic attacks and coronary heart disease, heart failure, and cardiac arrhythmias. These cardiovascular risks are likely due to the release of proinflammatory and prothrombotic factors that have been identified to be important in the development of atherosclerosis as a consequence of apnea events and by "downstream effects" of arousals that terminate apnea events.

Other consequences of the disorder include excessive daytime sleepiness, which can be relatively mild or may be severe enough to interfere with employment or driving an automobile. Several studies have documented an increased risk of automobile crashes in patients with OSA, such that it is considered a disorder associated with loss of consciousness in some states. Quality of life is demonstrably impaired in patients with OSA, including complaints of fatigue, memory impairment, reduced concentration, depressed mood, and irritability. Some patients may experience decreased libido or erectile dysfunction. These symptoms virtually always improve, and may resolve completely, with effective treatment.

Treatment

Nasal CPAP administered via a nasal mask or interface is the treatment of choice for moderate-to-severe OSA. The positive pressure generated by CPAP functions as a pneumatic stent for the upper airway, preventing the airway collapse that otherwise would occur as a consequence of negative inspiratory pressure.

Nasal CPAP therapy for sleep apnea was first described in 1981, but it was not initially widely accepted in treatment. CPAP is administered by a soft mask held in place against the face, usually covering only the nose (although some patients may need a "full face" mask covering the nose and mouth). Sufficient pressure is introduced to eliminate apneas, hypopneas, and snoring. At appropriate pressures, CPAP is almost always effective in treatment of OSA. Limitations have included the bulk and noise of early CPAP units and problems with early masks including poor fit and the need to use an adhesive to attach the mask to the face. Continuing technical improvements in the design of masks and CPAP units has led to dramatically increased acceptance of CPAP therapy.

Surgical therapy for sleep apnea includes a broad range of procedures. Although tracheostomy is curative of this disorder, it is associated with significant medical risks and lifestyle limitations and generally is reserved for patients with severe sleep apnea unable to use nasal CPAP in treatment.

The most widely used surgery for sleep apnea, uvulopalatopharyngoplasty (UPPP), was described in 1981 [8]. This procedure involves removal of redundant or excess tissue in the throat to improve airway patency, reduce snoring, and reduce apnea severity. It was seen initially as a viable and mildly invasive alternative to CPAP, initially perceived as burdensome and "a treatment, not a cure."

Outcome analyses for UPPP procedures suggested that significant improvement (defined as a $\geq 50\%$ reduction in the AHI) was seen in only about 50% of patients. Patients often complained of significant pain associated with the procedure, which required hospitalization for at least several days. In addition, complications such as altered speech and velopalatal incompetence were seen in some patients. These complications seemed to be more common in the early years in which this procedure was performed and in cases in which the surgery may have been more aggressive. As a consequence of these issues, the number of UPPP procedures has reduced dramatically in recent years.

A variant of this procedure, laser-assisted uvulopalatoplasty, was developed to provide a less invasive treatment alternative. Although it is often described as providing results comparable to UPPP, pain associated with the multiple (typically three to five) laser treatments needed to complete this procedure limited patient acceptance. Treatment outcome is not likely to be equal to that of UPPP because laser-assisted uvulopalatoplasty relies primarily on scarring of the airway and retraction of tissue as a consequence rather than removal of soft tissue in the airway as occurs with UPPP.

Radiofrequency ablation is another alternative to UPPP and laser-assisted uvulopalatoplasty that works by stiffening the soft palate and shrinking tissue in the airway. An advantage of radiofrequency ablation is that it is minimally invasive, with few treatment-associated complications. Although it has been shown to be a benefit in patients who snore, few data have been published suggesting benefit in patients with significant sleep apnea.

Weight reduction surgery must be mentioned among surgical options for the treatment of sleep apnea. Although many sleep apnea patients may be of normal weight, weight is an exacerbating factor for virtually all apnea patients, and a high proportion of morbidly obese patients have sleep apnea [9]. Patients with sleep apnea who undergo bariatric surgery typically have a progressive reduction in the apnea severity associated with weight loss and usually are able to reduce their CPAP pressure as they lose weight. Not all patients are "cured" of apnea as a consequence of weight loss, and continued use of nasal CPAP, use of an oral appliance, or surgical treatment of the upper airway may be required after maximal weight loss.

Alternative Approach

An alternative nonsurgical approach for patients who are not candidates for or who cannot tolerate CPAP is use of an oral appliance, also known as an airway dilator. These devices, at times similar in appearance to a "bite plate" or night guard used for bruxism or an athletic mouthpiece, are often beneficial in selected patients [10]. The therapeutic effect of these devices is presumed to be due to stimulation of muscles in the airway in sleep, reducing the tendency to collapse that otherwise occurs in association with the muscle flaccidity of sleep. The fabrication and fitting of these appliances is best performed by a dentist knowledgeable about sleep apnea and with significant experience in the use of these devices.

At present, no pharmacologic treatments have been shown to be effective in the treatment of sleep apnea. Although some limited treatment trials have supported the hypothesis that tricyclic antidepressants and some selective

narcolepsy suggests that an HLA-related autoimmune response of unknown origin may trigger damage to these hypocretin-secreting cells leading to the development of narcolepsy.

Consequences

The impact of narcolepsy on social and interpersonal function is dramatic and well documented. The excessive sleepiness that is a core symptom of the disorder is associated with school performance problems, often leading to limitations in educational achievement owing to the perception that the patient with narcolepsy is lazy or disinterested. The excessive daytime sleepiness of narcolepsy also generates a high automobile accident rate in patients with this disorder, leading to limitations on licensure to drive a car in some states. It has been shown to lead to a high socioeconomic burden, including increased risk of unemployment.

Compared with population norms, baseline quality-of-life scores for subjects in narcolepsy studies have shown substantial burdens in vitality, social functioning, and performance of usual activities. Consequences for patients with narcolepsy are dramatic [25], particularly because this condition often is not appropriately diagnosed until affected individuals have had their symptoms for many years. Even with treatment, patients may have problems functioning successfully in school or at work. The sleepiness that is beyond the narcoleptic's control may be interpreted as disinterest or laziness by family members or a spouse; cataplexy may be interpreted as behavior suspicious of sedative abuse. These patients may be referred for evaluation for depression as a consequence of misperceptions on the part of relatives that these symptoms are signs of depression. The risk of developing depression may be increased as a consequence of the social and interpersonal stresses these patients experience.

Treatment

The excessive sleepiness of narcolepsy historically has been treated using amphetamine and other stimulant agents, such as methylphenidate and pemoline (Table 1) [26]. These compounds all are centrally acting sympathomimetic agents that promote the release of monoamines and block their reuptake. The problems associated with these medications are well recognized and well described, including risks of abuse and diversion; provocation of or exacerbation of tendencies to psychosis; and other side effects, such as tremulousness, elevation of blood pressure, agitation, and motor restlessness. Pemoline has been withdrawn from the market because of hepatotoxicity.

Alternative treatments for excessive sleepiness in narcolepsy also have been developed. The wake-promoting compound modafinil was approved by the US Food and Drug Administration (FDA) for the treatment of excessive sleepiness in narcolepsy in 1998 and subsequently has received additional approvals for treatment of residual sleepiness in treated patients with sleep apnea and for the treatment of shift work sleep disorder [27,28]. Modafinil has a novel mechanism and is theorized to work in a localized manner, using hypocretin, histamine, epinephrine, γ-aminobutyric acid, and glutamate [29]. It is a well-tolerated medication with low propensity for abuse.

Table 1
Sleepiness: commonly used agents

Agent	Typical daily dosage	Side effects	FDA approved
Modafinil	100–400 mg	Headache, nausea, nervousness	Yes
Methylphenidate	10–60 mg	Nervousness, insomnia, anorexia, palpitations	Yes
Dextroamphetamine	10–60 mg	Palpitations, tachycardia, nervousness, insomnia, anorexia	Yes
Sodium oxybate (gamma hydroxybutyrate)	3–9 g	Headache, nausea, vomiting, dizziness, somnolence	Yes

Another primary symptom of narcolepsy, cataplexy, has been treated in the past with tricyclic antidepressants, most often protriptyline (Vivactil) (Table 2). More recently, use of newer selective serotonin reuptake inhibitor antidepressant agents has been supported in clinical reviews, although little research evidence supports their use in treatment.

A new treatment agent specifically indicated for the treatment of cataplexy, gamma hydroxybutyrate, was approved by the FDA in 2002. Known formally as sodium oxybate and marketed as Xyrem, this compound seems to work by promotion of slow-wave sleep. Although the mechanism of action is not clearly understood, it is presumed that the capacity of this agent to consolidate nocturnal sleep leads to a reduction in cataplexy. Additionally, this agent has been shown to improve residual sleepiness in patients with narcolepsy, leading to approval for treatment of excessive daytime sleepiness in patients with narcolepsy in 2005. Access to medication is restricted through use of a single, mail-order pharmacy, minimizing the prospect of diversion and abuse of this agent. Treatment with sodium oxalate has led to improved functioning and quality of life for many patients with narcolepsy [30].

Current research in the treatment of excessive sleepiness is focusing on various areas, including treatment with armodafinil, an active stereoisomer of modafinil [31], and compounds capable of crossing the blood-brain barrier and affecting hypocretin receptors. Research also is under way exploring the possible use of immunosuppression at the time of narcolepsy onset, based on the hypothesis that immunosuppression therapy during a period of pathologic immune response could prevent or reduce damage to the hypocretin system that otherwise would lead to development of narcolepsy.

Table 2
Cataplexy: commonly used agents

Agent	Typical daily dosage	Side effects	FDA approved
Tricyclic antidepressants			
Protriptyline	5–60 mg	Constipation, urinary retention, dry mouth, dizziness, orthostasis, anxiety	No
Imipramine	10–100 mg	Constipation, urinary retention, dry mouth, dizziness, orthostasis, sedation	No
Clomipramine	10–150 mg	Constipation, urinary retention, dry mouth, dizziness, orthostasis, sedation	No
Desipramine	25–200 mg	Constipation, urinary retention, dry mouth, dizziness, orthostasis, anxiety	No
Selective serotonin reuptable inhibitors			No
Fluoxetine	20–60 mg	Sexual dysfunction, disturbed sleep, nausea	No
Venlafaxine	75–300 mg	Sexual dysfunction, disturbed sleep, nausea	No
Sodium oxybate (gamma hydroxybutyrate)	3–9 g (divided in two doses)	Headache, nausea, vomiting, dizziness, somnolence	Yes

RESTLESS LEGS SYNDROME AND PERIODIC LIMB MOVEMENTS IN SLEEP

Restless legs syndrome (RLS) and periodic limb movements in sleep (PLMS) are related conditions that have escaped the attention of most practicing physicians until recent years. RLS is a diagnosed on the basis of symptomatic complaints; PLMS (also known as periodic limb movements disorder) is a sleep disorder, diagnosed through PSG studies. The two conditions overlap tremendously; most RLS patients, if studied in the sleep laboratory, exhibit periodic leg movement activity. When PLMS are noted as an "incidental finding" in a sleep study of a patient not known to have RLS, restless legs symptoms usually are present but may not have been reported.

The complaint of restless legs has been present throughout history, but the first description of this complaint as a specific condition was published by the Swedish neurologist Ekbom in 1945. This disorder, also known as Ekbom's syndrome, usually is described as a hard-to-define disorder of discomfort in the legs. A broad range of terms is used by patients to describe their symptoms: *pain, discomfort, creeping, crawling, tingling, pulling, twitching, tearing, aching, throbbing, prickling,* or *grabbing sensation* in the calves, legs, or arms. Symptoms typically are more severe during periods of inactivity or rest or while sitting or lying down.

These symptoms are distinct from complaints of akathisia, a complaint of motoric restlessness frequently experienced by psychiatric patients. Akathisia is seen most frequently in patients taking neuroleptic medications, but also may be reported as a consequence of use of selective serotonin reuptake inhibitors and tricyclic antidepressants.

Patients with RLS also are not experiencing symptoms of an anxiety disorder or attention-deficit/hyperactivity disorder. Although they are disturbed by the restlessness they experience, their mood state otherwise is usually normal, and they typically do not have the inattention, distractibility, or hyperactivity seen in attention-deficit/hyperactivity disorder.

Diagnosis

As noted previously, RLS is diagnosed on the basis of symptomatic complaints; PLMS must be diagnosed on the basis of PSG evaluation. It should not be assumed, however, that a complaint of restless legs and leg movement in sleep requires a PSG evaluation. RLS does not require PSG, and the finding of PLMS usually is associated with PSG evaluation of other complaints or conditions, including treatment-resistant RLS.

The second edition of the *International Classification of Sleep Disorders* (American Academy of Sleep Medicine) requires the presence of four diagnostic criteria, in the absence of other medical or psychiatric causes, as follows: (1) the urge to move the legs, accompanied by uncomfortable or unpleasant sensations in the legs; (2) worsening of symptoms in association with inactivity; (3) partial relief of symptoms with movement; and (4) the presence of symptoms only in the evening hours or worsening of symptoms at night or in the evening.

The International Restless Legs Syndrome Study Group, a body of professionals dedicated to the study of RLS, has developed a 10-point scale to measure RLS severity (Box 3). This scale has been validated in a large, multicenter study and frequently is used in clinical trials to assess the effects of pharmacologic treatments.

Box 3: Restless legs syndrome diagnosis per the International Restless Legs Syndrome Study Group

International Restless Legs Syndrome Study Group rating scale

1. Overall, how would you rate the RLS discomfort in your legs or arms?
2. Overall, how would you rate the need to move around because of your RLS symptoms?
3. Overall, how much relief of your RLS arm or leg discomfort do you get from moving around?
4. Overall, how severe is your sleep disturbance from your RLS symptoms?
5. How severe is your tiredness or sleepiness from your RLS symptoms?
6. Overall, how severe is your RLS as a whole?
7. How often do you get RLS symptoms?
8. When you have RLS symptoms, how severe are they on an average day?
9. Overall, how severe is the impact of your RLS symptoms on your ability to carry out your daily affairs (eg, living a satisfactory family, home, social, school, or work life)?
10. How severe is your mood disturbance from your RLS symptoms (eg, angry, depressed, sad, anxious, or irritable)?

- Each question (except question 3) has the following multiple choices: (4) Very severe, (3) Severe, (2) Moderate, (1) Mild, (0) None (sometimes with a more operational definition in parentheses)
- Question 3: (4) No relief, (3) Slight relief, (2) Moderate relief, (1) Either complete or almost complete relief, (0) No RLS symptoms and therefore question does not apply

Adapted from The International Restless Legs Syndrome Study Group: Validation of the International Restless Legs Syndrome Study Group rating scale for restless legs syndrome. Sleep Med 2003;4:121–32; with permission.

Epidemiology

Current estimates suggest that 5% to 10% of adults have RLS [32], with initial symptoms often appearing in the third decade of life. The disorder may appear in childhood, with estimates that 1% to 2% of the general pediatric population may be affected. In general, older patients are more likely to report restless legs complaints than younger ones, but patients historically have been unlikely to seek attention from primary care physicians leading to significant underdiagnosis of this problem. Patients may report symptoms present for 25 to 30 years without having had a diagnosis established or having received treatment.

Etiology

Primary and secondary forms of RLS exist. Strong historical evidence suggests that there is a genetic predisposition to the development of primary RLS, although the specific genetic basis for this disorder has not been elucidated. Not all patients report a family history for this disorder. Familial and spontaneous types likely exist.

Secondary RLS occurs in medical conditions associated with the symptom of restless legs, including end-stage renal disease, iron deficiency, and pregnancy, all of which may be associated with low iron stores. Ekbom first noted a relationship between RLS and impaired iron storage or iron metabolism in 1955, and impaired iron storage or metabolism is now recognized as a reversible cause of RLS. Evaluation of a patient with RLS complaints always should include measurement of iron, iron stores, and ferritin levels.

These abnormalities of iron storage and metabolism may play a central role in the cause of this disorder. Iron seems to play a role in normal dopaminergic function in the central nervous system, perhaps related to dopamine transport and to dopamine synthesis. Although a clear-cut link with iron metabolism has not been established, it is interesting to consider this relationship in the context of the role of dopaminergic agonists in the treatment of this disorder.

Consequences

The primary impact of RLS on health is mediated through the sleep disturbance that is characteristic of RLS. As would be expected, the inability to fall asleep, disrupted sleep through the night with inability to resume sleep after awakening, and insufficient hours of sleep are common among individuals with RLS. Individuals with RLS frequently report disturbance of daytime activities and function, however, and the risk of daytime symptoms is increased in association with greater chronicity.

Quality of life in RLS also has been evaluated using the Short Form–36 Health Survey (SF-36), an extensively tested and validated tool that assesses eight dimensions of health-related quality of life: physical functioning, physical limitations on normal role activities, bodily pain, general health, energy and vitality, social functioning, emotional limitations on normal role activities, and mental health. Based on SF-36 evaluation, patients with RLS are significantly different from the general population, with a quality of life comparable to that seen in patients with chronic medical conditions, such as type 2 diabetes and clinical depression.

Treatment

Various agents have been used to provide symptomatic relief for RLS and PLMS. In the 1950s, efforts at treatment of RLS with intravenous iron were undertaken, with significant improvement noted in small patient populations. Formal approval by the FDA of ropinirole in 2005 in treatment of RLS was accomplished as a consequence of multiple studies showing efficacy of this agent [33,34].

At the time of this writing (July 2006), another dopaminergic agonist approved for the treatment of Parkinson's disease, pramipexole, is awaiting word from the FDA with regard to possible approval for RLS treatment. Other dopaminergic agonist compounds, such as carbidopa-levodopa, bromocriptine, and pergolide, may be beneficial for some treatment-resistant patients.

Until the approval of ropinirole in treatment of RLS, all treatment was off-label. For many years, sedating agents such as the benzodiazepine clonazepam (Klonopin) were prescribed in treatment and were recommended in clinical reviews of the treatment of the complaint of restless legs and in sleep textbooks. Although it was recognized that these sedating agents did not alter the frequency of leg movement activity and might lead to residual sedation, patients often experienced a sense of relief, presumably on the basis of sleep consolidation. Opioids such as codeine, hydrocodone, oxycodone, propoxyphene, and methadone have been used in treatment and may be beneficial for patients whose complaints include severe pain, not affected by other treatment modalities.

Anticonvulsants such as carbamazepine and gabapentin are often used when dopamine agonists have failed. They may be useful in patients with coexisting peripheral neuropathy or when RLS discomfort is described as pain.

Iron treatment is indicated for patients with evidence of iron deficiency, typically for patients with serum ferritin levels less than 50 µg. Oral treatment usually is given as ferrous sulfate, 325 mg or its equivalent twice per day. Absorption of iron is improved by coadministration of vitamin C. For patients who have trouble absorbing iron or may have significant problems with side effects, such as indigestion or constipation, intravenous iron supplementation may be used.

Because some patients with RLS may be iron deficient on the basis of dietary iron intake, it is always necessary to ask patients about foods that they may avoid or not eat because of dietary restrictions. Patients may not eat red meat for "health reasons" and may have limited iron intake available from other sources. Although repletion of iron stores by increased dietary intake may not always be possible, patients should be educated about iron-rich foods that they may be able to eat (ie, beef, turkey, shrimp, sardines, tuna, iron-enriched breakfast cereals, green leafy vegetables) and encouraged to increase their intake of these foods.

SUMMARY

Sleep disorders, including RLS and periodic limb movements disorder, sleep apnea syndrome, and narcolepsy, are prevalent medical conditions, likely to be seen by practicing psychiatrists. Awareness of these conditions and their presentations, pathophysiology, and treatment allows psychiatrists to treat these conditions where appropriate, to minimize complications and health consequences associated with delayed diagnosis, and to reduce the burden of disease that these conditions may pace on patients already experiencing primary psychiatric disorders.

References
[1] Rosen R, Mahowald M, Chesson A, et al. The Taskforce 2000 Survey: medical education in sleep and sleep disorders. Sleep 1998;21:235–8.
[2] Kushida CA, Littner MR, Morgenthaler T, et al. Practice parameters for the indications for polysomnography and related procedures: an update for 2005. Sleep 2005;28:499–521.

[3] Flemons WW. Clinical practice: obstructive sleep apnea. N Engl J Med 2002;347: 498–504.

[4] Chesson AL Jr, Berry RB, Pack A. Practice parameters for the use of portable monitoring devices in the investigation of suspected obstructive sleep apnea in adults. Sleep 2003;26: 907–13.

[5] El-Ad B, Lavie P. Effect of sleep apnea on cognition and mood. Int Rev Psychiatry 2005;17: 277–82.

[6] Suhner AG, Darko DD, Erman MK, et al. Depressive symptoms in patients with OSA and the impact of nasal CPAP treatment. Sleep 2003;25:A225.

[7] Young T, Palta M, Dempsey J, et al. The occurrence of sleep-disordered breathing among middle-aged adults. N Engl J Med 1993;328:1230–5.

[8] Fujita S, Conway W, Zorick F, et al. Surgical correction of anatomic abnormalities in obstructive sleep apnea syndrome: uvulopalatopharyngoplasty. Otolaryngol Head Neck Surg 1981;89:923–34.

[9] Crookes PF. Surgical treatment of morbid obesity. Annu Rev Med 2006;57:243–64.

[10] Walker-Engstrom ML, Tegelberg A, Wilhelmsson B, et al. 4-year follow up of treatment with dental appliance or uvulopalatopharyngoplasty in patients with obstructive sleep apnea: a randomized study. Chest 2002;121:739–46.

[11] Hanzel DA, Proia NG, Hudgel DW. Response of obstructive sleep apnea to fluoxetine and protriptyline. Chest 1991;100:416–21.

[12] Daniels L. Narcolepsy. Medicine (Baltimore) 1934;13:1–22.

[13] Yoss RE, Daly DD. Criteria for the diagnosis of the narcoleptic syndrome. Mayo Clin Proc 1957;32:320–8.

[14] Vogel G. Studies in psychophysiology of dreams: III. the dream of narcolepsy. Arch Gen Psychiatry 1960;3:421–8.

[15] Carskadon MA, Dement WC, Mitler MM, et al. Guidelines for the multiple sleep latency test (MSLT): a standard measure of sleepiness. Sleep 1986;9:519–24.

[16] Scammell TE. The neurobiology, diagnosis, and treatment of narcolepsy. Ann Neurol 2003;53:154–66.

[17] Honda Y, Asake A, Tanaka Y, et al. Discrimination of narcolepsy by using genetic markers and HLA. Sleep Res 1983;12:254.

[18] Littner MR, Kushida C, Wise M, et al. Practice parameters for clinical use of the multiple sleep latency test and the maintenance of wakefulness test. Sleep 2005;28:113–21.

[19] American Academy of Sleep Medicine. International classification of sleep disorders: diagnostic and coding manual. 2nd edition. Westchester (IL): American Academy of Sleep Medicine; 2005.

[20] Mignot E. Genetic and familial aspects of narcolepsy. Neurology 1998;50(Suppl 1): S16–22.

[21] Juji T, Matsuki K, Tokunaga K, et al. Narcolepsy and HLA in the Japanese. Ann N Y Acad Sci 1988;540:106–14.

[22] Lin L, Faraco J, Li R, et al. The sleep disorder canine narcolepsy is caused by a mutation in the hypocretin (orexin) receptor 2 gene. Cell 1999;98:365–76.

[23] Chemelli RM, Sinton CM, Yanagisawa M. Polysomnographic characterization of orexin-2 receptor knockout mice. Sleep 2005;23:A296–7.

[24] Nishino S, Ripley B, Overeem S, et al. Hypocretin (orexin) deficiency in human narcolepsy. Lancet 2000;355:39–40.

[25] Goswami M. The influence of clinical symptoms on quality of life in patients with narcolepsy. Neurology 1998;50(Suppl 1):S31–6.

[26] Mitler M, Erman M, Hajdukovic R. The treatment of excessive somnolence with stimulant drugs. Sleep 1993;16:203–6.

[27] Thorpy M, Black J, Erman M, et al. Tolerability of modafinil in disorders of sleep and wakefulness. Sleep 2004;27:A130.

Table 2
Characteristics of parasomnias

Parasomnia	N-REM parasomnias				REM parasomnias		
	Confusional arousals	Sleep walking	Sleep terrors	SRED	RBD	Sleep paralysis	Nightmare disorder
Stage of arousal	II, III, IV	III, IV	III, IV	II, III, IV	REM	REM	REM
Typical time of night	Anytime	First 2 h	First 2 h	Anytime	Anytime	Anytime (first 2 h)	Anytime
EEG during event	NA	Mixed	Mixed	Mixed	REM pattern	Wake pattern	NA
EMG activity during event	↑	↑	↑	↑	↑	↓	NA
Decreased responsiveness during event	+	+	+	+	+	−	+
Autonomic hyperactivity	−	−	+	−	+	±	+
Amnesia	+	+	+	± (partial)	− (Dream recall)	− (Experience recall)	− (Dream recall)
Confusion post episode	+	+	+	+	−	−	−
Family history	+	+	+	+	−	±	−

sleep (and seldom from napping). Although they typically may arise from SWS, it is important to note that these parasomnias are disorders of arousal, not sleep per se. Physiologically, arousals are transient events (typically a few seconds in duration) during which the electroencephalogram (EEG) shifts from a deeper stage of sleep, to a higher frequency (often alpha rhythm). As these arousals are brief, they do not represent full wakefulness, and the limited duration of the arousal is not sufficient to change the stage of sleep (as they are only a fraction of the 30-second epoch typically used to score sleep stages). Behaviorally, arousals are events in which wakefulness has not been fully re-established, and in the case of a NREM parasomnia, behaviors (eg, walking, eating, and sexual behavior) and mood states (eg, fear and anger) are expressed that are not fully (or at all) under conscious control or remembered on awakening [6]. These behaviors occur without complex mentation, ordered judgment, or full integration of environmental feedback. NREM parasomnias commonly are seen in childhood and classically diminish with increasing age. There often is a family history of NREM parasomnias in individuals who present for evaluation, and these disorders likely are expressed when environmental factors affect genetically predisposed individuals [7]. In susceptible individuals, precipitating events can be either endogenous factors (eg, apnea, periodic limb movements, or pain) or exogenous factors (eg, sleep deprivation or medications) that disturb sleep [3].

As a result of commonalities, the categorization of NREM parasomnias typically is based on the type of behavior that occurs. In the following sections, these disorders are presented along a continuum of behavioral arousal while acknowledging that clinical overlap can exist between these disorders.

CONFUSIONAL AROUSALS

Confusional arousals typically are brief, simple motor behaviors that occur without significant affective expression or responsiveness to the environment. They are associated with mental confusion on arousal or awakening [8]. The motor behaviors are simple and may be accompanied by indistinct vocalization. The episodes are brief and because of dense amnesia for the episode, without collateral information from a bed partner or parent, they often are unnoticed. Although self-report data likely underestimate the prevalence of the disorder, prevalence is estimated at 4.2%, with comparable rates in men and women and prevalence that decreases with age [8].

A variant of confusional arouals is described as "sleep drunkenness" or excessive sleep inertia [9,10]. What distinguishes confusional arousals from excessive sleep inertia is that the latter traditionally is referred to as a phenomenon that stems from final awakening; however it remains similar to confusional arousals in regard to its immediate development from sleep, impaired mentation, automatic behavior, and relative unresponsiveness to the environment. The duration during which sleep inertia can affect individuals is debated, with studies in the literature ranging from a few minutes to 4 hours [10]. There are interindividual differences on the impact on daily life, depending on the severity and time course over which sleep inertia might deter desired activities or mental tasks. Excessive sleep inertia can occur from naps and full sleep periods, and its severity and duration likely are related to the depth of prior sleep. Studies that use self-report to explore the epidemiology of confusional arousals may in fact focus on excessive sleep inertia, because patients are more apt to recall these episodes as their mentation improves and they achieve full wakefulness. One such study finds that bipolar disorder was associated strongly with such self-reported confusional arousals, although the significance of this finding is unclear [8].

SLEEPWALKING

Sleepwalking, or somnambulism, exists along a continuum with confusional arousals; however, it is distinguished by greater complexity of behavior. Sleepwalking behaviors often enact simple motivations (eg, desire to urinate); however, these behaviors may become dangerous because of limited conscious control (eg, climbing out a window). Dreaming typically is not present, but sleepwalkers may recount limited mentation of their motivations for their behavior if awakened during an episode. Episodes typically arise from SWS during the first part of the sleep episode. Sleepwalkers typically have eyes open during an event and may be clumsy in their behavior [11,12]. If left alone, sleepwalkers often return to sleep, although they may do so in atypical places. If interrupted while sleepwalking, they may have a range of responses ranging from no response to agitation or violence. It is not uncommon for individuals to have somnambulism as children but not to present for evaluation until they are young adults, when their behavior becomes concerning to a bed partner. Further influencing presentation for evaluation is the frequency and dangerousness of the sleepwalking behaviors, which can vary widely from nightly severe episodes to rare benign events. As in other NREM parasomnias, full or partial amnesia for the episode is typical.

Somnambulism occurs in 10% to 20% of all children, with the greatest prevalence occurring between 3 and 10 years of age [13]. Because it is so common in young children and its prevalence tends to decrease with increasing age, sleepwalking often is considered to be a transiently disruptive phenomenon that resolves by adolescence. Sleepwalking occurs in 1% to 4% of adults, and within this population exist individuals who did not sleepwalk as children; however, approximately 80% of adults who have somnambulism have it as a continuation of childhood behavior [8]. The prevalence of sleepwalking does not seem to be associated with gender, race, or socioeconomic conditions [13]. There is significant evidence to suggest that there likely is a genetic component to this disorder, as evidenced by epidemiologic and twin studies [14]. In fact, the HLA gene, DQB1, may confer susceptibility to somnambulism [15]. Risk of sleepwalking is approximately double for individuals if one parent and triple if both parents have a history of sleepwalking.

The relationship between psychopathology and sleepwalking is a debated issue in the literature [16]. Although sleepwalking in childhood does not seem to be related directly to psychiatric pathology, it is observed that psychopathology may be associated with sleepwalking in adolescence and adulthood [8,17]. Still, sleepwalking behaviors do not seem to represent unconscious motivations acted out during sleep in the vast majority of patients, with the caveat that psychologic conflict may not be detected readily in such individuals unless they concurrently are in psychotherapy [18]. Psychotropic medications may raise the risk of adult somnambulism because of their effects on sleep and wakefulness [19]. Also, because disrupted sleep and subsequent sleep deprivation are common among psychiatric patients, this may increase the risk of sleepwalking in these individuals [20].

SLEEP TERRORS
Sleep terrors have many of the same characteristics of sleepwalking; however, they are distinguished by more intense motor and autonomic activity and affective expression. Rather than construing sleep terrors and somnambulism as distinct disorders, it is more appropriate to consider them as related entities that can, in fact, evolve from one to the other during an episode. Similar to somnambulism, sleep terrors tend to occur in the first third of the sleep period and are believed caused by a confluence of genetic susceptibility with precipitating factors [21]. The prevalence of sleep terrors is 5% in children and 1% to 2% in adults [8]. In children, the presentation of sleep terrors typically is dramatic: a piercing scream followed by fear, crying, and inconsolability [22]. In adults, agitation is common and often individuals who have sleep terrors' may injure themselves, others, or property during an episode. Dreaming typically is not reported; however, similar to somnambulism, simple thoughts may be recalled (eg, "I am in danger") that can be difficult to dispel even once awakened. If confronted during an episode, there is the real danger that individuals may incorporate the witness into the sleep terror leading to potential harm. Thus, it is recommended that individuals having a sleep terror be redirected gently in an attempt to raise their level of consciousness, although full or partial amnesia is typical.

SLEEP-RELATED SEXUAL BEHAVIOR AND SLEEP-RELATED VIOLENCE
Along the continuum of NREM parasomnias associated with disordered arousal are sleep-related sexual behavior and sleep-related violence. Both of these disorders are less well understood compared with those disorders discussed previously; however, their unique clinical dimensions merit brief discussion.

Sleep-related sexual behavior, or sexsomnia, is a recently described parasomnia in which sexual behavior occurs with limited awareness during the act, relative unresponsiveness to the external environment, and amnesia for the event [23]. The sexual behavior exhibited often may be distinct from that typical for the patient in terms of partner or type of sexual act (eg, forced sex with on a bed partner, repetitive masturbation, or anal intercourse) [24]. Although poorly understood, it is proposed that distinguishing features of sexsomnia that differentiate it from sleepwalking include more widespread autonomic activation, sexual arousal, and duration of behavior that occasionally can exceed 30 minutes [23]. Not surprisingly, patients who have this parasomnia may present for evaluation for myriad reasons, ranging from complaint of a bed partner to criminal charges.

Sleep-related violence is another parasomnia considered distinct from those discussed previously. In many respects, it can be conceived as an overlap disorder of sleep terrors after sleepwalking [25]. The violent behavior occurs in a state consistent with night terrors, with anger or fear as the primary emotion, agitated resistance to the environment, a slow return to normal levels of alertness, and amnesia for the event. Like sexsomnia, the violent behavior often is atypical for the patient (eg, stabbing or bludgeoning a bed partner or homicidal attacks on others). The majority of cases are young to middle-aged men who have a previous history of sleepwalking [26]. Because sleep-related sexual and violent behaviors are the subject of recent forensic proceedings, there is an urgency in establishing a more comprehensive understanding of these parasomnias.

EVALUATION AND TREATMENT OF NON–RAPID EYE MOVEMENT PARASOMNIAS

Polysomnography (PSG) often is unnecessary for the evaluation of NREM parasomnias and, in any case, attempts to document somnambulism and sleep terrors by PSG often are unsuccessful. It long has been acknowledged that even nightly sleepwalkers may not exhibit the behavior when monitored [27]. Thus, PSG markers of susceptibility have been studied for their diagnostic usefulness and potential insight into pathogenesis. The vast majority of PSG studies of sleepwalkers demonstrate increased brief arousals from SWS with a preserved sleeping EEG, accompanied by autonomic activation after the arousal [28,29]. Similarly, multiple brief arousals with autonomic hyperactivity may be observed as a marker of sleep terrors [30]. PSG may be indicated when there is no history of childhood parasomnias, as their emergence in adulthood may be due to other disorders that can cause arousal from SWS, such as sleep-related breathing disorder, periodic limb movements of sleep (PLMS), or nocturnal seizures. The treatment of the parasomia complaint in these instances entails the treatment of the underlying or precipitating sleep disorder.

In the evaluation of patients who have episodes of abnormal, unwanted nocturnal motor or affective behaviors, ideally, practicing psychiatrists consider a broad range of diagnoses and are able to refer to a sleep specialist when appropriate. Often the differential diagnosis may include nocturnal panic attacks, nocturnal dissociative episodes, frontal lobe seizures, delirium associated with medical or neurologic disorders, and REM sleep behavior disorder (RBD) (discussed later). Sleep-related dissociative disorders (SRDD) only recently have been considered a distinct sleep disorder, included and categorized as a parasomnia in the *ICSD-2*, thus meriting brief discussion [5]. SRDD occurs when individuals who have a dissociative disorder have nocturnal episodes of disso-ciation during EEG established wakefulness (ranging from the transition from sleep to wakefulness to several minutes after achieving wakefulness). Myriad behaviors may manifest during these episodes that may be complex, violent, self-mutilating, abuse re-enactments, or fugue [31]. Prevalence is not known; however, 7 of 100 consecutive patients referred to a sleep disorders center for sleep-related injury were found to have SRDD [32]. Although nocturnal dis-sociative episodes tend to arise from more clearly established wakefulness than other parasomnias, their undesirable behavior, relatedness to sleep, and im-paired awareness further challenge the delineation of sleep from wakefulness and consciousness from unconsciousness [33]. A history of similar daytime be-haviors (eg, dissociation or panic attacks) makes the diagnosis of a NREM par-asomnia less likely but does not rule out the diagnosis definitively. PSG may be indicated to rule out frontal lobe seizures or RBD or more clearly delineate a nocturnal dissociative episode.

The decision to treat NREM parasomnias is based on a risk-benefit analysis that considers the frequency of the parasomnia event, the risk of injury to self or others, and the distress the behavior is causing patients or family members [6]. The decision to treat also is complicated by the fact that the majority of par-asomnias occur infrequently in adult patients; however, their appearance is unpredictable. Thus, adults who have problematic or high-risk parasomnias must decide whether or not chronic treatment for an episodic illness is desired.

For the majority of children, parasomnias do not require treatment because the behavior may be self-limited, poses little risk of harm to the child, and may have limited daytime sequelae because of amnesia for the event. Keeping reg-ular sleep and waking times and avoidance of sleep deprivation often reduce the frequency of events. For children and young adults who sleepwalk, improv-ing the safety of the sleeping environment (eg, locking doors and windows, keeping hallways and stairs well lit, removing dangerous objects from sleep area, placing mattress on floor, and, if possible, having bedroom on first floor) is important.

When treatment of sleepwalking or sleep terrors in adults is indicated, it is done following a three-step model: (1) modifying predisposing and precipitat-ing factors, (2) improving the safety of the sleeping environment, and, if neces-sary, (3) using pharmacotherapy. As there are no controlled clinical trials that examine pharmacotherapy for NREM parasomnias, medication selection is based largely on anecdote and clinical experience. The agents used most com-monly in the treatment of NREM parasomnias are from classes of medications that affect the γ-aminobutyric acid (GABA)-ergic system, although it is unclear whether or not these medications work by suppressing arousals during sleep or by decreasing SWS. The most data regarding treatment of NREM parasomnias exist for benzodiazepines (primarily clonazepam [0.5–2.0 mg at bedtime] but also alprazolam and other benzodiazepines), which are used successfully in moderate-sized open label trials in the treatment of injurious parasomnias for greater than 6 months [32,34]. Although these studies are limited in their ability to detect tolerance, the majority of patients taking these agents do not have to escalate their dose to manage their parasomnia once at a therapeutic dose [34]. The long half-life of clonazepam increases the likelihood that patients may have lingering daytime effects of this medication; thus, if the parasomnia occurs in the first-half of the sleep period, selecting a shorter-acting benzodiazepine, such as triazolam (0.125–0.5 mg at bedtime), or benzodiazepine receptor agonist, such as zolpidem (5–10 mg at bedtime), may be tolerated better, keeping in mind that somnambulism-like behaviors can be rare side-effect of these medications and use of these medications is based largely on clinical experience and anecdote (Fig. 1).

SLEEP-RELATED EATING DISORDER

SRED is a NREM parasomnia that only recently has been described in the medical literature but has achieved notoriety in the popular media [35]. SRED is conceptualized best as a combination of the binge eating of bulimia nervosa with the disordered arousal, confusional behavior, and amnesia of a parasomnia [36,37]. SRED manifests as repetitive partial arousals from sleep, typically within 2 to 3 hours of sleep, with ingestion of food often in a hurried or "out-of-control" manner, despite frequent lack of hunger at the time of the episode. Foods consumed often are high-carbohydrate but also may consist of unusually combined foods, frozen foods, or non-nutritive substances. Patients often feel ashamed, gain weight as a result of the behaviors, and may attempt to

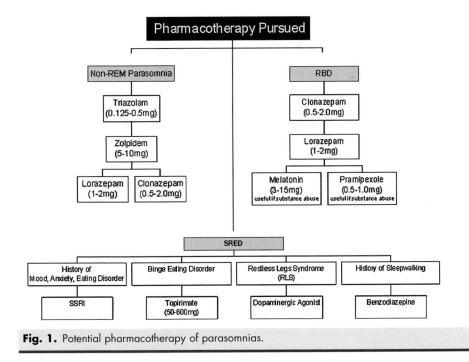

Fig. 1. Potential pharmacotherapy of parasomnias.

control their overall caloric intake forcibly via daytime anorexia. Many patients report reduced awareness at the time of the episode, stating they were mostly asleep or half-awake/half-asleep. Many patients who have SRED also report at least occasional amnesia for the episodes, and specifics may be elucidated via witnesses to the episodes or reconstructed from evidence on awakening (eg, food missing, messy eating place, or food in bed). The level of awareness may vary between episodes within the same night and from night to night over the longitudinal course of the disorder. Diminished awareness during an episode is what distinguishes SRED from nocturnal eating syndrome (NES), a disorder characterized by eating excessive amounts of food either before bed or during nocturnal awakenings while maintaining full consciousness [38]. Given that the criteria for SRED in the recently revised *ICSD-2* do not require impairment in consciousness during nocturnal eating episodes, but rather only "involuntary" eating, it is not clear whether or not NES and SRED are distinct disorders [5]. It may be most useful to consider NES and SRED as entities at opposite ends of a continuum of awareness during nocturnal eating. Although studies are limited, the prevalence of SRED is estimated to be 1% to 5% in the general population, to be 2 to 4 times more common in females, and tends to have onset in late adolescence or early adulthood; the prevalence of NES is found to be as high as 12.3% in psychiatric outpatients [39,40]. SRED seems to be a chronic disorder, so patients often do not present until years after they first develop symptoms. Patients who have SRED may have a history of sleepwalking; however, once eating behaviors during sleep become established, they tend to replace any other distinct sleepwalking behaviors. The pathophysiology of SRED and NES remains unclear; however, both theoretically could be related to abnormalities in the expression of hormones regulating appetite and the sleep-wake cycle [41,42]. Restless legs syndrome (RLS) may be comorbid with SRED in some patients, although the prevalence of co-occurrence is unknown, and treatment of RLS in these individuals may diminish nocturnal eating behaviors. There also are some case reports that benzodiazepine receptor agonists, and possibly atypical antipsychotics, can produce symptoms of SRED [43–45].

SRED seems to be more common in patients who have a daytime eating disorder; however, the vast majority of patients who have SRED do not have an eating disorder that manifests while awake [39,46]. Approximately one-third of patients who have SRED have a first-degree family member who has similar symptoms, comparable to familial patterns observed in sleepwalking and certain eating disorders [47,48]. PSG studies show that SRED behaviors can manifest from any time of night and from all states of NREM sleep [36]. The PSG features of SRED, however, are similar to other NREM parasomnias with frequent arousals from SWS [37].

Treatment of SRED is similar to other NREM parasomnias, with some notable exceptions. Besides avoidance of sleep deprivation and maintaining the safety of the sleeping environment, normalization of a daytime eating schedule is important. Pharmacotherapy should be tailored to individual patients. Those who have a history of sleepwalking can be given short to intermediate acting benzodiazepines; however, this approach can worsen dissociated eating and amnesia. Alternatively, selective serotonin reuptake inhibitors (SSRIs) or topiramate are effective in some case series [49–51]. Treatment of patients who have SRED (in particular those who have symptoms of RLS) with dopamine agonists also is shown useful in an uncontrolled case series [46].

RAPID EYE MOVEMENT–RELATED PARASOMNIAS
During REM sleep, the body undergoes specific physiologic and experiential phenomena, including atonia of the voluntary muscles (except extraocular), elevated autonomic activity, and dreaming. The following REM-related parasomnias involve either the incoordination of these processes or the inappropriate admixture of REM sleep and wakefulness.

RAPID EYE MOVEMENT SLEEP BEHAVIOR DISORDER
RBD is characterized by the loss of coordination of dreaming and paralysis of the skeletal muscles during sleep. With the body free to move during REM sleep, individuals who have RBD act out their dreams, which can include complex motor behaviors, including screaming, punching, kicking, and so forth. In RBD, patients exhibit behavior with eyes closed and unresponsive to the environment around them. When awakened while acting out a dream, individuals achieve rapid full alertness and often report a dream to which their behavior corresponds. The impetus that often brings patients who have RBD to a physician's office is agitated or violent behavior leading to self-injury or injury to a bed partner.

The prevalence of RBD is estimated to be between 0.04% and 0.5% of the population [52]. It often is useful to separate RBD into two clinical forms, acute and chronic. Acute RBD typically is associated with medications, drugs of abuse, or withdrawal (in particular alcohol) [53]. The chronic form is seen most commonly in men who are over 50 years of age. Chronic RBD typically is subdivided into two types, idiopathic and secondary to a neurologic process. The diseases associated most commonly with RBD are the α-synucleinopathies, including Parkinson's disease, dementia with Lewy bodies, and multiple system atrophy—all of which are characterized by pathologic accumulation of the protein α-synuclein [54]. The three largest cohorts of patients who have RBD suggest that approximately 60% of chronic RBD is idiopathic, with the remainder secondary to a neurologic disease [52]. Follow-up studies suggest, however, that idiopathic RBD may be a prodromal syndrome for an underlying condition, leading some to question the nosology of idiopathic RBD [52,55]. Still, many patients initially diagnosed with idiopathic RBD never develop other neurologic illness, even decades after the onset of RBD.

Although the pathophysiology of RBD is not clear, the extrapyramidal and REM sleep systems in the brainstem share specific neuronal connections, which may be central to RBD pathogenesis. Animal models of RBD in which lesions in the brainstem in the region of the locus coeruleus produced REM sleep without atonia, were developed many years before RBD was described clinically as a disorder in humans, implicating these brainstem areas in the control of motor activity during REM sleep [56]. Furthermore, reduced dopamine transporters in the striatum and diminished striatal dopaminergic innervation (using single photon emission CT and positron emission tomography, respectively) are demonstrated in RBD [57,58]. Similarly, a reduction of neurons in the peri-locus coeruleus is observed [59]. One intriguing hypothesis is that the pedunculopontine nucleus (PPN) may play a large role in the REM-atonia circuitry and its disruption in RBD, connecting clinical observations regarding the α-synucleinopathies/extrapyramidal system and RBD with observations in pontine-lesioned animal models [60].

Besides clinical history, PSG is necessary in confirming the diagnosis of RBD. PSG monitoring demonstrates elevated muscle tone or increased phasic muscle activity in the chin (submental) or limb (anterior tibialis) electromyogram during REM sleep [5]. At times, subtle or gross body movements may be recorded during the study. It is not unusual to see excess PLMS during REM and NREM sleep, but otherwise the PSG typically is normal. PSG may, however, be useful if another sleep disorder (eg, sleep-disordered breathing) is believed to contribute to the emergence of RBD. Nonspecific signs and symptoms that also may be found in RBD include general slowing of the waking EEG, subtle neuropsychologic dysfunction, autonomic dysfunction, subtle abnormalities of motor and gait speed, impairment in color discrimination, and olfactory dysfunction [61–64].

The management of RBD typically is behavioral and pharmacologic. From a behavioral standpoint, it is not uncommon for patients to devise their own home remedies to manage their behavior during sleep, such as sleeping in sleeping bags, tethering themselves to their beds, and so forth [53]. Although some of these may be problematic, they do adhere to management principles of other parasomnias—creating a safe sleeping environment for patients and bed partners.

First-line pharmacologic agents in the treatment of RBD are benzodiazepine receptor agonists (Fig. 1). The most commonly used of these agents is clonazepam (0.5 mg–2 mg), which is shown to decrease the frequency and extent of problematic dream-enacting behavior in open label trials [34,65]. In general, this agent is well tolerated; however, given that the majority of patients who have RBD are older individuals, the cognitive impairment and daytime sedation that may be associated with this long-acting benzodiazepine is of concern. In such instances, shorter-acting benzodiazepines (ie, lorazepam 1–2 mg) may be used. In cases where benzodiazepines are problematic because of daytime motor/cognitive effects or in patients who have substance abuse problems, small, uncontrolled case series suggest that melatonin (3–15 mg at bedtime) and pramipexole (0.5–1 mg at bedtime) may be efficacious in RBD [66,67].

Of particular importance to practicing psychiatrists is the role that REM-suppressing antidepressants (SSRIs), monamine oxidase inhibitors (MAOIs), and tricyclic antidepressants (TCAs) can play in exacerbating RBD, as these agents are reported to cause or worsen RBD [65]. Furthermore, subclinical

RBD, in which motor tone is disinhibited, is associated with acute and chronic use of serotonergic antidepressants [68]. Thus, we (the authors) recommend the discontinuation of SSRIs, MAOIs, and TCAs if clinically feasible in patients who have RBD, particularly if RBD emerges as a result of these medications.

SLEEP PARALYSIS

Sleep paralysis (SP) refers to a conscious state at the onset or offset of sleep with associated paralysis of the voluntary musculature. Episodes may last from seconds to minutes, can be associated with hypnogogic or hypnopompic hallucinations, and thus, can be quite distressing. SP is believed to result from inappropriate REM intrusion into wakefulness or, conversely, the failure to maintain sleep during REM periods [69]. SP can occur at any time of night but tends to be clustered in the first 2 hours of the sleep period or at final awakening and may be worsened by sleep deprivation and supine positioning [69–71]. Episodes typically last seconds to minutes, and may disappear either spontaneously or when touched (eg, by a bed partner). The lifetime prevalence of SP is unclear, as estimates in the literature vary widely between 2.3% and 40%, with multiple episodes occurring in 1% to 10% of the population [69]. Not surprisingly, myriad cultural factors may influence reporting, subjective experience, and explanation of SP [72].

Although many patients who have SP may have it in isolation, the symptom of SP should prompt practitioners to inquire about other symptoms of associated neuropsychiatric illness. Primarily, SP is a classic symptom of narcolepsy; thus, symptoms of excess daytime sleepiness, cataplexy, and sleep attacks should be elicited [73]. Unless narcolepsy is suspected by history, PSG typically is not indicated. Furthermore, although the vast majority of patients who have SP likely do not have associated psychiatric illness, large epidemiologic studies find significantly higher rates of bipolar, depressive, and anxiety disorders among individuals who have SP [74]. Furthermore, some small studies find higher rates of SP in posttraumatic stress disorder (PTSD) versus non-PTSD individuals in specific cultural cohorts [75]. Treatment of underlying neuropsychiatric illness, when indicated, is important in the management of secondary SP; however, often times, reassurance and education are most useful in isolated cases. If the frequency of SP is bothersome to patients, there is a suggestion that SSRIs may be of some benefit, likely because of their REM-suppressing properties [76].

NIGHTMARE DISORDER

Dreams represent recall of mental activity that occurs during sleep, and although dreaming tends to occur predominantly during REM sleep, dreams occur during REM and NREM sleep. Nightmare disorder is characterized by recurrent dreams, followed by awakening with full and often detailed recall of the dream. Typically, fear is the predominant associated emotion recalled; however, anger, embarrassment, and sorrow also might occur. Nightmares typically occur in the latter third of the night, which coincides with the increased proportion of REM sleep that occurs at this time [77]. Unlike RBD, nightmares typically are not associated with overt motor dream enactment. It often is difficult for individuals to return to sleep after a nightmare (unlike after sleep terrors), thus, frequent nightmares can lead to fear of going to sleep and subsequent insomnia.

Estimates of the epidemiology of nightmares and their association with psychiatric illness are hindered by inconsistent definitions. Still, it is estimated that 5% to 8% of adults in the general population have nightmares frequently enough to cause complaint, and nightmares are more common in women than men [78,79]. The majority of studies (but not all) find nightmares to be associated with myriad psychiatric diagnoses, including depression, substance abuse disorders, and personality disorders [80]. There also is some data to suggest a connection between nightmares and suicidality [81,82]. When distress and frequency of nightmares are assessed independently, distress seems to be tied more closely to psychopathology [83].

The psychiatric illness associated most commonly with nightmares is PTSD, as nightmares are a diagnostic feature of PTSD as part of the re-experiencing cluster [4]. It is notable that the *DSM-IV-TR* excludes the diagnosis of the parasomnia nightmare disorder if the nightmare is believed secondary to another psychiatric illness; however, the *ICSD-2* considers PTSD a predisposing factor for nightmare disorder [4,5]. The prevalence of nightmares in PTSD seems to be related in part to the study population and the specific trauma. Studies examining the general population, however, find individuals who have PTSD report nightmares at nearly fivefold higher rates relative to non-PTSD individuals [84]. Nightmares associated with PTSD often have similar thematic content or literal associations to the trauma history, and recurrent nightmares often occur [85]. A tendency to experience "bad dreams" and interrupted sleep preceding a trauma was found to be a risk factor for PTSD and depressive symptoms after Hurricane Andrew, which suggests premorbid nightmares may be a marker for posttrauma psychopathology [86].

The diagnosis of nightmare disorder is clinical, as PSG is generally of little value, unless needed to rule out another parasomnia. In PTSD, nightmares rarely are observed in sleep laboratories, but when seen, they occur from REM and NREM sleep. Several medications are found effective in the treatment of PTSD-related nightmares, including prazosin (small, controlled trial), topiramate (open-label, add-on trial), and atypical antipsychotics (case reports); however, the majority of studies are limited by small sample size [87–89]. The behavioral intervention of imagery rehearsal therapy, in which alternative versions of nightmares with better outcomes are rehearsed while awake, also shows benefit for the treatment of nightmares, trauma and nontrauma related [90].

SUMMARY

Parasomnias represent undesirable behaviors that arise from sleep but are not fully under voluntary control. Different classification schemas exist for the

[42] Allison KC, Ahima RS, O'Reardon JP, et al. Neuroendocrine profiles associated with energy intake, sleep, and stress in the night eating syndrome. J Clin Endocrinol Metab 2005;90: 6214–7.

[43] Morgenthaler TI, Silber MH. Amnestic sleep-related eating disorder associated with zolpidem. Sleep Med 2002;3:323–7.

[44] Lu ML, Shen WW. Sleep-related eating disorder induced by risperidone. J Clin Psychiatry 2004;65:273–4.

[45] Paquet V, Strul J, Servais L, Pelc I, et al. Sleep-related eating disorder induced by olanzapine. J Clin Psychiatry 2002;63:597.

[46] Schenck CH, Hurwitz TD, O'Connor KA, et al. Additional categories of sleep-related eating disorders and the current status of treatment. Sleep 1993;16:457–66.

[47] Hublin C, Kaprio J, Partinen M, et al. Prevalence and genetics of sleepwalking: a population-based twin study. Neurology 1997;48:177–81.

[48] Klump KL, Kaye WH, Strober M. The evolving genetic foundations of eating disorders. Psychiatr Clin North Am 2001;24:215–25.

[49] Winkelman JW. Treatment of nocturnal eating syndrome and sleep-related eating disorder with topiramate. Sleep Med 2003;4:243–6.

[50] O'Reardon JP, Allison KC, Martino NS, et al. A randomized, placebo-controlled trial of sertraline in the treatment of night eating syndrome. Am J Psychiatry 2006;163:893–8.

[51] Winkelman JW. Efficacy and tolerability of topiramate in the treatment of sleep-related eating disorder: An open-labe, retrospective case series. J Clin Psych, in press.

[52] Fantini ML, Ferini-Strambi L, Montplaisir J. Idiopathic REM sleep behavior disorder: toward a better nosologic definition. Neurology 2005;64:780–6.

[53] Schenck CH, Mahowald MW. REM sleep behavior disorder: clinical, developmental, and neuroscience perspectives 16 years after its formal identification in SLEEP. Sleep 2002;25: 120–38.

[54] Boeve BF, Silber MH, Parisi JE, et al. Synucleinopathy pathology and REM sleep behavior disorder plus dementia or parkinsonism. Neurology 2003;61:40–5.

[55] Schenck CH, Bundlie SR, Mahowald MW. REM behavior disorder (RBD): delayed emergence of parkinsonism and/or dementia in 65% of older men initially diagnosed with idiopathic RBD, and an analysis of the minimum & maximum tonic and/or phasic electromyographic abnormalities found during REM sleep. Sleep 2003;26:A316.

[56] Jouvet M, Delorme F. Locus coeruleus et sommeil paradoxal. C R Soc Biol 1965;159: 895–9.

[57] Eisensehr I, Linke R, Noachtar S, et al. Reduced striatal dopamine transporters in idiopathic rapid eye movement sleep behaviour disorder. comparison with parkinson's disease and controls. Brain 2000;123(Pt 6):1155–60.

[58] Albin RL, Koeppe RA, Chervin RD, et al. Decreased striatal dopaminergic innervation in REM sleep behavior disorder. Neurology 2000;55:1410–2.

[59] Turner RS, D'Amato CJ, Chervin RD, et al. The pathology of REM sleep behavior disorder with comorbid lewy body dementia. Neurology 2000;55:1730–2.

[60] Rye DB. Contributions of the pedunculopontine region to normal and altered REM sleep. Sleep 1997;20:757–88.

[61] Gagnon JF, Fantini ML, Bedard MA, et al. Association between waking EEG slowing and REM sleep behavior disorder in PD without dementia. Neurology 2004;62:401–6.

[62] Postuma RB, Lang AE, Massicotte-Marquez J, et al. Potential early markers of parkinson disease in idiopathic REM sleep behavior disorder. Neurology 2006;66:845–51.

[63] Ferini-Strambi L, Di Gioia MR, Castronovo V, et al. Neuropsychological assessment in idiopathic REM sleep behavior disorder (RBD): does the idiopathic form of RBD really exist? Neurology 2004;62:41–5.

[64] Ferini-Strambi L, Oldani A, Zucconi M, et al. Cardiac autonomic activity during wakefulness and sleep in REM sleep behavior disorder. Sleep 1996;19:367–9.

[65] Schenck CH, Mahowald MW. Rapid eye movement sleep parasomnias. Neurol Clin 2005;23:1107–26.

[66] Boeve BF, Silber MH, Ferman TJ. Melatonin for treatment of REM sleep behavior disorder in neurologic disorders: Results in 14 patients. Sleep Med 2003;4:281–4.

[67] Fantini ML, Gagnon JF, Filipini D, et al. The effects of pramipexole in REM sleep behavior disorder. Neurology 2003;61:1418–20.

[68] Winkelman JW, James L. Serotonergic antidepressants are associated with REM sleep without atonia. Sleep 2004;27:317–21.

[69] Girard TA, Cheyne JA. Timing of spontaneous sleep-paralysis episodes. J Sleep Res 2006;15:222–9.

[70] Takeuchi T, Fukuda K, Sasaki Y, et al. Factors related to the occurrence of isolated sleep paralysis elicited during a multi-phasic sleep-wake schedule. Sleep 2002;25:89–96.

[71] Cheyne JA. Situational factors affecting sleep paralysis and associated hallucinations: position and timing effects. J Sleep Res 2002;11:169–77.

[72] Hinton DE, Hufford DJ, Kirmayer LJ. Culture and sleep paralysis. Transcult Psychiatry 2005;42:5–10.

[73] Guilleminault C, Fromherz S. Narcolepsy: ciagnosis and management. In: Kryger MH, Roth T, Dement WC, editors. Principles and practice of sleep medicine. 4th ed. Philadelphia (PA): Elsevier Saunders; 2005. p. 780–90.

[74] Ohayon MM, Zulley J, Guilleminault C, et al. Prevalence and pathologic associations of sleep paralysis in the general population. Neurology 1999;52:1194–200.

[75] Hinton DE, Pich V, Chhean D, et al. 'The ghost pushes you down': sleep paralysis-type panic attacks in a khmer refugee population. Transcult Psychiatry 2005;42:46–77.

[76] Koran LM, Raghavan S. Fluoxetine for isolated sleep paralysis. Psychosomatics 1993;34:184–7.

[77] Pagel JF. Nightmares and disorders of dreaming. Am Fam Physician 2000;61:2037–42, 2044.

[78] Zadra A, Donderi DC. Nightmares and bad dreams: their prevalence and relationship to well-being. J Abnorm Psychol 2000;109:273–81.

[79] Ohayon MM, Morselli PL, Guilleminault C. Prevalence of nightmares and their relationship to psychopathology and daytime functioning in insomnia subjects. Sleep 1997;20:340–8.

[80] Nielsen TA, Laberge L, Paquet J, et al. Development of disturbing dreams during adolescence and their relation to anxiety symptoms. Sleep 2000;23:727–36.

[81] Agargun MY, Cilli AS, Kara H, et al. Repetitive and frightening dreams and suicidal behavior in patients with major depression. Compr Psychiatry 1998;39:198–202.

[82] Tanskanen A, Tuomilehto J, Viinamaki H, et al. Nightmares as predictors of suicide. Sleep 2001;24:844–7.

[83] Levin R, Fireman G. Nightmare prevalence, nightmare distress, and self-reported psychological disturbance. Sleep 2002;25:205–12.

[84] Ohayon MM, Shapiro CM. Sleep disturbances and psychiatric disorders associated with posttraumatic stress disorder in the general population. Compr Psychiatry 2000;41:469–78.

[85] Harvey AG, Jones C, Schmidt DA. Sleep and posttraumatic stress disorder: a review. Clin Psychol Rev 2003;23:377–407.

[86] Mellman TA, David D, Kulick-Bell R, et al. Sleep disturbance and its relationship to psychiatric morbidity after hurricane andrew. Am J Psychiatry 1995;152:1659–63.

[87] Raskind MA, Peskind ER, Kanter ED, et al. Reduction of nightmares and other PTSD symptoms in combat veterans by prazosin: a placebo-controlled study. Am J Psychiatry 2003;160:371–3.

[88] Berlant JL. Prospective open-label study of add-on and monotherapy topiramate in civilians with chronic nonhallucinatory posttraumatic stress disorder. BMC Psychiatry 2004;4:24.

[89] Ahearn EP, Krohn A, Connor KM, et al. Pharmacologic treatment of posttraumatic stress dis-order: a focus on antipsychotic use. Ann Clin Psychiatry 2003;15:193–201.
[90] Krakow B, Hollifield M, Johnston L, et al. Imagery rehearsal therapy for chronic nightmares in sexual assault survivors with posttraumatic stress disorder: a randomized controlled trial. JAMA 2001;286:537–45.

Circadian Rhythm Sleep Disorders and Phototherapy

Christopher D. Fahey, MD, Phyllis C. Zee, MD, PhD*

Department of Neurology, Northwestern University Feinberg School of Medicine, Abbott Hall, 11ᵗʰ Floor, 710 N. Lake Shore Drive, Chicago, IL 60611, USA

C ircadian rhythms are physiologic or behavioral cycles with a period of approximately 24 hours produced by an endogenous pacemaker. In humans, the most apparent function of the circadian system is the regulation of the sleep–wake cycle, and the system promotes both sleep and wakefulness at discrete points of the cycle [1]. Circadian rhythm sleep disorders are defined by an alteration of the phase relationship between the intrinsic circadian system and the extrinsic light–dark cycle resulting in an unconventional or abnormal sleep–wake pattern. Consequent symptoms of insomnia, excessive sleepiness, or impairment of occupational, academic, or social functioning may prompt the afflicted to seek medical evaluation.

Of the six recognized circadian rhythm sleep disorders, four are thought to involve a primary alteration of the patient's endogenous circadian system (delayed sleep phase syndrome, advanced sleep phase syndrome, non–24-hour sleep–wake syndrome, and irregular sleep–wake rhythm), whereas the other two involve a change in the timing of environmental light–dark or social/activity cycles relative to the patient's intrinsic circadian rhythm (shift work sleep disorder and jet lag disorder). In the last several decades, understanding of the anatomic and physiologic origins of circadian rhythmicity has expanded considerably, leading to greater insight into these disorders and novel treatment strategies. This article briefly describes circadian rhythms and their properties, explores the use of light and other agents as therapeutic tools, and concludes with a description of the six recognized circadian rhythm sleep disorders.

CIRCADIAN RHYTHMS

The suprachiasmatic nucleus within the anterior hypothalamus houses the overriding oscillator responsible for circadian rhythms in mammals [2–4]. When kept free from temporal cues, the endogenous period of circadian periods in humans has been found to be slightly longer than 24 hours, at approximately 24.2 hours [5]. Because of this discrepancy, there exists a need to

*Corresponding author. E-mail address: p-zee@northwestern.edu (P.C. Zee).

0193-953X/06/$ – see front matter
doi:10.1016/j.psc.2006.09.009

synchronize the endogenous pacemaker with the external environment. Synchronization of the endogenous period and the 24-hour day occurs by way of the process of entrainment by various external and internal stimuli, termed *zeitgebers* (German for "time givers") [6]. In humans and most other species, the foremost of these zeitgebers is the daily light–dark cycle. Measurement of the circadian phase (timing of the endogenous circadian rhythm relative to the entraining agent) itself and changes directed at this phase can be obtained through the assessment of assorted proxy markers of the circadian rhythm including core body temperature minimum and the dim light melatonin onset (DLMO) (the time at which endogenous melatonin begins to climb). The core body temperature minimum occurs approximately 2 hours before awakening from nocturnal sleep [7], while the DLMO takes place approximately 2 to 3 hours before the routine bedtime [8,9].

PHOTIC ENTRAINMENT AND THERAPY

As the most dependable gauge of the 24-hour day, light remains the most potent of entraining agents. As with other zeitgebers, the effect of light on the circadian pacemaker can be charted using a phase response curve (PRC), where the direction and magnitude of a change in the timing of circadian rhythms in response to a particular stimulus is plotted as a function of the circadian time in which that stimulus is delivered. Light delivered in the early evening tends to result in a phase delay (ie, a tendency toward later sleep and wake times, as well as later onset of other circadian rhythms), whereas light delivered in the early morning hours tends to result in a phase advance (ie, a tendency toward earlier sleep and wake times, as well as earlier other circadian rhythms) (Fig. 1). The peak of the phase-shifting properties of light actually occurs just before (phase delay) and just after (phase advancement) minimum core body temperature [10,11]. However, awakening the patient at either of these two points is generally considered impractical, and late evening and early morning administration times, though less potent, are typically used. Bright light at near daylight intensities clearly results in entrainment of circadian rhythms [10,11], but depending on the history of prior light exposure, much lower levels of lighting can also alter circadian rhythms [12]. After 3 consecutive days of 5 hours of light exposure given 1.5 hours after core body temperature minimum, a dose–response curve has been demonstrated with a phase advance of approximately 4.5 hours at an intensity of 9500 lux, a phase advance of approximately 2.7 hours at an intensity of 1260 lux, and a phase advance of about 1.2 hours at 180 lux [13]. Although clear guidelines for the precise optimal dosing of light do not exist, most of the research that has demonstrated efficacy of light therapy in humans has used light intensities between 2500 to 9500 lux [14], with 2500 to 10,000 lux commonly used in the clinical setting [15]. In addition to intensity, the wavelength of light may also be important in that the phase-shifting capabilities of light at a shorter wavelength of 460 nm (within the blue spectrum) are more powerful relative to other wavelengths [16–19].

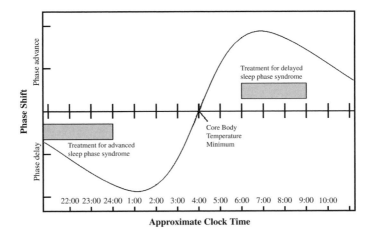

Fig. 1. General schematic of the phase-shifting properties of light as a function of circadian time delivered. Light delivered before the core body temperature minimum tends to result in a phase delay, with a greater magnitude of phase shift as the core body temperature minimum is approached. Conversely, light delivered after the core body temperature minimum tends to result in a phase advance. The core body temperature minimum occurs approximately 2 hours before habitual wake time. For an individual with a habitual wake time of 6:00 AM, the core body temperature minimum would fall around 4:00 AM. The gray bars represent common times for the use of light therapy in the treatment of advanced and delayed sleep phase syndrome.

The ideal duration of light therapy has not been studied, and a duration response curve is nonexistent. That being said, in clinical practice, often for reasons of patient convenience, light bursts of 1 to 2 hours are often used [15]. Phototherapy is expensive, with light boxes generally costing between $200 and $400 [20]. Rental units are also available. Light boxes filter UV rays and are generally felt to be safe. Side effects are generally mild and transient with headache, transient visual problems, nausea and vomiting, and hypomania being the most commonly reported [21]. Potential relative contraindications include mania, migraine headaches, and retinal photosensitivity, and patients who have ophthalmologic disease should be seen by an ophthalmologist before the initiation of treatment [22–24].

OTHER ENTRAINING AGENTS

Another important entraining agent is melatonin, a hormone produced by the pineal gland and released into the systemic circulation [25]. Its synthesis and secretion by the pineal gland are dictated by the suprachiasmatic nucleus through sympathetic efferents, while melatonin release is inhibited by exposure to bright light. Simplistically, melatonin can be thought of as an "internal dark signal," having the opposite PRC relative to light. Namely, exposure to melatonin early in the night results in a phase advance, whereas exposure in the early morning results in a phase delay [8]. The phase-delaying properties of melatonin may be of a lesser magnitude than its phase-advancing properties [26]. In sighted individuals, melatonin is thought to be a weaker zeitgeber relative to light [27]. Given its ability to reset circadian phases, exogenous melatonin has been used to treat various circadian rhythm sleep disorders [28–32].

The combination of exogenous melatonin and light therapy may be more effective in producing phase shifts than light therapy alone [33]. Melatonin has not been approved for use in circadian rhythm sleep disorders by the US Food and Drug Administration. The major side effect of melatonin is sleepiness, and patients should not drive after its use for at least several hours. Additionally, melatonin may potentially exacerbate asthma [34]. Given the lack of safety data, melatonin is not advised for pregnant or breastfeeding women or for patients taking warfarin or anticonvulsants [24].

Other than melatonin, the other nonphotic entraining agent for which there is substantial evidence is physical exercise, which, when performed nocturnally, results in a phase delay [35]. Alternative weaker proposed entraining agents include mealtimes [36], listening to music [37], social contact [38], and bedtime and other social cues [39].

DELAYED SLEEP PHASE SYNDROME

As first reported by Weitzman and colleagues [40], delayed sleep phase syndrome (DSPS) is characterized by a stable tendency toward later sleep onset and wake times (Fig. 2). Patients have a mean sleep onset time of 4:00 AM and a mean wake time of 10:30 AM [41]. Affected patients who attempt to

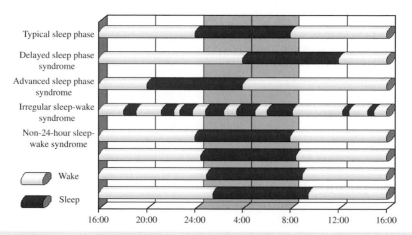

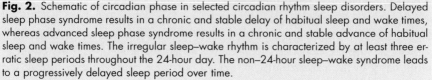

Fig. 2. Schematic of circadian phase in selected circadian rhythm sleep disorders. Delayed sleep phase syndrome results in a chronic and stable delay of habitual sleep and wake times, whereas advanced sleep phase syndrome results in a chronic and stable advance of habitual sleep and wake times. The irregular sleep–wake rhythm is characterized by at least three erratic sleep periods throughout the 24-hour day. The non–24-hour sleep–wake syndrome leads to a progressively delayed sleep period over time.

conform to a more conventional sleep–wake cycle will often report difficulty in the initiation of sleep, resulting in insomnia, and further difficulty awakening in the morning, resulting in excessive sleepiness. Impairment of daytime–especially morning–functioning may follow if the total sleep time is reduced. When permitted to sleep to their preferred schedule, the sleep itself has been traditionally described to be normal as evaluated by polysomnogram [42–44]. However, a recent controlled study has challenged that notion, noting an increase in stage 1 and 2 of sleep and a decrease in slow-wave sleep in DSPS patients [45]. In addition to the presence of the above symptoms, the *International Classification of Sleep Disorders: Diagnostic and Coding Manual, Second Edition* (ICSD-2), requires that a stable delay in the habitual sleep period be verified by at least 1 week of a sleep log or actigraphy [46]. A delay in the core body temperature minimum or in DLMO may also be useful in establishing the diagnosis [46]. Finally, other sleep, medical, or psychiatric disorders, medication usage, or substance use disorders ought not better account for the patient's disturbance in sleep [46]. The diagnostic criteria for DSPS within the text revision of the *Diagnostic and Statistical Manual for Mental Disorders, Fourth Edition*, shares many of the features of those within the ICSD-2. Namely, the pattern of later sleep onset and wake times must be persistent; must be secondary to a disparity between the environmentally required sleep–wake schedule and his or her current sleep–wake schedule; and must lead to symptoms of either excessive sleepiness or insomnia, as well as distress or functional impairment in a patient's social, occupational, or other important areas of life. Furthermore, the patient must have an inability to sleep and wake at the preferred earlier schedule, and the sleep disturbance should not occur exclusively in the presence of another sleep or mental disorder, nor should it be secondary to substance use or a medical condition [47].

Estimates of the prevalence of DSPS range between 0.13% and 3.1%, depending on the methodology employed [48–50]. Within the population of patients evaluated for insomnia at sleep disorder clinics, between 5% and 10% are estimated to have a diagnosis of DSPS [46], with some estimates being as high as 16% [41]. DSPS appears to be more common in adolescents and young adults, with a prevalence between 7% and 16% [41,51].

Several proposals exist as to the underlying pathophysiology of DSPS. One theory holds that an unusually long endogenous circadian period that otherwise maintains its entrainment to the light–dark cycle could lead to a tendency to later sleep onsets [41]. Another holds that a smaller magnitude of the advance portion of the PRC for light or a larger magnitude of the delay portion may lead to a delayed sleep phase over time [52]. Behavioral components may be important as well, with later wake times resulting in less early morning light exposure and less phase advancement, leading to a vicious cycle of a continually delayed sleep cycle. Although circadian changes currently maintain a role of primacy in the pathophysiology of DSPS, homeostatic factors are now also thought to play a significant role. Relative to controls, patients who have DSPS deprived of sleep for 24 hours show an inability to compensate with recovery sleep during the following day and early evening, suggesting the potential importance of impaired sleep recovery in the symptomatology of DSPS [53,54]. Finally, in a subset of patients, genetics undoubtedly plays an important role. Polymorphisms present within various circadian genes have been reported to be linked with DSPS, including human PER3 [55], 3111 CLOCK [56], and the arylalkylamine *N*-acetyltransferase gene [57], as well as a higher prevalence of HLA-DR1 [58]. Furthermore, a family with an autosomal dominant mode of inheritance for the DSPS phenotype has been reported [59].

As one of the most influential of entraining agents, light offers an important part of possible treatment strategies in patients who have DSPS. An initial 2-week trial of light therapy at 2500 lux given for 2 hours between 6:00 AM and 9:00 AM in combination with evening light restriction demonstrated an advancement of core body temperature minimum of 1.4 hours and an improvement in multiple sleep latencies [60]. A later study reported a 1.5-hour earlier sleep onset time after 5 days of 3 hours of phototherapy given 1.5 hours after core body temperature minimum [61]. One case report used 2500 lux upon awakening over 3 weeks to eventually stably advance the sleep onset time by 5 hours and the wake time by 4 hours in a single patient [62]. In a study using a "bright-light mask" during sleep, a 2700-lux light source was delivered 4 hours before habitual wakening [63]. A phase advance of approximately 1 hour was achieved after nearly 4 weeks of treatment. Although optimal timing, dosing, and duration has not clearly been established, exposure to light at an intensity of 2500 to 10,000 lux in the morning (6:00–8:00 AM) is commonly employed for a period of 1 to 2 hours [15]. One potential pitfall is that without specific knowledge of a particular patient's circadian phase, the delivery of light in the early morning to patients who have DSPS may actually fall before the minimum core body temperature, resulting in further delay of the sleep–wake schedule.

Another potential strategy to advance the sleep–wake schedule in these patients comes in the form of nighttime melatonin. In one trial of more than 60 DSPS patients, 5 mg of melatonin was given at 10:00 PM, 5 hours before mean sleep onset time, for a period of 6 weeks [64]. An overwhelming majority (97%) of patients reported that this regimen improved their symptoms, advanced their sleep onset by nearly 1.5 hours, and advanced their wake time by nearly 2 hours. Nevertheless, nearly all of these patients had reverted to their previous sleep schedule within 1 year of discontinuation of therapy. In a later study, only 40% of 30 DSPS patients were deemed responders (as defined by an "appropriate" sleep phase advance and wake time of before 9:00 AM) when given 0.3 mg of melatonin at 5 hours, 3 hours, and 1 hour before habitual sleep time for 3 months [65]. Finally, a 2005 study by Mundey and colleagues [66] demonstrated a greater magnitude of phase shift with melatonin given 6.5 hours before DLMO compared with 1.5 hours before DLMO. Dosages of 0.3 mg and 3.0 mg were used, without significant differences in outcome between the two. A separate study also failed to demonstrate differences in efficacy between lower versus higher dosages of melatonin [33], whereas others have suggested some degree of dose dependence [67,68]. After discontinuation of the drug, circadian rhythms, including sleep and wake times, tend to drift back to their previously preferred delayed schedule [64,69].

One of the original proposed treatments of DSPS was chronotherapy, a process by which bedtime and wake time were delayed by 3 hours each day until the ideal sleep schedule was obtained [52]. Although good results were reported, practical limitations limit chronotherapy's use in the clinical setting, and there may be a risk of developing non–24-hour sleep–wake syndrome [70]. Vitamin B_{12} has been reported as effective in advancing sleep phase in several uncontrolled case reports [71,72], but was shown to be ineffective in a larger placebo controlled study of DSPS patients [73].

Further recommendations for treatment of DSPS include a firm devotion to the new sleep schedule, an avoidance of napping to enhance homeostatic drive to sleep during the night, and the avoidance of bright light exposure in the evening hours. Addressing concurrent psychiatric pathology as well as social, work, or school stresses is another important aspect of treatment.

ADVANCED SLEEP PHASE SYNDROME

In contrast to DSPS, advanced sleep phase syndrome (ASPS) is typified by advanced sleep onsets and wake times compared with an individual's preferred sleep schedule (Fig. 2) [46]. Impairments in functioning occur not in the morning as with DSPS, but in the late afternoon and evening, when sleepiness begins. Patients awaken in the early morning, and often feel the most alert during this time. If patients attempt to delay their bedtime, they will frequently still wake in the early morning. When allowed to sleep at their preferred schedule, the sleep of these patients is otherwise stable and normal. Other diagnostic criteria include confirmation of the advanced timing of the sleep period with a sleep log or actigraphy for at least 7 days, as well as the exclusion of causative sleep, medical, mental, or substance use disorders, or medication use [46]. The core body temperature minimum and corresponding sleep phase occur earlier in these patients [74]. Patients generally complain of excessive sleepiness in the early evening or late afternoon as well as early morning awakenings. Not infrequently, however, individuals with an advanced phase of sleep are not particularly perturbed by their sleep schedule and rather enjoy their productive early mornings. Because these individuals lack the requisite distress or impairment in social, occupational, or other functioning characteristic of all circadian rhythm sleep disorders, they, by definition, do not have ASPS and may more accurately be described as "larks" or "morning types."

The prevalence of ASPS has been estimated to be approximately 1% in middle-aged individuals [50], although the prevalence of suggestive symptoms in this population has more recently been estimated to be approximately 7% [75]. ASPS appears to be more common with advancing age; however, cases in younger patients do occur [76–78].

As with DSPS, several theories exist as to the underlying pathophysiology of ASPS. Sleeping at earlier times leads to less exposure to early evening light, which may perpetuate an advancement in phase. Older individuals may be particularly vulnerable to a reduction in light transmission given a higher prevalence of various ophthalmologic conditions, including cataracts, glaucoma, and senile miosis [79]. An intrinsic circadian period of less than 24 hours may be an alternative explanation [80], as may a more or less prominent phase-advance or phase-delay region, respectively, in the light PRC. A weakening of the homeostatic drive toward sleep may be important as well in the development of ASPS, particularly in the elderly [81]. ASPS has been linked with genetic polymorphisms at human Per2 genes [82], and families with an ASPS phenotype inherited in an autosomally dominated fashion have been described [77,78,80].

Light therapy may be used in the evening to delay the circadian phase in patients who have ASPS. One study examining older women with ASPS used a 4000-lux artificial light source over 12 consecutive days from 7:00 PM to 9:00 PM [83]. Decreased awakenings and phase advancement were achieved in these patients. Another study also reported successful phase advancement using a 2500-lux light source over 4 hours (from 8:00 PM to 12:00 AM) over 2 days [84]. However, it must be noted that compliance with usage of the brighter light boxes may be an issue with older subjects [85]. A more recent study using a 265-lux light source for 2 to 3 hours in the evening was not effective in advancing sleep phase compared with placebo [86].

Given its PRC, melatonin taken in the morning ought to delay the sleep schedule in these patients. The known soporific effects of melatonin [87], however, may limit this use in certain patients. Chronotherapy to treat ASPS, in which sleep onset is advanced 3 hours at a time at an interval of 2 days until the desired sleep–wake cycle timing is obtained, is an efficacious treatment [76]; however, the same concerns of patient acceptance and practicality limit its usage.

NON–24-HOUR SLEEP–WAKE SYNDROME

Non–24-hour sleep–wake syndrome entails a circadian rhythm that free-runs at a period of its endogenous circadian clock (ie, longer than 24 hours) even in the presence of environmental time cues [46]. Therefore, the sleep–wake period gradually shifts to later in the day as time advances (Fig. 2) [88]. One of the hallmarks of the disorder is symptomatology (insomnia, excessive daytime sleepiness, and functional impairment) that occurs episodically depending upon the phase of the patient's circadian clock at any given particular time. If the phase is completely out of sync with the desired sleep–wake schedule, then symptoms are at their maximum. If the phase is identical to the desired sleep–wake schedule, symptoms may not be present at all. Other diagnostic criteria include verification with a sleep log or actigraphy of the progressively delayed sleep and wake times with a period of greater than 24 hours characteristic of the disorder. At least 7 days (and preferably more) of monitoring with either of these diagnostic tools should be used [46].

The majority of patients afflicted with this syndrome are blind, because transmission from the eyes to the suprachiasmatic nucleus fails, and the most dominant zeitgeber of light is thus incapable of entraining the circadian rhythm [89–91]. Conversely, of the blind, approximately 50% have a nonentrained circadian rhythm and 70% have complaints of abnormal sleep [89,91,92]. Non–24-hour sleep–wake syndrome has been infrequently reported in the sighted [93–95]. Within the sighted population, the disorder may be secondary to a diminished sensitivity to light as an entraining agent [96] or may be secondary to an exceedingly long intrinsic circadian rhythm that loses its capability to be entrained to the 24-hour day [97].

In the blind, melatonin is the treatment of choice, because it can entrain the circadian phase unbound from the antagonism from light. Dosages between 0.5 mg [32,98] and 10 mg [99] given at night (ideally within an hour of the model bedtime) have demonstrable efficacy in entraining the circadian pacemaker over the course of 1 to 3 weeks. In sighted individuals, artificial light given similarly to that delivered to patients who have DSPS may be effective in "slowing down" the patient's endogenous circadian clock. However, if the underlying pathology in these individuals is a diminished responsiveness to the entraining effects of light, the response to light therapy may not be as robust as one would otherwise expect. Finally, vitamin B_{12} has been reported to be effective in entraining the circadian clock both with [71] and without a simultaneous hypnotic [100]. This finding has yet to be verified with placebo-controlled trials.

IRREGULAR SLEEP–WAKE RHYTHM

Patients who have irregular sleep–wake rhythm complain of a lack of clearly distinct sleep–wake cycles resulting in symptoms of insomnia or sleepiness. Nighttime sleep demonstrates poor consolidation and is truncated. The daytime is characterized by frequent, irregular napping. The total amount of sleep over 24 hours is normal, but sleep tends to be divided among 3 or more erratic sleep periods (Fig. 2). Over the course of at least a week, actigraphy or sleep logs should demonstrate at least three irregular sleep bouts during the 24-hour period [46].

The precise prevalence of this disorder is uncertain, but is likely rare [101]. Irregular sleep–wake rhythm is often seen in institutionalized patients who have dementia [102] and can also be seen with other disorders of the neurologic system, including traumatic brain injury and in children with mental retardation [103, 104]. In patients without central nervous system dysfunction, the disorder is seen in those with extremely poor sleep hygiene and decreased exposure to light or decreased structured social and physical activities, with frequent napping leading to poor nocturnal sleep and poor nocturnal sleep leading to frequent napping [105]. If not readily obvious from the clinical history, it is said that patients who merely have poor sleep hygiene can be distinguished from those with organic brain disease by whether napping occurs with regularity during the "forbidden zone," that time during the late afternoon where normal circadian function dictates maximum alertness [105]. Patients who have organic disease and consequent disruption of the central originators of the circadian rhythm will nap during this forbidden zone, whereas those who have poor sleep hygiene will not.

Treatment of irregular sleep rhythm can be challenging with frequently mixed results. Typical strategies include increasing the intensity and duration of light exposure during the day and limiting evening light exposure. Results of light treatment studies in dementia indicate that increasing morning or evening light exposure can improve circadian rhythmicity and consolidate nocturnal sleep as measured by actigraphy [106–109]. Based on hourly recordings by nursing staff, morning bright light exposure (2 hours at 3000–5000 lux) for 4 weeks increased nocturnal sleep time and decreased daytime sleep time in patients who have dementia [107]. Therefore, behavioral interventions such as increasing light exposure and physical and social activities during the day and decreasing exposure to light and noise during the night are considered first-line approaches for all patients who have irregular sleep–wake rhythm.

In addition, nonphotic cues such as structured physical and social activity may be beneficial [110]. In children who have mental retardation and irregular sleep, 3 mg of melatonin given in the evening resulted in significantly increased nighttime sleep of 1.5 hours and an equivalent drop in daytime sleep [111]. However, in a large multicenter study, Singer and colleagues [112] could find no significant objective improvement in sleep in the use of melatonin in patients who have Alzheimer's disease and disturbed sleep. Finally, combination therapy with light therapy, hypnotics, chronotherapy, and vitamin B_{12} may lead to consolidated sleep [101].

SHIFT WORK SLEEP DISORDER

Unlike the previously described circadian rhythm sleep disorders, shift work sleep disorder does not involve a primary disturbance of the endogenous circadian rhythm. Instead, shift work involves a change in the desired sleep time to a time that is at odds with the normally functioning intrinsic circadian clock. Diagnostic criteria include symptoms of either insomnia or excessive sleepiness, temporal relationship of these symptoms with work that occurs during the normal sleep period, symptom presence associated with the work schedule for at least 1 month, and a 7-day sleep log or actigraph that reveals a disturbed circadian and sleep-time alignment [46]. Total sleep time is reduced with shift workers reporting approximately 10 fewer hours of total sleep time per week compared with those who work during the day [113]. Frequently, shift workers revert back to their naturally preferred sleep schedule on weekends or their days off. Once shift work is initiated, if they occur, phase changes take place slowly, at a rate of approximately 90 min/d [114]. However, many, if not most, shift workers fail to delay their circadian rhythm as measured by endogenous melatonin, potentially because of exposure to bright light in the morning [115,116]. Additionally, shift workers may have an increased risk of development of disease in a variety of organ systems, including cardiovascular disease, gastrointestinal disease, depression, reproductive disorders, as well as an increased accident rate [117].

[85] Suhner AG, Murphy PJ, Campbell SS. Failure of timed bright light exposure to alleviate age-related sleep maintenance insomnia. J Am Geriatr Soc 2002;50(4):617–23.

[86] Palmer CR, Kripke DF, Savage HC Jr, et al. Efficacy of enhanced evening light for advanced sleep phase syndrome. Behav Sleep Med 2003;1(4):213–26.

[87] Cajochen C, Krauchi K, Wirz-Justice A. The acute soporific action of daytime melatonin administration: effects on the EEG during wakefulness and subjective alertness. J Biol Rhythms 1997;12(6):636–43.

[88] Sack RL, Lewy AJ. Circadian rhythm sleep disorders: lessons from the blind. Sleep Med Rev 2001;5(3):189–206.

[89] Miles LE, Raynal DM, Wilson MA. Blind man living in normal society has circadian rhythms of 24.9 hours. Science 1977;198(4315):421–3.

[90] Okawa M, Nanami T, Wada S, et al. Four congenitally blind children with circadian sleep-wake rhythm disorder. Sleep 1987;10(2):101–10.

[91] Sack RL, Lewy AJ, Blood ML, et al. Circadian rhythm abnormalities in totally blind people: incidence and clinical significance. J Clin Endocrinol Metab 1992;75(1):127–34.

[92] Martens H, Endlich H, Hildebrandt G. Sleep/wake distribution in blind subjects with and without sleep complaints. Sleep Research 1990;9:398.

[93] Kokkoris CP, Weitzman ED, Pollak CP, et al. Long-term ambulatory temperature monitoring in a subject with a hypernychthemeral sleep–wake cycle disturbance. Sleep 1978;1(2):177–90.

[94] Weber AL, Cary MS, Connor N, et al. Human non-24-hour sleep-wake cycles in an every-day environment. Sleep 1980;2(3):347–54.

[95] McArthur AJ, Lewy AJ, Sack RL. Non-24-hour sleep-wake syndrome in a sighted man: circadian rhythm studies and efficacy of melatonin treatment. Sleep 1996;19(7):544–53.

[96] Klein T, Martens H, Dijk DJ, et al. Circadian sleep regulation in the absence of light percep-tion: chronic non-24-hour circadian rhythm sleep disorder in a blind man with a regular 24-hour sleep-wake schedule. Sleep 1993;16(4):333–43.

[97] Uchiyama M, Shibui K, Hayakawa T, et al. Larger phase angle between sleep propensity and melatonin rhythms in sighted humans with non-24-hour sleep-wake syndrome. Sleep 2002;25(1):83–8.

[98] Hack LM, Lockley SW, Arendt J, et al. The effects of low-dose 0.5-mg melatonin on the free-running circadian rhythms of blind subjects. J Biol Rhythms 2003;18(5):420–9.

[99] Sack RL, Brandes RW, Kendall AR, et al. Entrainment of free-running circadian rhythms by melatonin in blind people. N Engl J Med 2000;343(15):1070–7.

[100] Kamgar-Parsi B, Wehr TA, Gillin JC. Successful treatment of human non-24-hour sleep-wake syndrome. Sleep 1983;6(3):257–64.

[101] Yamadera H, Takahashi K, Okawa M. A multicenter study of sleep-wake rhythm disorders: clinical features of sleep-wake rhythm disorders. Psychiatry Clin Neurosci 1996;50(4):195–201.

[102] Bliwise DL. Sleep in normal aging and dementia. Sleep 1993;16(1):40–81.

[103] Witting W, Kwa IH, Eikelenboom P, et al. Alterations in the circadian rest-activity rhythm in aging and Alzheimer's disease. Biol Psychiatry 1990;27(6):563–72.

[104] Hoogendijk WJ, van Someren EJ, Mirmiran M, et al. Circadian rhythm-related behavioral disturbances and structural hypothalamic changes in Alzheimer's disease. Int Psychoger-iatr 1996;8(Suppl 3):245–52 [discussion: 69–72].

[105] Richardson GS, Malin HV. Circadian rhythm sleep disorders: pathophysiology and treat-ment. J Clin Neurophysiol 1996;13(1):17–31.

[106] Van Someren EJ, Kessler A, Mirmiran M, et al. Indirect bright light improves circadian rest-activity rhythm disturbances in demented patients. Biol Psychiatry 1997;41(9):955–63.

[107] Mishima K, Okawa M, Hishikawa Y, et al. Morning bright light therapy for sleep and be-havior disorders in elderly patients with dementia. Acta Psychiatr Scand 1994;89(1):1–7.

[108] Ancoli-Israel S, Martin JL, Kripke DF, et al. Effect of light treatment on sleep and circadian rhythms in demented nursing home patients. J Am Geriatr Soc 2002;50(2):282–9.

[109] Ancoli-Israel S, Gehrman P, Martin JL, et al. Increased light exposure consolidates sleep and strengthens circadian rhythms in severe Alzheimer's disease patients. Behav Sleep Med 2003;1(1):22–36.

[110] van Someren EJ, Hagebeuk EE, Lijzenga C, et al. Circadian rest-activity rhythm disturbances in Alzheimer's disease. Biol Psychiatry 1996;40(4):259–70.

[111] Pillar G, Shahar E, Peled N, et al. Melatonin improves sleep-wake patterns in psychomotor retarded children. Pediatr Neurol 2000;23(3):225–8.

[112] Singer C, Tractenberg RE, Kaye J, et al. A multicenter, placebo-controlled trial of melatonin for sleep disturbance in Alzheimer's disease. Sleep 2003;26(7):893–901.

[113] Tasto DL, Colligan MJ, Polly SJ. Health consequences of shift work. Menlo Park (CA): SRI, Intl.; 1978.

[114] Barnes RG, Deacon SJ, Forbes MJ, et al. Adaptation of the 6-sulphatoxymelatonin rhythm in shiftworkers on offshore oil installations during a 2-week 12-h night shift. Neurosci Lett 1998;241(1):9–12.

[115] Dumont M, Benhaberou-Brun D, Paquet J. Profile of 24-h light exposure and circadian phase of melatonin secretion in night workers. J Biol Rhythms 2001;16(5):502–11.

[116] Sack RL, Blood ML, Lewy AJ. Melatonin rhythms in night shift workers. Sleep 1992;15(5):434–41.

[117] Knutsson A. Health disorders of shift workers. Occup Med (Lond) 2003;53(2):103–8.

[118] US Congress OoTA. Biological rhythms: implications for the worker. OTA-BA-463. Washington (DC): US Government Printing Office; 1991.

[119] Akerstedt T, Torsvall L. Shift work. Shift-dependent well-being and individual differences. Ergonomics 1981;24(4):265–73.

[120] Drake CL, Roehrs T, Richardson G, et al. Shift work sleep disorder: prevalence and consequences beyond that of symptomatic day workers. Sleep 2004;27(8):1453–62.

[121] Monk TH, Folkard S. Individual differences in shiftwork adjustment. In: Folkard S, Monk TH, editors. Hours of work. New York: John Wiley; 1985. p. 227–37.

[122] Campbell SS. Effects of timed bright-light exposure on shift-work adaptation in middle-aged subjects. Sleep 1995;18(6):408–16.

[123] Folkard S, Monk TH, Lobban MC. Short and long-term adjustment of circadian rhythms in 'permanent' night nurses. Ergonomics 1978;21(10):785–99.

[124] Tepas DI, Monk TH. Work schedules. In: Salvendy G, editor. Handbook of human factors. New York: John Wiley & Sons; 1987. p. 819–43.

[125] Boivin DB, James FO. Circadian adaptation to night-shift work by judicious light and darkness exposure. J Biol Rhythms 2002;17(6):556–67.

[126] Czeisler CA, Johnson MP, Duffy JF, et al. Exposure to bright light and darkness to treat physiologic maladaptation to night work. N Engl J Med 1990;322(18):1253–9.

[127] Eastman CI, Stewart KT, Mahoney MP, et al. Dark goggles and bright light improve circadian rhythm adaptation to night-shift work. Sleep 1994;17(6):535–43.

[128] Dawson D, Campbell SS. Timed exposure to bright light improves sleep and alertness during simulated night shifts. Sleep 1991;14(6):511–6.

[129] Dawson D, Encel N, Lushington K. Improving adaptation to simulated night shift: timed exposure to bright light versus daytime melatonin administration. Sleep 1995;18(1):11–21.

[130] Baehr EK, Fogg LF, Eastman CI. Intermittent bright light and exercise to entrain human circadian rhythms to night work. Am J Physiol 1999;277(6 Pt 2):R1598–604.

[131] Crowley SJ, Lee C, Tseng CY, et al. Combinations of bright light, scheduled dark, sunglasses, and melatonin to facilitate circadian entrainment to night shift work. J Biol Rhythms 2003;18(6):513–23.

[132] Martin SK, Eastman CI. Medium-intensity light produces circadian rhythm adaptation to simulated night-shift work. Sleep 1998;21(2):154–65.

[133] Campbell SS, Dijk DJ, Boulos Z, et al. Light treatment for sleep disorders: consensus report. III. Alerting and activating effects. J Biol Rhythms 1995;10(2):129–32.

[134] Folkard S, Arendt J, Clark M. Can melatonin improve shift workers' tolerance of the night shift? Some preliminary findings. Chronobiol Int 1993;10(5):315–20.

[135] Jorgensen KM, Witting MD. Does exogenous melatonin improve day sleep or night alertness in emergency physicians working night shifts? Ann Emerg Med 1998;31(6): 699–704.

[136] James M, Tremea MO, Jones JS, et al. Can melatonin improve adaptation to night shift? Am J Emerg Med 1998;16(4):367–70.

[137] Jockovich M, Cosentino D, Cosentino L, et al. Effect of exogenous melatonin on mood and sleep efficiency in emergency medicine residents working night shifts. Acad Emerg Med 2000;7(8):955–8.

[138] Walsh JK, Muehlbach MJ, Schweitzer PK. Acute administration of triazolam for the daytime sleep of.rotating shift workers. Sleep 1984;7(3):223–9.

[139] Czeisler CA, Walsh JK, Roth T, et al. Modafinil for excessive sleepiness associated with shift-work sleep disorder. N Engl J Med 2005;353(5):476–86.

[140] Czeisler CA, Dinges DF, Walsh JK, et al. Absence of detectable effect of modafinil on daytime sleep after a simulated night shift in SWSD patients [abstract 0284.E]. Sleep 2003;26:A115.

[141] Walsh JK, Muehlbach MJ, Schweitzer PK. Hypnotics and caffeine as countermeasures for shiftwork-related sleepiness and sleep disturbance. J Sleep Res 1995;4(S2):80–3.

[142] Leger D, Badet D, De la Glicais B. The prevalence of jet-lag among 507 traveling businessmen. Sleep Res 1993;22:239.

[143] Burgess HJ, Crowley SJ, Gazda CJ, et al. Preflight adjustment to eastward travel: 3 days of advancing sleep with and without morning bright light. J Biol Rhythms 2003;18(4): 318–28.

[144] Herxheimer A, Petrie KJ. Melatonin for the prevention and treatment of jet lag. Cochrane Database Syst Rev 2002;2:CD001520.

[145] Jamieson AO, Zammit GK, Rosenberg RS, et al. Zolpidem reduces the sleep disturbance of jet lag. Sleep Med 2001;2(5):423–30.

[146] Beaumont M, Batejat D, Pierard C, et al. Caffeine or melatonin effects on sleep and sleepiness after rapid eastward transmeridian travel. J Appl Physiol 2004;96(1):50–8.

[147] Herxheimer A. Jet lag. Clin Evid 2005;13:2178–83.

Sleep in Mood Disorders

Michael J. Peterson, MD, PhD, Ruth M. Benca, MD, PhD*

Department of Psychiatry, University of Wisconsin-Madison, Madison, WI, USA

INTRODUCTION AND EPIDEMIOLOGY

Prevalence and Types of Sleep Problems in Mood Disorders

Sleep disturbance is a common complaint in patients who have mood disorders, and changes in sleep are a diagnostic criterion of each of the major mood disorders in the *Diagnostic and Statistical Manual of Mental Disorders, Fourth Edition, Text Revision (DSM-IV-TR)* [1], reflecting their importance and prevalence in the presentation of these disorders. Insomnia is present in approximately 10% to 16% of the general population but is much more common in patients who have mood disorders. Complaints of sleep disruptions are common preceding and during major depressive or manic episodes. At least 65% of patients who have major depressive disorder report at least one of the following sleep complaints: difficulty falling asleep (initial insomnia, 38%), frequent awakenings (middle insomnia, 39%), or early morning awakening (terminal insomnia, 41%) [2]. Other common complaints include more frequent nocturnal awakenings, nonrestorative sleep, disturbing dreams, or decreased total sleep. During manic periods, patients usually report reductions in total sleep, often with a sense of decreased sleep need. Patients who have bipolar affective disorder may report insomnia while depressed but also may report fatigue and hypersomnia [3]. Hypersomnia, generally defined as daily sleep in excess of 9 to 10 hours and reported in 3% to 8% of the general population [4,5], also is reported commonly in major depression with atypical features or a seasonal pattern. A subset of patients may have complaints of insomnia and hypersomnia, perhaps suggesting a more severe pathophysiology [2,5].

Epidemiology of Sleep Disturbance and Mood Disorders

People who have sleep complaints are more likely to have a concurrent mood disorder. Population surveys indicate that adults who have insomnia are up to 9 times more likely to have major depression at the time of the interview than those who do not have insomnia [6–8]. Young adults who have a history of insomnia, hypersomnia, or both show a 10- to 20-fold increase in the lifetime

*Corresponding author. Department of Psychiatry, 6001 Research Park Boulevard, Madison, WI 53719. E-mail address: rmbenca@wisc.edu (R.M. Benca).

0193-953X/06/$ – see front matter

doi:10.1016/j.psc.2006.09.003

prevalence of major depression compared with those who have no sleep problems [5]. Additionally, the degree and duration of insomnia are associated with more severe or recurrent major depression [6,7]. In a survey of the general population, those who had insomnia at baseline and at 1-year follow-up had a relative risk of 39.8 for major depression compared with those who did not have insomnia [4].

The correlation between sleep and mood seems even higher in medical populations. In outpatients at general medical clinics, sleep and fatigue symptoms had the highest positive predictive value for major depression (61% and 69%, respectively) [9]. More than three quarters of patients who had insomnia evaluated in a multicenter study also met criteria for psychiatric disorders, including mood disorders [10]. The prevalence of major depression in patients who had insomnia in general medical (31%) [11] or sleep center clinics (32.3%) [10] was much higher than patients who did not have insomnia (4%).

Predictive Value and Specificity of Sleep Disturbance for Mood Disorders

Insomnia and hypersomnia also are associated with an increased risk for a new onset of major depressive or manic episodes [12,13]. Subjects reporting insomnia at an initial assessment were 2 to 5.4 times more likely than those who did not have insomnia to develop major depression during follow-up periods of 3.5 to 34 years [5,14]. Similarly, hypersomnia was associated with a relative risk of 2.9 for developing major depression [5]. Notably, two of these studies were longitudinal studies of young adults [5,14], demonstrating that insomnia at a young age confers a lifetime risk for developing mood disorders.

Insomnia and fatigue are the symptoms reported most frequently preceding a recurrent depressive episode [13,15]. In approximately half of new-onset or recurrent depressive episodes and in approximately three quarters of manic episodes, insomnia preceded the appearance of mood changes [12,16]. More ominously, an increase or decrease of 3 hours or more of sleep suggests imminent onset of a recurrent mood episode in patients diagnosed with bipolar disorder [17]. Moreover, major depression combined with insomnia confers an increased risk for suicide in adolescents [18,19] and adults [20,21].

Interepisodic Persistence of Subjective Sleep Disruption

Subjective reports of insomnia may improve, but not necessarily normalize, with remission from major depression [22]. Insomnia is the residual symptom reported most commonly in patients who have remitted major depression [23] and persists in patients who are euthymic and have bipolar affective disorder [24]. Persistence of sleep disturbances is shown predictive of increased severity and recurrence of major depression [25,26].

Other Comorbidities Associated with Sleep and Mood Disorders

The presence of sleep and mood disorders also is associated with an increased risk for other comorbid medical and psychiatric conditions. Abuse of and dependence on nicotine, alcohol, and other drugs seem more common when insomnia or hypersomnia is present. Adolescents who have sleep disturbance have an odds ratio (OR) of 1.5 to 3.8 for nicotine, alcohol, or other drug abuse, with higher OR for increased drug use. Adults who have insomnia also are more likely to develop nicotine or drug abuse or dependence during a follow-up period (OR 2.4 or 7.2) [5]. Additionally, hypersomnia conferred an even higher risk for nicotine, alcohol, or drug abuse (OR 2.3, 3.9, or 13.4) [5]. Some of these associations between sleep and substance use, however, may have been related to comorbid psychiatric disorders [27].

Conditions, such as obstructive sleep apnea (OSA) and restless legs syndrome (RLS), generally considered primary sleep disorders, also seem more prevalent in patients who have mood disorders than the general population [28–30]. This relationship is bidirectional, as approximately 18% of patients who had OSA also were diagnosed with major depression, and nearly 18% of patients who had major depression were diagnosed with OSA [28]. The relationship between major depression and RLS is complex but suggests that the presence of one diagnosis increases the risk for the other [30].

CLASSIFICATION OF MOOD AND DISORDERS

Mood disorders are among the most common categories of psychiatric diagnoses, second only to anxiety disorders [31], and are responsible for tremendous socioeconomic costs worldwide (including eventual suicide in 15% of persons who have major depression, increased morbidity and mortality from other illnesses, and economic impacts from associated disability [32]. Mood disorders are diagnosed based on the pattern of depressive or manic episodes. Major depressive or manic episodes are categorized as psychotic or nonpsychotic, based on the presence or absence of delusions and hallucinations. Major depression is subcategorized further based on common symptom clusters. Melancholic features may include an almost complete loss of interest in pleasurable activities, a failure to respond to normally pleasurable stimuli, a diurnal variation of mood (typically worse in the morning), and early-morning awakening (terminal insomnia). In contrast, patients who are depressed and have atypical features often retain mood reactivity to positive events, show significant weight gain, and have hypersomnia. Major depression with catatonic features is defined by significant psychomotor disturbance, ranging from catalepsy, stupor, and mutism to excessive, purposeless motor activity. Depression, in major depression and bipolar affective disorder, can show a seasonal pattern, with a typical onset in the fall or winter. Additionally, remission of depression or even (hypo)manias have a peak incidence in the spring.

SLEEP FINDINGS IN MOOD DISORDERS
Subjective Sleep Complaints
Some reports suggest that there is a discrepancy between subjective and objective sleep measurements in patients who have mood disorders. For example, in many patients who were depressed and who reported sleep complaints, no abnormalities were identified by polysomnographic (PSG) recordings [33,34].

Similarly, a recent study of adolescents who had major depression found subjective, but not objective, sleep disturbances [35]. Several studies have investigated the under- or overestimation of sleep parameters, including sleep-onset latency, number of awakenings, sleep depth, and total sleep time [36–41]. The study designs and results vary, however, and there is no clear consensus on the topic. Subjects who are depressed do not differ from controls in their self-report accuracy in some reports but substantially over- or under-estimate sleep parameters in others. Similarly, although less studied, objective measures of hypersomnia and daytime sleepiness often correlate poorly with subjective reports [37,42,43].

Insomnia, like major depression, is a clinical diagnosis based on patients' reported symptoms. Nevertheless, general trends suggest that in patients who have major depression, increased stage 1 sleep correlates with subjective reports of poor sleep quality, and with treatment, increased amounts of slow wave sleep (SWS) (stages 3 and 4) correlate with reports of deeper or more satisfying sleep [36,44]. This objective and subjective decrease in SWS is reflected consistently in the PSG recordings of patients who have major depression [45]. Correspondingly, in an 8-week treatment response study of patients who had major depression, increases in SWS correlated with subjective scores of sleep depth and satisfaction [36].

Objective measures from PSG recordings may be better biologic markers, but based on epidemiologic studies discussed previously, subjective measures do seem to have a value in the clinical assessment and treatment of major depression and may be a better indication of predicting onset and measuring initial treatment response. This is relevant particularly as reports of insomnia improve, but do not normalize, with remission of depression [22]. Ideally, however, subjective and objective measures are used because they relate to different clinical aspects of sleep and mood.

Polysomnographic and Architectural Sleep Changes

Sleep electroencephalogram (EEG) changes have been studied extensively as biologic markers of major depression since the late 1960s. Most patients who have major depression have some objective findings of sleep disturbance [45], but these findings not always are specific for depression and can vary with age and other factors.

Sleep architecture abnormalities in major depression can be grouped into three general categories (summarized in Table 1) [46]:

1. Sleep continuity disturbances. Patients who have major depression often show prolonged sleep-onset latency (time from lights out to first appearance of sleep), increased number and duration of waking periods during sleep, and early morning awakening. These disturbances are reflected by increased sleep fragmentation and decreased sleep efficiency.
2. SWS deficits. Stages 3 and 4 of nonrapid eye movement (NREM) sleep are considered SWS, colloquially referred to as deep sleep, because arousal threshold is high in this state. Patients who are depressed often have

Table 1
Sleep abnormalities in depression (and mania)

Subjective complaints	Polysomnographic findings
Insomnia	Sleep continuity disturbances
Difficulty falling asleep (initial insomnia)	Prolonged sleep-onset latency
Increased awakening at night/restless	Increased wake time during sleep
sleep (middle insomnia)	Increased early morning wake time
Early morning awakening (terminal	Decreased total sleep time
insomnia)	SWS deficits
Decreased amounts of sleep	Decreased SWS amount
Sleep less "deep" or less satisfying	Decreased SWS percentage of total sleep
Disturbing dreams	REM sleep abnormalities
	Reduced REM sleep latency
	Prolonged first REM sleep period
	Increased REM activity (total number of
	eye movements during the night)
	Increased REM density (REM activity/total
	REM sleep time)
	Increased REM sleep percentage of total
	sleep

a reduction of SWS, as the percentage of total sleep and as actual minutes of SWS. Furthermore, an abnormal temporal distribution of sleep is identified in some studies of this population. Subjects who are healthy have a peak in SWS time during the first sleep cycle, with a gradual decline through subsequent cycles. Subjects who are depressed often have less SWS during the first cycle and a relative peak during the second cycle [47]. Recently, computerized analysis has led to further descriptions of these patterns (discussed later).

3. Rapid eye movement (REM) sleep abnormalities. Changes in REM sleep parameters long have been believed the most consistent and relatively specific sleep abnormalities in major depression [45,46]. Decreased time to the onset of REM sleep (ie, reduced REM sleep latency) is the sleep finding reported and studied most commonly in major depression. Other abnormalities include a prolonged first REM sleep period, increased rapid eye movements during REM sleep periods (increased REM density), and increased percentage of REM sleep.

Similar findings also are documented in patients who had bipolar disorder with depression or mania, although these populations are studied far less. During manic episodes, disrupted sleep continuity, shortened REM sleep latency, and increased REM density were reported in PSG studies [48–50]. Patients who had bipolar depression and hypersomnia did not consistently have decreased REM sleep latency and also did not show decreased sleep latency despite complaints of daytime sleepiness, although these results are from a single study [51].

As with bipolar disorder, few studies have investigated sleep patterns in dysthymia, and the results are variable. Some studies lacked control or comparison groups with major depression, limiting the comparability of this small pool of studies. In these studies in general, however, there is some suggestion that patients who have dysthymia may have some of the sleep findings characteristic of major depression but not to the same extent [52]. Similarly, in a study of patients who showed some symptoms of depression but did not meet criteria for major depressive disorder, significant sleep EEG abnormalities were not observed [53]. Although the EEG changes described previously occur frequently in depression, they are not specific to depression. Some studies also found similar changes in REM sleep or SWS in schizophrenia and anxiety disorders [45].

Attempts have been made to correlate PSG findings in major depression with specific symptoms, symptom severity, or course of illness. Giles and colleagues show that terminal insomnia, decreased appetite, anhedonia, and decreased mood reactivity are associated more strongly with reduced REM sleep latency [54]. Another multivariate analysis identified 15 core depressive symptoms that correlate with nine sleep variables, suggesting a biologic relationship between core mood and sleep findings [2]. Some sleep changes, including increased REM density and reduced sleep efficiency, seem more correlated with illness severity and seem to normalize with remission from depression [55]. Reduced REM sleep latency and decreased SWS can persist, however, for long periods of time, even when patients are asymptomatic [55,56]. These results lend support to the hypothesis that sleep findings may reflect the "state" (current level of symptoms) and "trait" (biologic disposition) of major depression. The severity of these persistent findings may reflect a more pronounced biologic subtype of illness [57] and an increased risk for recurrence. The hypothesis that REM sleep latency is a trait marker for major depression also is supported by evidence from family studies; first-degree relatives of patients who have major depression tend to have shortened REM sleep latency, whether or not they have a personal history of depression [58,59].

EEG sleep variables in depression also are affected by gender and age. Studies show that loss of SWS in major depression is more prominent in men than women, both adults [60,61] and adolescents [62]. This may suggest differing biologic effects of depression between women and men, perhaps related in part to endocrine or developmental differences.

Age effects also may interact with depression-related changes in sleep. Some studies show clear differences between older adults (up to the seventh decade of life) who have major depression and age-matched controls [61]. Another study suggests that no differences in SWS were identified between depressed and control subjects until the middle of the fourth decade of life, and these differences remained until the seventh decade [63].

In contrast to adults, younger patients who have major depression often are indistinguishable from age-matched controls [64,65]. Amount of SWS is greatest in children and adolescents, and it decreases to adult amounts by the end of puberty. This shift likely is related to synaptic pruning and maturation of the prefrontal cortex. The maturation of endocrine systems (including the hypothalamic-pituitary-adrenal [HPA] axis) is involved in this process and also is changing dynamically during this time [46,64,65]. Overall, sleep changes associated with mood disorders are characterized best and identified most easily in adult subjects, particularly compared with children and adolescents. The relationships between gender, age, major depression, and sleep, however, are not yet elucidated fully.

Advanced Sleep Electroencephalogram Analysis

Recent advances in EEG recording, including digital recording and increased availability of powerful computational analyses, have provided new tools to study sleep in relation to mood disorders. Techniques include quantitative analysis of EEG activity across a broad range of frequencies (power spectral analysis); the automated detection and investigation of specific EEG waveforms, such as slow waves, spindles, and REMs; and measures of EEG synchronization across brain regions (synchrony and coherence). The use of high-density (hd) EEG, with the application of 60 or more recording electrodes to the scalp, also has facilitated topographic analysis of sleep-related waveforms, allowing for identification of the brain regions involved in their generation.

Power Spectral Analysis

Analysis of the EEG power spectra (also known as power density) allows quantification of EEG activity changes during sleep in different frequency ranges. Power spectra for individual subjects are extremely consistent between nights [66] and show characteristic changes when comparing patient and control groups. An advantage of power spectral analysis over traditional sleep scoring is that activity can be quantified over sleep cycles or whole nights independent of staging. Because sleep EEG waveforms, such as slow waves, are not restricted to single stages (slow waves are present in stage 2 and in SWS), power spectral analysis within this frequency band (the delta frequency band, 0.5–4.5 Hz) allows a more complete assessment of slow wave activity (SWA or delta band EEG power). Total minutes of SWS for the night are decreased in most studies of patients who are depressed [45]. Borbely and colleagues [67] used power spectral analysis to characterize SWA in control subjects and subjects who were depressed, confirming that SWS reductions in major depression are correlated with decrements in SWA and validating the use of EEG power spectra to quantify SWS. A similar study of bipolar depression did not identify SWA differences and speculates it could be the result of differences between the biologic basis of uni- and bipolar depression [68]. Kupfer and colleagues extended their findings to demonstrate that delta band power is a stable finding between acute depression and remission and more likely is a trait marker of major depression [69]. Additionally, SWA was predictive of response to antidepressant treatments. Depressed subjects who responded to antidepressant medication had a higher relative amount of SWA compared to nonresponders [70]. Furthermore, subjects who had major depression and who had an acute increase of SWA over the whole night after antidepressant administration were more likely to respond to subsequent treatment [71]. In contrast, Buysse and colleagues did not identify differences in SWA between responders or non-responders to interpersonal psychotherapy (IPT) [72]. They speculated that the severity of depression, gender, and responsiveness to psychotherapy in their subjects could account for the difference. Also, these differences across studies highlight a difficulty inherent in psychiatric research: illnesses based on patient and clinician descriptions may reflect a diverse spectrum of biologic illness. In contrast, they also reflect the importance of objective measures, such as sleep EEG findings, that might identify biologic subtypes of illness and could be important in selecting study populations.

The majority of studies of sleep and major depression using power spectral analysis has focused on differences in the delta frequency range because of its relationship to slow waves. A few studies have identified differences in other frequency ranges, however, including an increase in 12- to 20-Hz power [71] between patients in remission compared the same subjects when acutely depressed and increases from 20 to 35 Hz (beta2) and 35 to 45 Hz (gamma) ranges in subjects who were depressed compared with controls [67,69,73]. The significance of these findings is not as clear because they do not correlate with predominant sleep waveforms; however, these investigators speculate that higher frequency EEG activity could reflect changes in overall levels of arousal or integrative processing associated with the depressive state.

Automated Slow Wave Analysis

The technique of computerized slow wave counts using automated algorithms also has advanced slow wave analysis. This technology has allowed for more sensitive detection of slow waves and a more quantifiable measure of slow waves than from sleep staging alone [46].

In addition to a reduction of total minutes of SWS, an altered distribution of SWS during the night is shown in subjects who have major depression [74]. Minutes of SWS generally are greatest in the first NREM sleep period and decrease linearly through subsequent periods. Many subjects who are depressed show increased or equal minutes of SWS in the second compared with the first period. This difference is defined more clearly by automated slow wave counts. Kupfer and colleagues defined the delta sleep ratio as the ratio of the average slow (delta) wave counts per minute in the first NREM sleep period to the average counts per minute in the second NREM sleep period [75]. In control subjects, this ratio (typically >1.6) reflects the higher density of slow waves in the first NREM sleep period. Subjects who are depressed typically have a lower ratio (≤1.1), reflecting this abnormal distribution. The delta sleep ratio is believed to reflect an abnormal homeostatic regulation of sleep in depression (deficient Process S) [76].

With prolonged wakefulness, there is an increase in SWS at the beginning of the night and delay in REM sleep onset, reflecting a homeostatic increase in SWS during the first NREM sleep period. In major depression, REM sleep onset is earlier, and there is less SWS during the first NREM sleep period, the opposite of the normal homeostatic pattern. One article suggests that a higher ratio of SWA in the first to second NREM sleep periods (delta sleep EEG power, not slow wave counts) predicts a more robust antidepressant response effect of sleep deprivation [77]. The delta sleep ratio, as with other SWA markers, is shown to predict treatment response and likelihood of recurrence [55,56,75]. Although reduced SWA in the first NREM sleep period also is found in subjects who have schizophrenia, only subjects who have depression showed a reduced delta sleep ratio, suggesting this measure may be more specific for major depression [78,79].

Coherence of Sleep Electroencephalogram Rhythms

Coherence is a measure of the similarity of EEG rhythms at different cortical locations and measures of EEG coherence are believed to reflect the functional relationships between different cortical regions. Functional cortical connections may be impaired in psychiatric disorders, including major depression. Both intra- and interhemispheric coherence are shown to be lower in subjects with major depression compared with controls [80–81]. Decreased coherence is identified primarily in the delta (0.5–4 Hz) and beta (16–32 Hz) frequency ranges, in adolescents and adults who have major depression [61,80–85]. Reduced coherence also seems to be present in offspring at risk for developing major depression [82,84] and correlates with risk for recurrence in children and adolescents who have major depression [81], suggesting it may be a biologic marker of illness. Most reports suggest that coherence changes are more prominent in girls and women who have major depression in contrast with reduced numbers of slow waves that tend to be more prominent in men [86]. Fewer studies have investigated coherence changes in adults who have major depression, and the relationship of coherence to age and other sleep measures, such as SWA, should be delineated further.

Topography of Sleep Electroencephalogram Activity

Sleep EEG patterns classically have been recorded from one or two central electrodes. EEG recordings from different scalp locations can vary significantly, however, and analyses of EEG patterns across the scalp can yield substantial additional information. The use of hd EEG (generally greater than 20–256 electrodes) has facilitated the description of normal sleep EEG topography and how it varies over the course of the night. Topographic patterns seem stable between nights, despite differences in sleep architecture [87–89]. Additionally, different frequency ranges have characteristic distributions of activity, likely related to different cortical sources of rhythm generation [88,89]. SWA, in particular, shows a characteristic frontal distribution, with an increased power density, but stable topography, after sleep deprivation, consistent with the homeostatic increase in SWS [76,87,89,90]. Despite the potential advantages of hd EEG, few studies have applied this technology to psychiatric populations. Given the convergence of imaging data demonstrating regional differences in brain activity (see previous and later sections summarizing this research) and the clear associations of altered SWS/SWA during depression, hd-EEG studies of sleep likely will yield important information to further the understanding of the common biologic bases of sleep and mood disorders.

BIOLOGIC MECHANISMS OF SLEEP CHANGES IN MOOD DISORDERS

The high coincidence and overlapping symptoms of major depression and insomnia suggest common neurobiology. Reflecting their common clinical presentations, many of the criteria in the recently published American Academy of Sleep Medicine research diagnostic criteria for insomnia [91] are shared with the *DSM-IV-TR* criteria for major depressive episodes (asterisked items) (Table 2). This raises the question as to which is the primary or secondary disorder or if they are manifestations of the same underlying process representing a spectrum disorder. Despite the prevalence and impact of mood disorders, the exact etiologies still are not understood fully. Similarly, there are many speculations about the mechanisms of sleep changes in mood disorders and correlations with other biologic abnormalities identified in depression. At a more fundamental level, the regulation of and biologic need for sleep still are defined incompletely (see article elsewhere in this issue). The close association of mood and sleep suggests that the neurobiology is intertwined closely; it is likely that advances in the understanding of either component will lead to a more complete explanation of the other. The following sections discuss some, but certainly not all, of the hypotheses explaining this association.

Neurotransmitters

The classic neurotransmitter hypothesis of mood regulation was based on the discovery that increases or decreases in monoaminergic neurotransmitters (such as serotonin, norepinephrine, and dopamine) correlated with improved or worsened depression, respectively. In fact, the majority of pharmaceutical

---

Table 2
Insomnia research diagnostic criteria

One or more
    *Difficulty initiating sleep
    *Difficulty maintaining sleep
    *Waking up too early
    *Nonrestorative sleep
Sleep difficulty occurs despite adequate opportunity for sleep
At least one of the following
    *Fatigue/malaise
    *Attention, concentration, or memory impairment
    Social/vocational dysfunction or poor school performance
    *Mood disturbance/irritability
    Daytime sleepiness
    *Motivation/energy/initiative reduction
    Proneness for errors/accidents
    Tension headaches or gastrointestinal symptoms
    Concerns or worries about sleep

Adapted from Edinger JD, Bonnet MH, Bootzin RR, et al. Derivation of research diagnostic criteria for insomnia: report of an American Academy of Sleep Medicine Work Group. Sleep 2004;27:1567–96.

agents (including tricyclic antidepressants (TCAs), monoamine oxidase inhibitors (MAOIs), and SRIs) used to treat depression primarily increase synaptic levels of these neurotransmitters. Conversely, the same medications can trigger manic episodes in susceptible individuals, suggesting that the other pole of the mood spectrum relates to excessive monoamine transmission. Recent evidence continues to support this hypothesis and has identified alterations in neurotransmitter levels, in activity of brain areas associated primarily with monoaminergic activity, and of candidate genes associated with serotonin levels and function [92].

Normal regulation of sleep also is tied closely to these systems–REM sleep requires a decrease in monoaminergic tone (including serotonin and norepinephrine) and increased cholinergic tone [93]. Most antidepressant medications increase serotonin and, correspondingly, increase REM sleep latency, decrease REM sleep amount, and increase SWS–reversing the typical architectural abnormalities of sleep in depression [94,95]. Although this is proposed as the primary mechanism for antidepressant effect, some antidepressants do not alter REM sleep or serotonin levels [95].

More recently, investigations have suggested roles for additional neurotransmitter systems in mood disorders. Amino acid neurotransmitters, such as glutamate acting via α-amino-3-hydroxy-5-methyl-4-isoxazolepropionic acid (AMPA) receptors signaling pathways, increasingly are found to play a role in depression [96–98]. Particularly relevant are the associations of glutamate signaling with plasticity (via increased brain-derived neurotrophic factor [BDNF] levels) and learning [99–101]. A decrease in neurotrophic factors, such as BDNF, related to depression could result in decreased neurogenesis, or even neural cell loss, in brain regions critical to mood regulation and responsiveness.

The glutamate system also is tied intimately to REM and NREM sleep regulation. Glutamate interacts with cholinergic neurons to increase activity of the reticular system associated with REM sleep onset. During NREM sleep, excitatory glutamate neurotransmission has a prominent role in the thalamocortical generation of sleep EEG oscillations [93]. Additionally, sleep increasingly is shown necessary for plastic processes, such as learning and memory, and affects the expression of plasticity-related genes [102]. The intertwined processes of mood, sleep, and plasticity, and their modulation through factors such as glutamate and BDNF, make them appealing targets for future therapies [99].

Evidence indicates that conventional serotonergic antidepressants indirectly may potentiate AMPA receptors, possibly relating to their efficacy [96]. The evidence for involvement of neuroplasticity and other signaling cascades perhaps explains the therapeutic lag between drug initiation and clinical effect. Similarly, overlapping signaling pathways that regulate cell death and survival may be long-term targets for mood stabilizers and antidepressants [100,101]. As one of such pathways, the glutamate system and downstream signaling cascades also may provide a therapeutic target for future generations of antidepressants [96,100].

Neuroimaging

A growing body of literature has started to identify the brain regions involved in regulation of sleep and how their activity is altered in mood disorders with sleep disturbances. Imaging studies are identifying brain areas involved in the sleep disturbances, such as reduced SWS and increased REM sleep, in patients who are depressed. During normal NREM sleep, compared with waking levels, metabolic activity is decreased broadly in the frontal, temporal, and parietal cortexes. Nofzinger and colleagues [103,104] demonstrate that subjects who have current major depression have a smaller decrease in these cortical regions from waking to sleep and a relative hypoactivity in waking. It is possible that the waking hypofrontality could reflect a deficit in a sleep-wake related process present in major depression, such as decreased synaptic potentiation (during waking) or decreased downscaling (during sleep) [90]. Other brain areas involved in emotional regulation (anterior cingulate cortex, amygdala, parahippocampal cortex, and thalamus) (reviewed in Ref. [105]) also had a smaller decline in metabolic level from waking to NREM sleep. Relative to control subjects, however, these areas have elevated metabolic levels during sleep. Altered function in these regions could relate to a failure of arousal mechanisms to decline from waking to sleep and changes in cognition, attention, and emotional regulation in depression [106]. In two studies on increased REM sleep (which correlates with depression severity and clinical outcomes), depressed subjects demonstrated increased metabolic activity during REM sleep in diffuse cortical and subcortical structures as compared to controls [107,108]. As there is a shift from predominantly monoaminergic activity during waking to cholinergic activity during REM sleep, these alterations also could reflect an imbalance of monoaminergic/cholinergic systems in altered mood states. A relative state of arousal with lower monoaminergic activity in depression could explain the increased REM sleep, decreased REM sleep latency, and decreased SWS.

Other imaging studies have focused on changes in brain activity in patients who are depressed after total sleep deprivation (TSD) or partial sleep deprivation (PSD), which results in an antidepressant response in approximately 50% of patients who have major depression (discussed later and reviewed in Refs. [109–111]). These studies suggest that there is a biologic subtype of depression with deficits that can be corrected by sleep deprivation, lending further support to the hypothesis that sleep and mood regulation are controlled by overlapping brain regions. Several studies show consistency with this hypothesis, in that sleep deprivation responders had increased metabolic activity in the amygdala, orbital prefrontal cortex, and inferior temporal and anterior cingulate before sleep deprivation that normalized afterwards [112–115]. Volk and colleagues demonstrate predeprivation perfusion levels correlating with the reduction of depressive symptoms [112]. Functional imaging studies with single photon emission CT suggest that sleep deprivation responders may have a particular deficit in monoaminergic systems involved with attention, arousal, and affect–particularly in dopaminergic and serotonergic systems [113,116].

Endocrine Changes

Neuroendocrine dysregulation, in particular overactivation of the HPA axis, also has been recognized as playing a key role in the genesis of mood disorders and potentially could lead to sleep disturbance (reviewed in Refs. [117,118]). Elevations of corticotropin releasing hormone (CRH) and cortisol are associated with major depression and could play a role in atrophy of hippocampal neurons, in turn reducing their inhibition of ACTH secretion, thus exacerbating the elevation of HPA activity.

Abnormalities of the HPA axis are found in almost half of patients who have major depression. The most common abnormality is hypercortisolemia, which classically has been assessed by the dexamethasone suppression test. Elevated levels of cortisol are also associated with stress and can lead to more fragmented sleep and hippocampal damage. Coincident with cortisol elevations, CRH is also secreted based on circadian rhythms and is elevated in patients who are depressed. Increased nocturnal CRH actually may be responsible for increased awakenings with HPA hyperactivity [119]. Supporting this hypothesis, administration of a CRH receptor antagonist was reported to improve sleep EEG patterns of patients who were depressed [120]. Growth hormone releasing hormone (GHRH) has a reciprocal relationship with CRH and promotes sleep. GHRH and growth hormone also may be decreased in some patients who have depression, contributing further to SWS decrements [118].

Genetic Polymorphisms

Genetic factors likely account for at least 33% of the risk for major depression and more than 85% of the risk for bipolar affective disorder [121,122]. Both of these disorders likely are polygenic, heterogeneous, and the result of a combination of genetic and environmental factors. Based on understanding of the neurobiology of these disorders, there are several candidate genes and possible associations of polymorphisms that could partially account for some cases of mood disorders. A handful of genes is implicated in mood disorders and sleep regulation.

Genes that regulate monoamine levels (in particular serotonin and norepinephrine) are particularly intriguing candidates, given the importance of these neurotransmitters in the response to most antidepressant medications. The gene for monoamine oxidase A (MAO-A) and the serotonin transporter gene linked polymorphic region (5-HTTLPR) are implicated in depression and suggested to correlate with insomnia scores (MAO-A) or treatment response to sleep deprivation (5-HTTLPR) [123,124].

There recently are reports that the angiotensin I–converting enzyme gene and mineralocorticoid receptor gene expression are altered in major depression and bipolar disorder, respectively [125,126]. Both genes are candidates to explain, at least partially, abnormalities of the HPA axis in mood and sleep disturbances.

Recent years have seen rapid advances in identifying clock genes involved in regulating circadian rhythms. No specific circadian genes are linked clearly to depression or bipolar disorder, but several of them are implicated and may help explain treatment responses and some aspects of these disorders. A recent report suggests a link between the genotype of the *CLOCK* gene and presence of insomnia in patients who are depressed [127]. Lithium, the prototypic pharmacologic mood stabilizer, is shown to inhibit glycogen synthase kinase 3 (GSK3), which also is a circadian regulator. The GSK3 gene is under intense scrutiny as a possible candidate gene for bipolar disorder, but several studies reveal only a moderate linkage in relatively small populations [128–130]. More importantly, the polymorphism in question is not shown to have an effect on gene expression or activity. Yin and colleagues recently demonstrated that lithium also affects stability of the Rev-erbα protein, which in turn regulates the activation of other clock genes [131]. This is an intriguing possible link between bipolar disorder and circadian genes, but an involvement in patients is not yet demonstrated.

Plasticity-related cascades are a developing area of investigation for identifying candidate genes and novel molecular targets for therapeutics (reviewed in Refs. [100,101]). These include genes involved in regulation of DNA replication, such as histone deacetylase, and others that are members of signal transduction cascades. Glutamate-AMPA receptor cascades are particularly interesting targets, and several experimental therapeutic agents affect this system [97,100]. Plasticity is linked closely to learning, sleep, and hormonal (cortisol) regulation. Supporting this connection, molecular investigations of the genes regulated by sleep and sleep deprivation identified a number of plasticity-related gene targets [102,132]; genes related to plasticity and synaptic potentiation tend to be expressed during wakefulness, and genes related to synaptic downscaling expressed during sleep [90]. It is feasible that sleep is required for the downscaling of synapses on a daily basis and that alterations in sleep or mood disorders could affect this normal process. Conversely, sleep deprivation could strengthen synapses in brain regions involved in affect regulation, potentially explaining some of the acute effects of sleep deprivation therapy.

Although anatomic, neurochemical, neuroendocrine, and genetic evidence seems to be converging, it remains unknown which abnormalities are responsible for initiating mood disorders and sleep disturbance. Nevertheless, approaches to identifying gene linkages and molecular targets potentially involved in illness will continue to be critical for understanding and treating the overlapping disturbances of mood and sleep.

TREATMENT OF SLEEP DISTURBANCE AND MOOD DISORDERS
Pharmacologic Treatments

Because of the high comorbidity of mood disorders and insomnia (or hypersomnia) (discussed previously), patients presenting with complaints of one must be assessed for the other. Specific treatment modalities for insomnia are discussed in articles elsewhere in this issue; however, a few specific topics regarding mood disorders deserve attention.

Almost all of the available antidepressant medications, including TCAs, MAOIs, trazodone and nefazodone, SRIs or serotonin-norepinephrine reuptake inhibitors, bupropion, and mirtazapine can exacerbate insomnia or hypersomnia, impair or improve sleep quality, and affect EEG measures of sleep architecture [94,133]. Exacerbation of insomnia or a further decrement in sleep quality could lead to additional sleep loss or worsened depression and could contribute to medication noncompliance. Increased hypersomnia, similarly, could impair the ability of patients further to carry out daily activities. Alternatively, although not Food and Drug Administration (FDA) approved specifically for this purpose, sedating medications, such as TCAs, trazodone, and mirtazapine, sometimes are used to treat insomnia associated with depression. Stimulants often are used as an adjunctive, but not FDA-approved, treatment for depression, and have a well-known association with decreased sleep and insomnia. It is critical to monitor insomnia and hypersomnia when treating depression. Even in patients who are "adequately treated" and are in remission from mood symptoms, sleep disturbance is the most common residual symptom [134]. As discussed previously, insomnia is a strong predictor for recurrent episodes of depression. Whether or not treatment of residual insomnia will prevent recurrence, however, is not clear.

The use of the antidepressant trazodone deserves particular mention, as it is one of the most prescribed agents to improve sleep. Trazodone is not FDA approved for treating insomnia, but it is used far more frequently for sleep than as an antidepressant. Despite its prevalent use, few objective data on its effect on sleep are available, although some studies suggest it may improve insomnia in depression [135]. The doses used for insomnia are far below the therapeutic dose for depression and likely provide little benefit for depressed mood.

Just as the standard of care for treating a mood disorder with psychotic features requires specific interventions for mood and psychosis, treatment of mood disorder with sleep disturbance should address both aspects of illness. A recent study suggests that coadministration of a GABA-A hypnotic (eszopiclone) with an SRI could lead to a more rapid and robust improvement in depression [136]. Other studies show that adding zolpidem or lorazepam does not slow antidepressant response or cause adverse drug interactions and can improve symptoms of insomnia [137–139]. Second-generation antipsychotics, including risperidone, olanzapine, and clozapine, have been studied for effects on sleep in depression [140–143]. These studies, although with only small numbers (n = 8–15) of subjects, suggest that antipsychotics may improve sleep measures and could be useful adjunctive treatments to SRIs in treatment-resistant depression (risperidone or olanzapine) [140–142] or in the treatment of bipolar disorder (clozapine) [143]. In addition to pharmacologic interventions, increasing evidence supports the efficacy of cognitive behavioral therapy for insomnia for improvement of sleep associated with mood disorders [144].

At the other end of the spectrum, treatment of (seasonal or atypical) depression with fatigue or hypersomnia can be improved with the addition of modafinil [145–151]. In these studies, antidepressant response seemed to have a more rapid onset, and there was a clear improvement in fatigue.

Sleep Deprivation Therapy

One of the most rapid, but perhaps least frequently used, treatments for depression is sleep deprivation. TSD, preventing any sleep during the night, can reduce depressive symptoms (a 50% reduction of Hamilton Depression Rating Scale scores) within hours in 30% to 60% of patients who have major depression [152]. PSD, particularly during the latter part of the night, is shown in some studies to provide a similar improvement and is easier to implement. The effect of TSD or PSD often is short-lived, and a relapse of symptoms may occur after even short periods of sleep in at least 50% to 80% of responders. Sleep deprivation is combined with other treatment modalities (including medications, sleep phase advance, light therapy, and transcranial magnetic stimulation) as an attempt to combine the rapid response with sustained improvements from other modalities.

The response to sleep deprivation provides another clear link between the neurobiology of mood disorders and sleep regulation. Although neither TSD nor PSD has become a widely used therapy, both provide opportunities to simultaneously investigate rapidly occurring changes in mood and other biologic variables [109,153,154]. The antidepressant response to sleep deprivation is correlated with other biologic markers in sleep EEG [77], imaging [112–116], and genetic [123] studies (discussed previously). Additionally, response to sleep deprivation may serve as a biologic marker of a major depression subtype and the basis for designing novel antidepressants.

Sleep Loss and Bipolar Disorder

Sleep loss has long been recognized as a trigger for manic episodes in patients who have bipolar disorder [17,155–158]. Although it can be difficult to separate insomnia's possible role as a prodromal symptom of mania, studies have used various designs to demonstrate that sleep loss may be a risk factor for mania, independent of prodromal mood symptoms. Additionally, laboratory-based experiments suggest that sleep loss induced by forced wakefulness, medication, or other factors can trigger mania in the absence of other changes [156–159]. Sleep loss also is associated, although not as strongly, with bipolar depression [15,17,155]. Sleep loss in bipolar patients often is followed by the onset of mood episodes in the following 24-hour period, and the magnitude of sleep change seems to correlate with the likelihood of a subsequent mood change [17,155]. These findings stress the importance of closely monitoring sleep patterns in patients who have bipolar disorder and aggressively treating the first signs of sleep loss and insomnia.

Clinical Use of Polysomnography

Despite the numerous EEG abnormalities of sleep associated with mood disorders, none currently is considered specific or sensitive enough to warrant the use of routine PSG recordings in the diagnosis of mood disorders. Recent reports suggest, however, that the incidence of OSA is higher in a cohort of subjects who have major depression, and mood disorders are more common in patients who have OSA than in controls [28,29]. Combined with the increasing prevalence of obesity and other risk factors in the general population, assessing and treating OSA is becoming increasingly important in the psychiatric setting. Additionally, psychiatrists need to be vigilant for iatrogenic sleep disorders caused or exacerbated by psychopharmacologic agents. Weight gain associated with antipsychotics, mood stabilizers, and antidepressants can contribute to OSA. Additionally, serotonergic antidepressants can induce or worsen several primary sleep disorders, such as RLS, periodic leg movements, and REM sleep behavior disorder [159,160].

Summary and Future Directions
Because of the close association between mood and sleep disorders, it is critical to assess all patients who have sleep complaints for mood disorders and vice versa. The presence of sleep disturbance alone also is strongly predictive of on-set of mood problems in the future. Simultaneous treatment of insomnia and major depression often is helpful, as insomnia is the most frequent residual symptom and its persistence is an important predictor of future illness.

Ongoing studies of the relationship between sleep disturbances and mood disorders should provide a better understanding of their neurobiologic under-pinnings—and more importantly for those suffering from these conditions, safer and more effective treatments. As with many other examples in medicine, an understanding of the disorder hopefully will lead to an understanding of nor-mal sleep and mood.

References
[1] American Psyciatric Association. Diagnostic and statistical manual of mental disorders. 4th ed., text revision. Washington (DC): American Psychiatric Association; 2000.
[2] Perlis ML, Giles DE, Buysse DJ, et al. Which depressive symptoms are related to which sleep electroencephalographic variables? Biol Psychiatry 1997;42:904–13.
[3] Detre T, Himmelhoch J, Swartzburg M, et al. Hypersomnia and manic-depressive disease. Am J Psychiatry 1972;128:1303–5.
[4] Ford DE, Kamerow DB. Epidemiologic study of sleep disturbances and psychiatric disor-ders. An opportunity for prevention? JAMA 1989;262:1479–84.
[5] Breslau N, Roth T, Rosenthal L, et al. Sleep disturbance and psychiatric disorders: a longi-tudinal epidemiological study of young adults. Biol Psychiatry 1996;39:411–8.
[6] Taylor DJ, Lichstein KL, Durrence HH, et al. Epidemiology of insomnia, depression, and anx-iety. Sleep 2005;28:1457–64.
[7] Kaneita Y, Ohida T, Uchiyama M, et al. The relationship between depression and sleep dis-turbances: a Japanese nationwide general population survey. J Clin Psychiatry 2006;67:196–203.
[8] Ohayon MM, Hong SC. Prevalence of major depressive disorder in the general population of South Korea. J Psychiatr Res 2006;40:30–6.
[9] Gerber PD, Barrett JE, Barrett JA, et al. The relationship of presenting physical complaints to depressive symptoms in primary care patients. J Gen Intern Med 1992;7:170–3.
[10] Buysse DJ, Reynolds CF 3rd, Kupfer DJ, et al. Clinical diagnoses in 216 insomnia patients using the International Classification of Sleep Disorders (ICSD), DSM-IV and ICD-10 cate-gories: a report from the APA/NIMH DSM-IV field trial. Sleep 1994;17:630–7.
[11] Simon GE, VonKorff M. Prevalence, burden, and treatment of insomnia in primary care. Am J Psychiatry 1997;154:1417–23.
[12] Jackson A, Cavanagh J, Scott J. A systematic review of manic and depressive prodromes. J Affect Disord 2003;74:209–17.

[13] Perlis ML, Giles DE, Buysse DJ, et al. Self-reported sleep disturbance as a prodromal symptom in recurrent depression. J Affect Disord 1997;42:209–12.

[14] Chang PP, Ford DE, Mead LA, et al. Insomnia in young men and subsequent depression. The Johns Hopkins Precursors Study. Am J Epidemiol 1997;146:105–14.

[15] Perlman CA, Johnson SL, Mellman TA. The prospective impact of sleep duration on depression and mania. Bipolar Disord 2006;8:271–4.

[16] Ohayon MM, Roth T. Place of chronic insomnia in the course of depressive and anxiety disorders. J Psychiatr Res 2003;37:9–15.

[17] Bauer M, Grof P, Rasgon N, et al. Temporal relation between sleep and mood in patients with bipolar disorder. Bipolar Disord 2006;8:160–7.

[18] Liu X. Sleep and adolescent suicidal behavior. Sleep 2004;27:1351–8.

[19] Barbe RP, Williamson DE, Bridge JA, et al. Clinical differences between suicidal and non-suicidal depressed children and adolescents. J Clin Psychiatry 2005;66:492–8.

[20] Agargun MY, Beisoglu L. Sleep and suicidality: do sleep disturbances predict suicide risk? Sleep 2005;28:1039–40.

[21] Hall RC, Platt DE, Hall RC. Suicide risk assessment: a review of risk factors for suicide in 100 patients who made severe suicide attempts. Evaluation of suicide risk in a time of managed care. Psychosomatics 1999;40:18–27.

[22] Reynolds CF 3rd, Hoch CC, Buysse DJ, et al. Sleep in late-life recurrent depression. Changes during early continuation therapy with nortriptyline. Neuropsychopharmacology 1991;5:85–96.

[23] Nierenberg AA. Do some antidepressants work faster than others? J Clin Psychiatry 2001;62(Suppl 15):22–5.

[24] Harvey AG, Schmidt DA, Scarna A, et al. Sleep-related functioning in euthymic patients with bipolar disorder, patients with insomnia, and subjects without sleep problems. Am J Psychiatry 2005;162:50–7.

[25] Dew MA, Reynolds CF 3rd, Houck PR, et al. Temporal profiles of the course of depression during treatment. Predictors of pathways toward recovery in the elderly. Arch Gen Psychiatry 1997;54:1016–24.

[26] Reynolds CF 3rd, Frank E, Houck PR, et al. Which elderly patients with remitted depression remain well with continued interpersonal psychotherapy after discontinuation of antidepressant medication? Am J Psychiatry 1997;154:958–62.

[27] Johnson EO, Breslau N. Sleep problems and substance use in adolescence. Drug Alcohol Depend 2001;64:1–7.

[28] Ohayon MM. The effects of breathing-related sleep disorders on mood disturbances in the general population. J Clin Psychiatry 2003;64:1195–200 [quiz: 1274–96].

[29] Sharafkhaneh A, Giray N, Richardson P, et al. Association of psychiatric disorders and sleep apnea in a large cohort. Sleep 2005;28:1405–11.

[30] Picchietti D, Winkelman JW. Restless legs syndrome, periodic limb movements in sleep, and depression. Sleep 2005;28:891–8.

[31] Kessler RC, Berglund P, Demler O, et al. Lifetime prevalence and age-of-onset distributions of DSM-IV disorders in the National Comorbidity Survey Replication. Arch Gen Psychiatry 2005;62:593–602.

[32] World Health Organization. Health Topics: Depression. Available at: http://www.who.int/topics/depression/en/. Accessed October 6, 2006.

[33] Reynolds CF 3rd, Kupfer DJ. Sleep research in affective illness: state of the art circa 1987. Sleep 1987;10:199–215.

[34] Feinberg M, Carroll BJ, Greden JF, et al. Sleep EEG, depression rating scales, and diagnosis. Biol Psychiatry 1982;17:1453–8.

[35] Bertocci MA, Dahl RE, Williamson DE, et al. Subjective sleep complaints in pediatric depression: a controlled study and comparison with EEG measures of sleep and waking. J Am Acad Child Adolesc Psychiatry 2005;44:1158–66.

[36] Argyropoulos SV, Hicks JA, Nash JR, et al. Correlation of subjective and objective sleep measurements at different stages of the treatment of depression. Psychiatry Res 2003;120:179–90.

[37] Matousek M, Cervena K, Zavesicka L, et al. Subjective and objective evaluation of alertness and sleep quality in depressed patients. BMC Psychiatry 2004;4:14.

[38] Mayers AG, van Hooff JC, Baldwin DS. Quantifying subjective assessment of sleep and life-quality in antidepressant-treated depressed patients. Hum Psychopharmacol 2003; 18:21–7.

[39] Rotenberg VS, Indursky P, Kayumov L, et al. The relationship between subjective sleep estimation and objective sleep variables in depressed patients. Int J Psychophysiol 2000;37: 291–7.

[40] Armitage R, Trivedi M, Hoffmann R, et al. Relationship between objective and subjective sleep measures in depressed patients and healthy controls. Depress Anxiety 1997;5: 97–102.

[41] Lee JH, Reynolds CF 3rd, Hoch CC, et al. Electroencephalographic sleep in recently remitted, elderly depressed patients in double-blind placebo-maintenance therapy. Neuropsychopharmacology 1993;8:143–50.

[42] Billiard M, Dolenc L, Aldaz C, et al. Hypersomnia associated with mood disorders: a new perspective. J Psychosom Res 1994;38(Suppl 1):41–7.

[43] Reynolds CF 3rd, Coble PA, Kupfer DJ, et al. Application of the multiple sleep latency test in disorders of excessive sleepiness. Electroencephalogr Clin Neurophysiol 1982;53: 443–52.

[44] Tsuchiyama K, Nagayama H, Kudo K, et al. Discrepancy between subjective and objective sleep in patients with depression. Psychiatry Clin Neurosci 2003;57:259–64.

[45] Benca RM, Obermeyer WH, Thisted RA, et al. Sleep and psychiatric disorders. A meta-analysis. Arch Gen Psychiatry 1992;49:651–68 [discussion: 669–70].

[46] Kupfer DJ. Sleep research in depressive illness: clinical implications—a tasting menu. Biol Psychiatry 1995;38:391–403.

[47] Kupfer DJ, Reynolds CF 3rd, Ulrich RF, et al. Comparison of automated REM and slow-wave sleep analysis in young and middle-aged depressed subjects. Biol Psychiatry 1986;21: 189–200.

[48] Knowles J, Waldron J, et al. Sleep preceding the onset of a manic episode. Biol Psychiatry 1979;14:671–5.

[49] Hudson JI, Lipinski JF, Keck PE Jr, et al. Polysomnographic characteristics of young manic patients. Comparison with unipolar depressed patients and normal control subjects. Arch Gen Psychiatry 1992;49:378–83.

[50] Hudson JI, Lipinski JF, Frankenburg FR, et al. Electroencephalographic sleep in mania. Arch Gen Psychiatry 1988;45:267–73.

[51] Nofzinger EA, Thase ME, Reynolds CF 3rd, et al. Hypersomnia in bipolar depression: a comparison with narcolepsy using the multiple sleep latency test. Am J Psychiatry 1991;148:1177–81.

[52] Howland RH, Thase ME. Biological studies of dysthymia. Biol Psychiatry 1991;30: 283–304.

[53] Cohen DB. Dysphoric affect and REM sleep. J Abnorm Psychol 1979;88:73–7.

[54] Giles DE, Roffwarg HP, Schlesser MA, et al. Which endogenous depressive symptoms relate to REM latency reduction? Biol Psychiatry 1986;21:473–82.

[55] Thase ME, Fasiczka AL, Berman SR, et al. Electroencephalographic sleep profiles before and after cognitive behavior therapy of depression. Arch Gen Psychiatry 1998;55: 138–44.

[56] Jindal RD, Thase ME, Fasiczka AL, et al. Electroencephalographic sleep profiles in single-episode and recurrent unipolar forms of major depression: II. Comparison during remission. Biol Psychiatry 2002;51:230–6.

[57] Thase ME, Buysse DJ, Frank E, et al. Which depressed patients will respond to interpersonal psychotherapy? The role of abnormal EEG sleep profiles. Am J Psychiatry 1997;154:502–9.

[58] Lauer CJ, Schreiber W, Holsboer F, et al. In quest of identifying vulnerability markers for psychiatric disorders by all-night polysomnography. Arch Gen Psychiatry 1995;52:145–53.

[59] Giles DE, Kupfer DJ, Rush AJ, et al. Controlled comparison of electrophysiological sleep in families of probands with unipolar depression. Am J Psychiatry 1998;155:192–9.

[60] Reynolds CF 3rd, Kupfer DJ, Thase ME, et al. Sleep, gender, and depression: an analysis of gender effects on the electroencephalographic sleep of 302 depressed outpatients. Biol Psychiatry 1990;28:673–84.

[61] Armitage R, Hoffmann R, Trivedi M, et al. Slow-wave activity in NREM sleep: sex and age effects in depressed outpatients and healthy controls. Psychiatry Res 2000;95:201–13.

[62] Robert JJ, Hoffmann RF, Emslie GJ, et al. Sex and age differences in sleep macroarchitecture in childhood and adolescent depression. Sleep 2006;29:351–8.

[63] Lauer CJ, Riemann D, Wiegand M, et al. From early to late adulthood. Changes in EEG sleep of depressed patients and healthy volunteers. Biol Psychiatry 1991;29:979–93.

[64] Ivanenko A, Crabtree VM, Gozal D. Sleep and depression in children and adolescents. Sleep Med Rev 2005;9:115–29.

[65] Dahl RE. The development and disorders of sleep. Adv Pediatr 1998;45:73–90.

[66] Buckelmuller J, Landolt HP, Stassen HH, et al. Trait-like individual differences in the human sleep electroencephalogram. Neuroscience 2006;138:351–6.

[67] Borbely AA, Tobler I, Loepfe M, et al. All-night spectral analysis of the sleep EEG in untreated depressives and normal controls. Psychiatry Res 1984;12:27–33.

[68] Mendelson WB, Sack DA, James SP, et al. Frequency analysis of the sleep EEG in depression. Psychiatry Res 1987;21:89–94.

[69] Kupfer DJ, Ehlers CL, Frank E, et al. Electroencephalographic sleep studies in depressed patients during long-term recovery. Psychiatry Res 1993;49:121–38.

[70] Luthringer R, Minot R, Toussaint M, et al. All-night EEG spectral analysis as a tool for the prediction of clinical response to antidepressant treatment. Biol Psychiatry 1995;38:98–104.

[71] Kupfer DJ, Ehlers CL, Pollock BG, et al. Clomipramine and EEG sleep in depression. Psychiatry Res 1989;30:165–80.

[72] Buysse DJ, Hall M, Begley A, et al. Sleep and treatment response in depression: new findings using power spectral analysis. Psychiatry Res 2001;103:51–67.

[73] Tekell JL, Hoffmann R, Hendrickse W, et al. High frequency EEG activity during sleep: characteristics in schizophrenia and depression. Clin EEG Neurosci 2005;36:25–35.

[74] Borbely AA, Wirz-Justice A. Sleep, sleep deprivation and depression. A hypothesis derived from a model of sleep regulation. Hum Neurobiol 1982;1:205–10.

[75] Kupfer DJ, Frank E, McEachran AB, et al. Delta sleep ratio. A biological correlate of early recurrence in unipolar affective disorder. Arch Gen Psychiatry 1990;47:1100–5.

[76] Borbely AA. The S-deficiency hypothesis of depression and the two-process model of sleep regulation. Pharmacopsychiatry 1987;20:23–9.

[77] Nissen C, Feige B, Konig A, et al. Delta sleep ratio as a predictor of sleep deprivation response in major depression. J Psychiatr Res 2001;35:155–63.

[78] Hoffmann R, Hendrickse W, Rush AJ, et al. Slow-wave activity during non-REM sleep in men with schizophrenia and major depressive disorders. Psychiatry Res 2000;95:215–25.

[79] Ganguli R, Reynolds CF 3rd, Kupfer DJ. Electroencephalographic sleep in young, never-medicated schizophrenics. A comparison with delusional and nondelusional depressives and with healthy controls. Arch Gen Psychiatry 1987;44:36–44.

[80] Armitage R, Roffwarg HP, Rush AJ. Digital period analysis of EEG in depression: periodicity, coherence, and interhemispheric relationships during sleep. Prog Neuropsychopharmacol Biol Psychiatry 1993;17:363–72.

[81] Armitage R, Hoffmann RF, Emslie GJ, et al. Sleep microarchitecture as a predictor of recurrence in children and adolescents with depression. Int J Neuropsychopharmacol 2002;5: 217–28.

[82] Morehouse RL, Kusumakar V, Kutcher SP, et al. Temporal coherence in ultradian sleep EEG rhythms in a never-depressed, high-risk cohort of female adolescents. Biol Psychiatry 2002;51:446–56.

[83] Armitage R, Hoffmann R, Emslie G, et al. Sleep microarchitecture in childhood and adolescent depression: temporal coherence. Clin EEG Neurosci 2006;37:1–9.

[84] Fulton MK, Armitage R, Rush AJ. Sleep electroencephalographic coherence abnormalities in individuals at high risk for depression: a pilot study. Biol Psychiatry 2000;47: 618–25.

[85] Armitage R, Hoffmann RF, Rush AJ. Biological rhythm disturbance in depression: temporal coherence of ultradian sleep EEG rhythms. Psychol Med 1999;29:1435–48.

[86] Armitage R, Hoffmann RF. Sleep EEG, depression and gender. Sleep Med Rev 2001;5: 237–46.

[87] De Gennaro L, Ferrara M, Vecchio F, et al. An electroencephalographic fingerprint of human sleep. Neuroimage 2005;26:114–22.

[88] Finelli LA, Borbely AA, Achermann P. Functional topography of the human nonREM sleep electroencephalogram. Eur J Neurosci 2001;13:2282–90.

[89] Tinguely G, Finelli LA, Landolt HP, et al. Functional EEG topography in sleep and waking: state-dependent and state-independent features. Neuroimage 2006;32:283–92.

[90] Tononi G, Cirelli C. Sleep function and synaptic homeostasis. Sleep Med Rev 2006;10: 49–62.

[91] Edinger JD, Bonnet MH, Bootzin RR, et al. Derivation of research diagnostic criteria for insomnia: report of an American Academy of Sleep Medicine Work Group. Sleep 2004;27: 1567–96.

[92] Adrien J. Neurobiological bases for the relation between sleep and depression. Sleep Med Rev 2002;6:341–51.

[93] Pace-Schott EF, Hobson JA. The neurobiology of sleep: genetics, cellular physiology and subcortical networks. Nat Rev Neurosci 2002;3:591–605.

[94] Thase ME. Depression, sleep, and antidepressants. J Clin Psychiatry 1998;59(Suppl 4): 55–65.

[95] Argyropoulos SV, Wilson SJ. Sleep disturbances in depression and the effects of antidepressants. Int Rev Psychiatry 2005;17:237–45.

[96] Alt A, Nisenbaum ES, Bleakman D, et al. A role for AMPA receptors in mood disorders. Biochem Pharmacol 2006;71:1273–88.

[97] Choudary PV, Molnar M, Evans SJ, et al. Altered cortical glutamatergic and GABAergic signal transmission with glial involvement in depression. Proc Natl Acad Sci USA 2005;102:15653–8.

[98] Kugaya A, Sanacora G. Beyond monoamines: glutamatergic function in mood disorders. CNS Spectr 2005;10:808–19.

[99] Manji HK, Moore GJ, Rajkowska G, et al. Neuroplasticity and cellular resilience in mood disorders. Mol Psychiatry 2000;5:578–93.

[100] Manji HK, Quiroz JA, Sporn J, et al. Enhancing neuronal plasticity and cellular resilience to develop novel, improved therapeutics for difficult-to-treat depression. Biol Psychiatry 2003;53:707–42.

[101] Zarate CA Jr, Singh J, Manji HK. Cellular plasticity cascades: targets for the development of novel therapeutics for bipolar disorder. Biol Psychiatry 2006;59:1006–20.

[102] Cirelli C. A molecular window on sleep: changes in gene expression between sleep and wakefulness. Neuroscientist 2005;11:63–74.

[103] Nofzinger EA, Buysse DJ, Germain A, et al. Alterations in regional cerebral glucose metabolism across waking and non-rapid eye movement sleep in depression. Arch Gen Psychiatry 2005;62:387–96.

[104] Germain A, Nofzinger EA, Kupfer DJ, et al. Neurobiology of non-REM sleep in depression: further evidence for hypofrontality and thalamic dysregulation. Am J Psychiatry 2004;161:1856–63.

[105] Davidson RJ, Pizzagalli D, Nitschke JB, et al. Depression: perspectives from affective neuroscience. Annu Rev Psychol 2002;53:545–74.

[106] Nofzinger EA, Buysse DJ, Germain A, et al. Functional neuroimaging evidence for hyperarousal in insomnia. Am J Psychiatry 2004;161:2126–8.

[107] Germain A, Buysse DJ, Wood A, et al. Functional neuroanatomical correlates of eye movements during rapid eye movement sleep in depressed patients. Psychiatry Res 2004;130: 259–68.

[108] Nofzinger EA, Buysse DJ, Germain A, et al. Increased activation of anterior paralimbic and executive cortex from waking to rapid eye movement sleep in depression. Arch Gen Psychiatry 2004;61:695–702.

[109] Berger M, van Calker D, Riemann D. Sleep and manipulations of the sleep-wake rhythm in depression. Acta Psychiatr Scand Suppl 2003;83–91.

[110] Giedke H, Schwarzler F. Therapeutic use of sleep deprivation in depression. Sleep Med Rev 2002;6:361–77.

[111] Riemann D, Voderholzer U, Berger M. Sleep and sleep-wake manipulations in bipolar depression. Neuropsychobiology 2002;45(Suppl 1):7–12.

[112] Volk SA, Kaendler SH, Hertel A, et al. Can response to partial sleep deprivation in depressed patients be predicted by regional changes of cerebral blood flow? Psychiatry Res 1997;75:67–74.

[113] Wu JC, Buchsbaum M, Bunney WE Jr. Clinical neurochemical implications of sleep deprivation's effects on the anterior cingulate of depressed responders. Neuropsychopharmacology 2001;25(5 Suppl):S74–8.

[114] Clark CP, Brown GG, Archibald SL, et al. Does amygdalar perfusion correlate with antidepressant response to partial sleep deprivation in major depression? Psychiatry Res 2006;146:43–51.

[115] Clark CP, Brown GG, Frank L, et al. Improved anatomic delineation of the antidepressant response to partial sleep deprivation in medial frontal cortex using perfusion-weighted functional MRI. Psychiatry Res 2006;146:213–22.

[116] Ebert D, Berger M. Neurobiological similarities in antidepressant sleep deprivation and psychostimulant use: a psychostimulant theory of antidepressant sleep deprivation. Psychopharmacology (Berl) 1998;140:1–10.

[117] Nestler EJ, Barrot M, DiLeone RJ, et al. Neurobiology of depression. Neuron 2002;34: 13–25.

[118] Steiger A. Neurochemical regulation of sleep. J Psychiatr Res 2006;12 (in press).

[119] Buckley TM, Schatzberg AF. On the interactions of the hypothalamic-pituitary-adrenal (HPA) axis and sleep: normal HPA axis activity and circadian rhythm, exemplary sleep disorders. J Clin Endocrinol Metab 2005;90:3106–14.

[120] Held K, Kunzel H, Ising M, et al. Treatment with the CRH1-receptor-antagonist R121919 improves sleep-EEG in patients with depression. J Psychiatr Res 2004;38:129–36.

[121] Fava M, Kendler KS. Major depressive disorder. Neuron 2000;28:335–41.

[122] McGuffin P, Rijsdijk F, Andrew M, et al. The heritability of bipolar affective disorder and the genetic relationship to unipolar depression. Arch Gen Psychiatry 2003;60:497–502.

[123] Benedetti F, Colombo C, Serretti A, et al. Antidepressant effects of light therapy combined with sleep deprivation are influenced by a functional polymorphism within the promoter of the serotonin transporter gene. Biol Psychiatry 2003;54:687–92.

[124] Du L, Bakish D, Ravindran A, et al. MAO-A gene polymorphisms are associated with major depression and sleep disturbance in males. Neuroreport 2004;15:2097–101.

[125] Baghai TC, Schule C, Zwanzger P, et al. Influence of a functional polymorphism within the angiotensin I-converting enzyme gene on partial sleep deprivation in patients with major depression. Neurosci Lett 2003;339:223–6.

[126] Xing GQ, Russell S, Webster MJ, et al. Decreased expression of mineralocorticoid receptor mRNA in the prefrontal cortex in schizophrenia and bipolar disorder. Int J Neuropsychopharmacol 2004;7:143–53.

[127] Serretti A, Cusin C, Benedetti F, et al. Insomnia improvement during antidepressant treatment and CLOCK gene polymorphism. Am J Med Genet B Neuropsychiatr Genet 2005;137:36–9.

[128] Benedetti F, Serretti A, Colombo C, et al. A glycogen synthase kinase 3-beta promoter gene single nucleotide polymorphism is associated with age at onset and response to total sleep deprivation in bipolar depression. Neurosci Lett 2004;368:123–6.

[129] Benedetti F, Serretti A, Pontiggia A, et al. Long-term response to lithium salts in bipolar illness is influenced by the glycogen synthase kinase 3-beta -50 T/C SNP. Neurosci Lett 2005;376:51–5.

[130] Iitaka C, Miyazaki K, Akaike T, et al. A role for glycogen synthase kinase-3beta in the mammalian circadian clock. J Biol Chem 2005;280:29397–402.

[131] Yin L, Wang J, Klein PS, et al. Nuclear receptor Rev-erbalpha is a critical lithium-sensitive component of the circadian clock. Science 2006;311:1002–5.

[132] Cirelli C, Gutierrez CM, Tononi G. Extensive and divergent effects of sleep and wakefulness on brain gene expression. Neuron 2004;41:35–43.

[133] Tsuno N, Besset A, Ritchie K. Sleep and depression. J Clin Psychiatry 2005;66:1254–69.

[134] Nierenberg AA, Keefe BR, Leslie VC, et al. Residual symptoms in depressed patients who respond acutely to fluoxetine. J Clin Psychiatry 1999;60:221–5.

[135] Mendelson WB. A review of the evidence for the efficacy and safety of trazodone in insomnia. J Clin Psychiatry 2005;66:469–76.

[136] Fava M, McCall WV, Krystal A, et al. Eszopiclone co-administered with fluoxetine in patients with insomnia coexisting with major depressive disorder. Biol Psychiatry 2006;59:1052–60.

[137] Buysse DJ, Reynolds CF 3rd, Houck PR, et al. Does lorazepam impair the antidepressant response to nortriptyline and psychotherapy? J Clin Psychiatry 1997;58: 426–32.

[138] Asnis GM, Chakraburtty A, DuBoff EA, et al. Zolpidem for persistent insomnia in SSRI-treated depressed patients. J Clin Psychiatry 1999;60:668–76.

[139] Allard S, Sainati SM, Roth-Schechter BF. Coadministration of short-term zolpidem with sertraline in healthy women. J Clin Pharmacol 1999;39:184–91.

[140] Sharpley AL, Bhagwagar Z, Hafizi S, et al. Risperidone augmentation decreases rapid eye movement sleep and decreases wake in treatment-resistant depressed patients. J Clin Psychiatry 2003;64:192–6.

[141] Sharpley AL, Attenburrow ME, Hafizi S, et al. Olanzapine increases slow wave sleep and sleep continuity in SSRI-resistant depressed patients. J Clin Psychiatry 2005;66: 450–4.

[142] Ostroff RB, Nelson JC. Risperidone augmentation of selective serotonin reuptake inhibitors in major depression. J Clin Psychiatry 1999;60:256–9.

[143] Armitage R, Cole D, Suppes T, et al. Effects of clozapine on sleep in bipolar and schizoaffective disorders. Prog Neuropsychopharmacol Biol Psychiatry 2004;28:1065–70.

[144] Smith MT, Huang MI, Manber R. Cognitive behavior therapy for chronic insomnia occurring within the context of medical and psychiatric disorders. Clin Psychol Rev 2005;25: 559–92.

[145] Ninan PT, Hassman HA, Glass SJ, et al. Adjunctive modafinil at initiation of treatment with a selective serotonin reuptake inhibitor enhances the degree and onset of therapeutic effects in patients with major depressive disorder and fatigue. J Clin Psychiatry 2004;65: 414–20.

[146] Fava M, Thase ME, DeBattista C. A multicenter, placebo-controlled study of modafinil augmentation in partial responders to selective serotonin reuptake inhibitors with persistent fatigue and sleepiness. J Clin Psychiatry 2005;66:85–93.

[147] Schwartz TL, Azhar N, Cole K, et al. An open-label study of adjunctive modafinil in patients with sedation related to serotonergic antidepressant therapy. J Clin Psychiatry 2004;65: 1223–7.

[148] Thase ME, Fava M, DeBattista C, et al. Modafinil augmentation of SSRI therapy in patients with major depressive disorder and excessive sleepiness and fatigue: a 12-week, open-label, extension study. CNS Spectr 2006;11:93–102.

[149] DeBattista C, Doghramji K, Menza MA, et al. Adjunct modafinil for the short-term treatment of fatigue and sleepiness in patients with major depressive disorder: a preliminary double-blind, placebo-controlled study. J Clin Psychiatry 2003;64:1057–64.

[150] Lundt L. Modafinil treatment in patients with seasonal affective disorder/winter depression: an open-label pilot study. J Affect Disord 2004;81:173–8.

[151] Nasr S. Modafinil as adjunctive therapy in depressed outpatients. Ann Clin Psychiatry 2004;16:133–8.

[152] Wu JC, Bunney WE. The biological basis of an antidepressant response to sleep deprivation and relapse: review and hypothesis. Am J Psychiatry 1990;147:14–21.

[153] Gillin JC, Buchsbaum M, Wu J, et al. Sleep deprivation as a model experimental antidepressant treatment: findings from functional brain imaging. Depress Anxiety 2001;14: 37–49.

[154] Wirz-Justice A, Van den Hoofdakker RH. Sleep deprivation in depression: what do we know, where do we go? Biol Psychiatry 1999;46:445–53.

[155] Leibenluft E, Albert PS, Rosenthal NE, et al. Relationship between sleep and mood in patients with rapid-cycling bipolar disorder. Psychiatry Res 1996;63:161–8.

[156] Wehr TA. Sleep loss: a preventable cause of mania and other excited states. J Clin Psychiatry 1989;50(Suppl):8–16 [discussion: 45–7].

[157] Wehr TA. Sleep-loss as a possible mediator of diverse causes of mania. Br J Psychiatry 1991;159:576–8.

[158] Wehr TA, Sack DA, Rosenthal NE. Sleep reduction as a final common pathway in the genesis of mania. Am J Psychiatry 1987;144:201–4.

[159] Yang C, White DP, Winkelman JW. Antidepressants and periodic leg movements of sleep. Biol Psychiatry 2005;58:510–4.

[160] Schenck CH, Mahowald MW. Rapid eye movement sleep parasomnias. Neurol Clin 2005;23:1107–26.

Sleep in Schizophrenia: Impairments, Correlates, and Treatment

Kathleen L. Benson, PhD

P. O. Box 335, Barnstable, MA 02630-0335, USA

The worldwide prevalence rate of schizophrenia is approximately 1%, with approximately 3 million affected individuals living in the United States. It is perhaps the most devastating neuropsychiatric illness, with the age of onset typically occurring in late adolescence. It seems that we can neither cure this disorder nor prevent its occurrence.

For the majority of schizophrenics, the prognosis is poor. Most experience life-long mental disability, emotional distress, and social and economic marginalization. For some, there are episodic flare-ups and repeated hospitalization; for others, there is permanent institutionalization. Schizophrenics also face a higher mortality rate from suicide and poor health.

Despite many and vigorous efforts to unmask the pathophysiology and etiology of the illness, the disease remains an enigma. The current consensus views schizophrenia as a neurodevelopmental disorder involving the interplay of multiple susceptibility genes and environmental factors. Multiple genetic and environmental factors are consonant with the clinical heterogeneity of schizophrenia and with the wide and diverse array of presenting clinical symptoms. With no disease-specific laboratory abnormality, the diagnosis of schizophrenia is based entirely on clinical findings and is guided by criteria defined in the *Diagnostic and Statistical Manual of Mental Disorders, Fourth Edition* [1]. Characteristic symptoms are organized into two main categories: positive and negative symptoms. Positive symptoms may include hallucinations, delusions, unusual thought content, disorganized speech, and gross disorganization or catatonic behavior. Negative symptoms include affective flattening, avolition, and poverty of speech. Cognitive impairment, or thought disorder, is believed to be the fundamental defining symptom of the illness.

One of the human costs associated with schizophrenia is severe insomnia and related sleep abnormalities. This article describes those sleep abnormalities and their significance. It also reviews the clinical, neurophysiologic, and cognitive correlates of these abnormalities. Finally, it addresses sleep-related treatment issues with particular emphasis on associated or emergent sleep disorders.

E-mail address: be97@stanford.edu

0193-953X/06/$ – see front matter
doi:10.1016/j.psc.2006.08.002

THE ABNORMALITIES OF SLEEP IN SCHIZOPHRENIA

Subjective Complaints

In patients who have schizophrenia, complaints of poor sleep quality are related directly to negative assessments of quality of life [2]. Poor sleep in schizophrenics who are in a state of active psychosis can range from periods of total sleeplessness to nights of significant insomnia. This insomnia is experienced as difficulty falling asleep, a loss of total sleep time (TST), multiple awakenings, and a degraded quality of sleep. Sleep also may be restless and agitated, and nightmares are not uncommon. Broadly speaking, treatment with antipsychotics (APs) ameliorates the severity of this insomnia. Even among patients who are clinically stable and treated with APs, however, complaints of sleep disturbance are common, in particular early and middle insomnia [3]. AP-treated patients also have a greater likelihood, relative to community controls, of sleeping during the day and wakefulness at night. This sleep-wake reversal is associated with subjective complaints of poor sleep quality [4].

Objective Assessment

Measures of sleep maintenance

A systematic review [5] of research studies and two meta-analyses [6,7] firmly support these complaints of insomnia. Multiple objective studies using overnight polysomnography (PSG) document poor sleep efficiency (SE) that is associated with reductions in TST and early, middle, and late insomnia. This review and the two meta-analyses concur in finding that early insomnia, or difficulty reaching a state of persistent sleep, is highly characteristic of the disturbed sleep in schizophrenia. It is important that clinicians know that severe insomnia is one of the prodromal symptoms of psychotic decompensation or relapse after the discontinuation of AP medication [8–10].

REM time and REM sleep eye movement activity

Shortly after the discovery of rapid eye movement (REM) sleep and its association with dream reports, there was much speculation about a possible linkage between hallucinations in schizophrenia and an abnormality of REM sleep allowing dream intrusion into waking. The review cited previously [5] concludes that REM sleep is neither systematically augmented nor reduced in schizophrenics. Furthermore, a cross-sectional study finds little difference in REM time between hallucinating and nonhallucinating schizophrenics [11]. Finally, a study of unmedicated schizophrenics and healthy controls observes no abnormal leakage of REM sleep phasic events into non-REM sleep [12].

Studies also have examined REM sleep eye movements (EMs), both raw frequencies and density measures, to correct for differences in stage REM time. EMs have been counted visually or scored by computerized EM detection software. In AP-naive and unmedicated patients, visual and computerized scoring find no difference in REM sleep EM activity between patients who are schizophrenic and control subjects [13–17].

Non–REM sleep and latency to the first REM period (REM latency)
Documented sleep abnormalities in schizophrenics also may include a foreshort-
ening of the latency to the onset of the first REM period, or REM latency
(REML). Many studies have examined this issue [13,14,16,18–24], and the majority report significantly shorter REMLs in schizophrenics relative to healthy
controls. Heterogeneity between patient samples and methodologic differences,
including prior exposure to AP treatment, may explain the lack of consistency
among these findings.

REML could be influenced by one or more mechanisms: first, a primary alteration or active enhancement of REM sleep mechanisms; or second, a slow
wave sleep (SWS) inhibitory effect (during the first non-REM cycle) on
REM mechanisms. Consequently, the finding of short REML is consistent
with and potentially related to another sleep abnormality frequently observed
in schizophrenics (ie, SWS deficits). SWS deficits would permit the passive advance of the first REM period, producing a shorted REML. SWS deficits or
stage 4 deficits frequently, but not consistently, are observed in PSG recordings
of patients who are schizophrenic [13–15,18–22,24–27]. Although it is suggested that prior exposure to or withdrawal from APs might explain this inconsistency, stage 4 deficits are observed in first-episode, neuroleptic-naive
schizophrenics [24].

SWS deficits play a key role in Feinberg's neurodevelopmental model of
schizophrenia [28]. According to this model, schizophrenia develops during adolescence because of some dysfunction in the normal maturational process of
synaptic elimination during the second decade of life. Excess synaptic pruning
would result in less synchronous EEG slow wave activity and observed SWS
deficits. In healthy subjects, SWS peaks during the first non-REM period and
declines throughout the remainder of the night. The amount of SWS during
a sleep period is a function of the amount of prior waking; total sleep deprivation increases the amount of waking before the next sleep period and is associated with a significant increase in SWS during the first recovery night. It is
believed that this homeostatic or dynamic response may serve a restorative
role in the central nervous system. Consequently, the restoration of SWS in patients who have schizophrenia may have important implications for their clinical and neurocognitive outcome.

CLINICAL AND NEUROPSYCHOLOGIC CORRELATIONS
Clinical Correlates
Global symptom severity is associated with increased waking, reduced REM
sleep time, SWS deficits, and short REML [20,21,29]. Studies find that prolonged SL [30], impaired SE [31], short REML [13,21,24,32], and increased
REM sleep EM density [16,17] correlate with positive symptoms, one constit-
uent of global severity. Positive symptoms also are associated with EEG high
frequency activity during the sleep of schizophrenics [33]. Negative symptoms,
another aspect of global severity, are associated with short REML [21,23] and
SWS deficits [19,34–37]. Cognitive dysfunction, or thought disorder, is

considered the core element of schizophrenia; it too correlates with SWS deficits, perhaps indicative of frontal lobe dysfunction [38]. Additionally, SWS deficits [39] and short REML [23,40] are linked to poor clinical and psychosocial outcome. Finally, three studies demonstrate sleep-related cognitive impairment in schizophrenics relative to healthy controls. Manoach and colleagues [41] observed impairment of sleep-dependent consolidation of procedural learning. Forest and coworkers [42] demonstrated a negative correlation between the amount of stage 4 sleep and reaction time in a selective attention task. A third study by Göder and coworkers [43] found that SWS deficits and impaired SE correlated significantly with impaired performance on a test of declarative memory.

In summary, these studies of the correlates of sleep abnormalities in schizophrenia suggest that insomnia and increased REM sleep EM activity are associated with psychosis, positive symptoms, and emotionality; SWS deficits seem to be related to negative symptoms and cognitive dysfunction. These studies suffer from a diversity of rating scales and clinical instruments, different algorithms to quantify sleep parameters, small sample sizes, differences in medication status and history, and the heterogeneity of patients who are schizophrenic. These contribute to results that are variable and potentially inconsistent across studies. Studies of clinical correlates also are limited by protocol design. Most of these studies are cross-sectional in nature, whereas a within-patient, longitudinal assessment of sleep patterns across changing clinical states might yield more consistent information.

Neurophysiologic Correlates
Structural and functional neuroimaging
Using brain-imaging technology, SWS deficits in schizophrenia are associated with structural dysmorphology (eg, increased ventricular system volume) [34,44] and functional impairment (eg, decreased brain anabolic processes) [35]. Sleep maintenance deficits also are associated with brain morphologic features. The size of the third ventricle correlates negatively with measures of TST [34] and sleep maintenance [45]. Finally, measures of awakening in drug-naive patients who are schizophrenic are associated with ventricular-brain ratio [13]. Neuroanatomic correlates of sleep abnormalities might suggest a stable or trait-like impairment.

Neurochemical abnormalities
Dopamine (DA) dysfunction has assumed a key role in the pathophysiology of schizophrenia. Unfortunately, there are no systematic studies of sleep abnormalities in schizophrenia in relationship to the DA system, although such studies would be difficult to interpret in the case of long-term exposure to APs with strong DA antagonism.

With regard to other neurotransmitter systems, cholinergic supersensitivity is suggested as a mechanism underlying short REMLs in schizophrenia [46]. Serotonergic (5-HT) mechanisms are implicated in SWS deficits by a report finding a positive correlation between SWS time and cerebrospinal fluid

(CSF) levels of the 5-HT metabolite, 5-hydroxyindole acetic acid, in unmedicated schizophrenics [47]. Norepinephrine (NE) is associated with psychotic decompensation; increased CSF levels of NE and its metabolite, 3-methoxy-4-hydroxyphenylglycol (MHPG), have accompanied relapse-related insomnia [8]. Finally, the characteristic insomnia of schizophrenia has been investigated in relationship to hypocretin. Hypocretin (orexin) is a major wake-promoting neurotransmitter of hypothalamic origin; in humans, hypocretin deficiency is associated with the sleep disorder narcolepsy [48]. In unmedicated schizophrenics, CSF hypocretin levels correlate positively with sleep latency, suggesting a possible relationship between hypocretin and hyperarousal in schizophrenia [49].

TREATMENT ISSUES
Antipsychotics: First and Second Generation
Although a minority of patients who have schizophrenia have a full recovery after an initial psychotic episode, the majority require long-term treatment with antipsychotic medications. APs can be differentiated by their neurotransmitter receptor profiles. APs have unique effects on DA, 5-HT, α-adrenergic, cholinergic and histaminic receptors, and their many subtypes [50,51]. Their primary mechanism of action involves receptor blockade; however, they also can achieve their therapeutic effects by acting as partial agonists and re-uptake blockers. As discussed later, the differential receptor binding profiles of APs are associated with a wide range of potentially adverse effects.

The first generation: traditional or typical antipsychotics
A strong affinity for the DA D_2 postsynaptic receptor characterizes traditional APs and is credited with their therapeutic efficacy. Unfortunately, this strong binding with D_2 receptors in the striatum is associated with extrapyramidal side effects (EPS), such as akathisia, dystonia, and parkinsonism. DA receptor blockade also is associated with a more damaging, and potentially irreversible consequence, namely tardive dyskinesia (TD). TD occurs in approximately 20% of patients who are schizophrenic and are receiving first-generation APs.

The second generation: novel or atypical antipsychotics
Currently, second-generation APs are first-line treatment for schizophrenia. Motivation for their development came from several sources. Relative to novel APs, first-generation APs were associated with a higher rate of treatment resistance, inadequate treatment of negative symptoms, and poorer compliance owing to adverse side effects, such as EPS and TD. Clozapine was the first novel AP to demonstrate good clinical efficacy with no EPS. At present, the atypical APs include other agents in common clinical use: risperidone, olanzapine, quetiapine, ziprasidone, and aripiprazole. Each has a unique receptor binding profile; however, all are associated with weaker affinity for the DA D_2 receptor (relative to first-generation APs), and strong affinity for serotonin $5\text{-}HT_2$ receptors [51].

In an extensive review of the second-generation APs, Lublin and colleagues [52] note that the novel APs improve negative symptoms and cognitive functioning more than traditional APs. Although the novel APs are associated with fewer EPS, risperidone, olanzapine, and ziprasidone show dose-related increases in EPS not shown by clozapine, quetiapine, and aripiprazole [52]. Of potentially greater clinical importance than the rate of EPS are observations linking second-generation APs to increased morbidity, such as weight gain, dyslipidemias, impaired glucose regulation, and type 2 diabetes [53]. Weight gain varies appreciably across second-generation APs with clozapine and olanzapine associated with the greatest weight gain, risperidone and quetiapine moderate gain, and ziprasidone and aripiprazole minimal gain. Although glucose dysregulation may be a direct effect of second-generation APs, this review suggests that the risk of adverse metabolic changes across the novel APs can be explained, at least in part, by their relative weight gain potential.

Antipsychotics: Sleep-Related Side Effects

As a general rule, sedation, as a side effect of first-generation APs, is associated with high-milligram, low-potency agents, such as chlorpromazine and thioridazine. Low-milligram, high-potency agents, such as fluphenazine, haloperidol, and thiothixene, are associated with lower sedation rates. The second-generation APs are associated with varying amounts of sedation. The National Institute of Mental Health–sponsored Clinical Antipsychotic Trials of Intervention Effectiveness (CATIE) study [54] reports on the prevalence of adverse effects in large samples of schizophrenics assigned to one first-generation AP (perphenazine) or one of four second-generation APs (olanzapine, risperidone, quetiapine, and ziprasidone). Within each of these five treatment groups, 10% to 20% of enrollees discontinued treatment because of adverse side effects. The CATIE study also examined the rates of somnolence and insomnia in the five treatment groups. Across the five treatment groups, rates of somnolence ranged from 24% to 31% but were not significantly different. Residual insomnia also was identified as an adverse side effect, and, across the five treatment groups, rates of insomnia ranged from 16% to 30%. These rates did vary significantly from group to group with ziprasidone associated with the highest rate (30%) and olanzapine the lowest rate (16%). In a separate study of outpatient schizophrenics and their attitudes toward APs, from among the range of side effects sedation was the most highly correlated with negative feelings [55]. Because compliance with therapy relies in part on patients' attitudes toward APs, significant somnolence may contribute to noncompliance and ultimately to poor outcome.

Antipsychotics: Effects on Sleep Patterns

As a general rule, first-generation APs improve sleep maintenance, increasing TST and SE and reducing SL and waking after sleep onset, although their effects on REML, REM time, and REM EM density differ [56–61]. Chlorpromazine increases SWS time, an effect consistent with a related increase in REML [56].

Schizophrenics, when switched from first-generation to second-generation APs, have expressed significant improvements in subjective sleep quality

[62]. With regard to objectively measured effects of atypical APs on sleep patterns in patients who are schizophrenic, PSG studies of clozapine note increased TST, SE, and stage 2 and decreased SWS, SL, and waking [61,63,64]. Schizophrenics treated with olanzapine show increased TST, stage 2, and EM density and decreased wake and stage 1 sleep; a significant increase in SWS also is noted [65]. A significant enhancement of SWS time also is observed in risperidone-treated schizophrenics [66]. PSG studies of schizophrenics treated with quetiapine, ziprasidone and aripiprazole are not available; however, in a double-blind, placebo-controlled, randomized crossover study, healthy controls given quetiapine revealed significant improvements in sleep induction and sleep continuity [67].

Although AP-related clinical improvement lags behind the initiation of AP treatment, positive improvement in sleep maintenance and structure has followed acute or short-term dosing. Improvements in sleep maintenance and architecture, secondary to AP-treatment, may be a positive contribution to AP efficacy and tolerance, not mere by-products of clinical improvement.

Adjunct Medications

Although studies of AP-treated schizophrenics show documented improvements in sleep maintenance and structure, in many cases there remains some degree of residual insomnia [54]. Benzodiazepine tranquilizers and hypnotics may be added to address issues of residual insomnia, but they should be used with discretion, particularly in the case of schizophrenics comorbid for a sleep-related breathing disorder or a comorbid history of alcohol or drug abuse. In addition to APs, mood stabilizers and antidepressants may be prescribed for patients who have schizoaffective disorder, concomitant depression, or impulse control problems; these adjuncts also should improve sleep maintenance.

Melatonin

As discussed previously, schizophrenics may demonstrate a positive clinical response to APs but continue to present with some degree of insomnia. These patients pose a problem for treating clinicians. A more sedating AP could be added or substituted or an adjunct hypnotic could be prescribed. These alternatives could increase patient exposure to an adverse event. A novel response to this dilemma is suggested by the assessment of neuroendocrine systems in schizophrenia. Melatonin is the chief hormonal product of the pineal gland. In healthy controls, melatonin displays a well-defined circadian rhythm, with low plasma concentrations during the circadian day and high plasma concentrations during the circadian night. Several studies show that the nocturnal rise of melatonin is blunted markedly in schizophrenia [68–70]. To follow-up on these observations, Shamir and colleagues [71] conducted a randomized, double-blind, crossover study to test the effect of melatonin replacement (2 mg) on sleep disturbances in patients who have schizophrenia. They found that melatonin replacement improved SE significantly as measured by actigraphy. These results are encouraging and argue strongly for replication.

Modafinil
In contrast to residual insomnia, many patients who are schizophrenic clearly are sedated by their prescribed AP dosage. Some case studies show that methylphenidate can be an effective treatment for persistent clozapine-related sedation [72], but methylphenidate is not Food and Drug Administration indicated for this use. More recent studies have turned their attention to modafinil, an agent known to promote wakefulness in narcolepsy. Case studies [73] and an open-label pilot study [74] show that modafinil, as an adjunct to AP treatment, can increase wake time, reduce fatigue and TST, and improve quality of life. Stimulant drugs that promote wakefulness may, however, in the case of schizophrenia, increase the risk of relapse or exacerbation of psychosis [75]. Although the degree of this risk may be dependent on the amount of modafinil and repeated dosing [76], off-label use of modafinil to control AP-related sedation in schizophrenia requires more extensive and controlled investigations.

Antipsychotics: Associated Sleep Disorders
In addition to the sleep impairments characteristically associated with schizophrenia, many schizophrenics also are comorbid for a variety of dyssomnias regularly seen in sleep disorder clinics. These may include inadequate sleep hygiene, irregular sleep-wake patterns, parasomnias, sleep-related movement disorders, and sleep-related breathing disorders. Some of these dyssomnias are associated directly or indirectly with schizophrenia per se. Unfortunately, others may be enhanced by, or possibly even induced by, AP treatment (discussed later). Because there are no prevalence studies of sleep disorders in AP-naive or unmedicated schizophrenics, their baseline rates for common sleep disorders are unknown.

Somnambulism
Treatment-emergent somnambulism is associated with first-generation APs, in particular the combination of APs with lithium [77]. Sleepwalking also is observed in patients started on olanzapine, a second-generation AP [78]. As discussed previously, olanzapine is associated with enhanced SWS, which may increase the risk of impaired arousal mechanisms.

Sleep-related movement disorders
DA deficiency is linked to the pathophysiology of sleep-related movement disorders, such as restless legs syndrome (RLS) and periodic limb movement disorder (PLMD) [79]. Because of the long-standing relationship of AP-associated movement disorders to DA receptor blockade, the question arises, can APs induce or augment RLS or PLMD because they diminish DA activity? For samples in which the majority of patients who were schizophrenic had been exposed to first-generation APs, a PLM index greater than 5 events (5 or more leg jerks causing arousal per hour of sleep) was observed in 13% [80] of patients AP free for 2 or more weeks and 14% [81] of patients currently treated with APs. With regard to second-generation APs, two case reports link second-generation APs to the development of RLS and a clinically significant PLMS index in patients who were schizophrenic. The first case was associated with olanzapine

treatment [82], the second case with risperidone treatment [83]. Both cases resolved on switching to a different atypical AP. Finally, quetiapine is associated with a dose-dependent induction of PLMS in healthy controls [67] and with the induction of RLS in a patient who had bipolar I disorder [84].

Sleep-disordered breathing
In a review of a predominantly male, Veterans Health Administration sample, approximately 4.5% of patients diagnosed with psychosis also were diagnosed with sleep apnea [85]. Higher prevalence rates are suggested by studies that enrolled patients who were schizophrenic in sleep research protocols and tested them for the presence of obstructive sleep apnea. These studies, which varied in terms of sample size, age, gender, inpatient/outpatient status, APs, and measurement instrument (oximetry, ambulatory apnea monitor, or PSG), reported the following estimates of sleep-disordered breathing: 17% with a respiratory disturbance index (RDI) greater than 5 events per hour of sleep [80], 48% with an RDI greater than 10 events per hour of sleep [81], and 19% with a desaturation index greater than 5 events per hour [86]. But in a study of patients who were schizophrenic referred to a sleep clinic for a suspected sleep disorder, more than 46% had a respiratory disturbance index greater than 10 events per hour; the mean RDI was 64.8 events per hour [87]. In this study, the strongest predictor of sleep-disordered breathing was obesity. Obesity is common among schizophrenics. Broadly speaking, weight gain is associated with AP treatment, and, as previously presented, weight gain (and glucose dysregulation) occurring secondary to treatment with second-generation APs has become a serious morbidity risk. A case study reporting on the development of moderate to severe sleep apnea in two schizophrenics treated with clozapine and risperidone, respectively, finds that the former was associated with a 40-lb weight gain and the latter with a 65-lb weight gain [88]. The possibility of comorbid sleep-disordered breathing must be given serious consideration for any schizophrenic who presents with daytime somnolence and who is obese by history or who has undergone weight gain secondary to treatment with atypical APs. Patients who are comorbid for schizophrenia and sleep-disordered breathing can be treated effectively with nasal continuous positive airway pressure; they also can demonstrate relatively good compliance and significant clinical improvement [89].

In summary, patients who have schizophrenia and who are comorbid for dyssomnias, such as a sleep-related breathing disorders and sleep-related movement disorders, must be approached with the same or even greater vigor shown to any other patient presenting with a suspected sleep disorder. Normalization of sleep and its restorative process may be a prerequisite for a positive clinical outcome.

References

[1] American Psychiatric Association. Diagnostic and statistical manual of mental disorders. 4th edition. Washington, DC: American Psychiatric Press; 1994. p. 273–90.
[2] Ritsner M, Kurs R, Ponizovsky A, et al. Perceived quality of life in schizophrenia: relationships to sleep quality. Qual Life Res 2004;13:783–91.

[3] Haffmans PM, Hoencamp E, Knegtering HJ, et al. Sleep disturbance in schizophrenia. Br J Psychiatry 1994;165:697–8.

[4] Hofstetter JR, Mayeda AR, Happel CG, et al. Sleep and daily activity preferences in schizophrenia: associations with neurocognition and symptoms. J Nerv Ment Dis 2003;191: 408–10.

[5] Benson KL, Zarcone VP. Schizophrenia. In: Kryger MH, Roth T, Dement WC, editors. Principles and practice of sleep medicine. 4th edition. Philadelphia: Elsevier Saunders; 2005. p. 1327–36.

[6] Benca RM, Obermeyer WH, Thisted RA, et al. Sleep and psychiatric disorders: a meta-analysis. Arch Gen Psychiatry 1992;49:651–68.

[7] Chouinard S, Poulin J, Stip E, et al. Sleep in untreated patients with schizophrenia: a meta-analysis. Schizophr Bull 2004;30:957–67.

[8] Van Kammen DP, van Kammen WB, Peters JL, et al. CSF MHPG, sleep and psychosis in schizophrenia. Clin Neuropharmacol 1986;9(Suppl 4):575–7.

[9] Dencker SJ, Malm U, Lepp M. Schizophrenic relapse after drug withdrawal is predictable. Acta Psychiatr Scand 1986;73:181–5.

[10] Chemerinski E, Ho B, Flaum M, et al. Insomnia as a predictor for symptom worsening following antipsychotic withdrawal in schizophrenia. Compr Psychiatry 2002;43:393–6.

[11] Koresko R, Snyder F, Feinberg I. "Dream time" in hallucinating and non-hallucinating schizophrenic patients. Nature 1963;199:1118–9.

[12] Benson KL, Zarcone VP. Testing the REM phasic event intrusion hypothesis of schizophrenia. Psychiatry Res 1985;15:163–73.

[13] Lauer CJ, Schreiber W, Pollmächer T, et al. Sleep in schizophrenia: a polysomnographic study on drug-naive patients. Neuropsychopharmacology 1997;16:51–60.

[14] Keshavan MS, Reynolds CF III, Miewald JM, et al. Delta sleep deficits in schizophrenia. Arch Gen Psychiatry 1998;55:443–8.

[15] Hoffman R, Hendrickse W, Rush AJ, et al. Slow-wave activity during non-REM sleep in men with schizophrenia and major depressive disorders. Psychiatry Res 2000;95:215–25.

[16] Feinberg I, Koresko RL, Gottlieb F. Further observations on electrophysiological sleep patterns in schizophrenia. Comp Psychiatry 1965;6:21–4.

[17] Benson KL, Zarcone VP. REM sleep eye movement activity in schizophrenia and depression. Arch Gen Psychiatry 1993;50:474–82.

[18] Zarcone VP, Benson KL, Berger PA. Abnormal rapid eye movement latencies in schizophrenia. Arch Gen Psychiatry 1987;44:45–8.

[19] Ganguli R, Reynolds CF III, Kupfer DJ. EEG sleep in young, never medicated, schizophrenic patients: a comparison with delusional and nondelusional depressives and with healthy controls. Arch Gen Psychiatry 1987;44:36–45.

[20] Kempenaers C, Kerkhofs M, Linkowski P, et al. Sleep EEG variables in young schizophrenic and depressive patients. Biol Psychiatry 1988;24:833–8.

[21] Tandon R, Shipley JE, Taylor S, et al. Electroencephalographic sleep abnormalities in schizophrenia: relationship to positive/negative symptoms and prior neuroleptic treatment. Arch Gen Psychiatry 1992;49:185–94.

[22] Hiatt JF, Floyd TC, Katz PH, et al. Further evidence of abnormal NREM sleep in schizophrenia. Arch Gen Psychiatry 1985;42:797–802.

[23] Taylor SF, Tandon R, Shipley JE, et al. Sleep onset REM periods in schizophrenic patients. Biol Psychiatry 1991;30:205–9.

[24] Poulin J, Daoust A, Forest G, Stip E, et al. Sleep architecture and its clinical correlates in first episode and neuroleptic-naive patients with schizophrenia. Schizophr Res 2003;62:147–53.

[25] Feinberg I, Braum N, Koresko RL, et al. Stage 4 sleep in schizophrenia. Arch Gen Psychiatry 1969;21:262–6.

[26] Caldwell DF, Domino EF. Electroencephalographic and eye movement patterns during sleep in chronic schizophrenic patients. Electroencephalogr Clin Neurophysiol 1967;22: 414–20.

[27] Traub AC. Sleep stage deficits in chronic schizophrenia. Psychol Rep 1972;31:815–20.

[28] Feinberg I. Schizophrenia: caused by a fault in programmed synaptic elimination during adolescence? J Psychiatr Res 1983;17:319–34.

[29] Thaker GK, Wagman AMI, Tamminga CA. Sleep polygraphy in schizophrenia: methodological issues. Biol Psychiatry 1990;28:240–6.

[30] Zarcone VP, Benson KL. BPRS symptom factors and sleep variables in schizophrenia. Psychiatry Res 1997;66:111–20.

[31] Neylan TC, van Kammen DP, Kelley ME, et al. Sleep in schizophrenic patients on and off haloperidol therapy. Arch Gen Psychiatry 1992;49:643–9.

[32] Howland RH. Sleep-onset rapid eye movement periods in neuropsychiatric disorders: implications for the pathophysiology of psychosis. J Nerv Ment Dis 1997;185: 730–8.

[33] Tekell JL, Hoffman R, Hendrickse W, et al. High frequency EEG activity during sleep: characteristics in schizophrenia and depression. Clin EEG Neurosci 2005;36:25–35.

[34] Van Kammen DP, van Kammen WM, Peters J, et al. Decreased slow-wave sleep and enlarged lateral ventricles in schizophrenia. Neuropsychopharmacology 1988;1:265–71.

[35] Keshavan MS, Pettegrew JW, Reynolds CF III, et al. Biological correlates of slow wave sleep deficits in functional psychoses: ^{31}P-magnetic resonance spectroscopy. Psychiatry Res 1995;57:91–100.

[36] Keshavan MS, Miewald J, Haas G, et al. Slow-wave sleep and symptomatology in schizophrenia and related psychotic disorders. J Psychiatry Res 1995;29:303–14.

[37] Kato M, Kajimura N, Okuma T, et al. Association between delta waves during sleep and negative symptoms in schizophrenia. Neuropsychobiology 1999;39:165–72.

[38] Yang C, Winkelman J. Clinical significance of sleep EEG abnormalities in chronic schizophrenia. Schiz Res 2006;82:251–60.

[39] Keshavan MS, Reynolds CF, Miewald J, et al. Slow-wave sleep deficits and outcome in schizophrenia and schizoaffective disorder. Acta Psychiatr Scand 1995;91:289–92.

[40] Goldman M, Tandon R, DeQuardo JR, et al. Biological predictors of 1-year outcome in schizophrenia in males and females. Schizophr Res 1996;21:65–73.

[41] Manoach DA, Cain MS, Vangel MG, et al. A failure of sleep-dependent procedural learning in chronic, medicated schizophrenia. Biol Psychiatry 2004;56:951–6.

[42] Forest G, Poulin J, Daoust A-M, et al. Attention and non-REM sleep in neuroleptic-naive persons with schizophrenia and control participants. Psychiatry Res, in press.

[43] Göder R, Boigs M, Braun S, et al. Impairment of visuospatial memory is associated with decreased slow wave sleep in schizophrenia. J Psychiatr Res 2004;38:591–9.

[44] Benson KL, Sullivan EV, Lim KO, et al. Slow wave sleep and CT measures of brain morphology in schizophrenia. Psychiatry Res 1996;60:125–34.

[45] Keshavan MS, Reynolds CF III, Ganguli R, et al. Electroencephalographic sleep and cerebral morphology in functional psychosis: a preliminary study with computed tomography. Psychiatry Res 1991;39:293–301.

[46] Riemann D, Hohagen F, Krieger S, et al. Cholinergic REM induction test: muscarinic supersensitivity underlies polysomnographic findings in both depression and schizophrenia. J Psychiat Res 1994;28:195–210.

[47] Benson KL, Faull KF, Zarcone VP. Evidence for the role of serotonin in the regulation of slow wave sleep in schizophrenia. Sleep 1991;14:133–9.

[48] Mignot E. A commentary on the neurobiology of the hypocretin/orexin system. Neuropsychopharmacology 2001;25:S5–13.

[49] Nishino S, Ripley B, Mignot E, et al. CSF Hypocretin-1 levels in schizophrenia and controls: relationship to sleep architecture. Psychiatry Res 2002;110:1–7.

[50] Bymaster FP, Calligaro DO, Falcone JF, et al. Radioreceptor binding profile of the atypical antipsychotic olanzapine. Neuropsychopharmacology 1996;14:87–96.

[51] Meltzer HY, Li Z, Kaneda Y, et al. Serotonin receptors: their key role in drugs to treat schizophrenia. Prog Neuropsychopharmacol Biol Psychiatry 2003;27:1159–72.

[52] Lublin H, Eberhard J, Levander S. Current therapy issues and unmet clinical needs in the treatment of schizophrenia: a review of the new generation antipsychotics. Int Clin Psychopharmaol 2005;20:183–98.

[53] Newcomer JW. Second-generation (atypical) antipsychotics and metabolic effects: a comprehensive literature review. CNS Drugs 2005;19(Suppl 1):1–93.

[54] Lieberman JA, Stroup TS, McEvoy JP, et al. Effectiveness of antipsychotic drugs in patients with chronic schizophrenia. N Engl J Med 2005;353:1209–23.

[55] Hofer A, Kemmler G, Eder U, et al. Attitudes toward antipsychotics among outpatient clinic attendees with schizophrenia. J Clin Psychiatry 2002;63:49–53.

[56] Kaplan J, Dawson S, Vaughan T, et al. Effect of prolonged chlorpromazine administration on the sleep of chronic schizophrenics. Arch Gen Psychiatry 1974;31:62–6.

[57] Taylor SF, Tandon R, Shipley JE, et al. Effect of neuroleptic treatment on polysomnographic measures in schizophrenia. Biol Psychiatry 1991;30:904–12.

[58] Nofzinger EA, van Kammen DP, Gilbertson MW, et al. Electroencephalographic sleep in clinically stable schizophrenic patients: two-weeks versus six-weeks neuroleptic free. Biol Psychiatry 1993;33:829–35.

[59] Keshavan MS, Reynolds CF III, Miewald JM, et al. A longitudinal study of EEG sleep in schizophrenia. Psychiatry Res 1996;59:203–11.

[60] Maixner S, Tandon R, Eiser A, et al. Effects of antipsychotic treatment on polysomnographic measures in schizophrenia: a replication and extension. Am J Psychiatry 1998;155:1600–2.

[61] Wetter TC, Lauer CJ, Gillich G, et al. The electroencephalographic sleep pattern in schizophrenic patients treated with clozapine or classical antipsychotic drugs. J Psychiat Res 1996;30:411–9.

[62] Yamashita H, Mori K, Nagao M, et al. Effects of changing from typical to atypical antipsychotic drugs on subjective sleep quality in patients with schizophrenia in a Japanese population. J Clin Psychiatry 2004;65:1525–30.

[63] Hinze-Selch D, Mullington J, Orth A, et al. Effects of clozapine on sleep: a longitudinal study. Biol Psychiatry 1997;42:260–6.

[64] Lee JH, Woo JI, Meltzer HY. Effects of clozapine on sleep measures and sleep-associated changes in growth hormone and cortisol in patients with schizophrenia. Psychiatry Res 2001;103:157–66.

[65] Salin-Pascual RJ, Herrera-Estrella M, Galicia-Polo L, et al. Olanzapine acute administration in schizophrenic patients increases delta sleep and sleep efficiency. Biol Psychiatry 1999;46:141–3.

[66] Yamashita H, Morinobu S, Yamawaki S, et al. Effect of risperidone on sleep in schizophrenia: a comparison with haloperidol. Psychiatry Res 2002;109:137–42.

[67] Cohrs S, Rodenbeck A, Guan Z, et al. Sleep-promoting properties of quetiapine in healthy subjects. Psychopharmacology (Berl) 2004;174:421–9.

[68] Monteleone P, Maj M, Fusco M, et al. Depressed nocturnal plasma melatonin levels in drug-free paranoid schizophrenics. Schizophr Res 1992;7:77–84.

[69] Vigano D, Lissoni P, Rovelli F, et al. A study of light/dark rhythm of melatonin in relation to cortisol and prolactin secretion in schizophrenia. Neuroendocrinol Lett 2001;22:137–41.

[70] Robinson S, Rosca P, Durst R, et al. Serum melatonin levels in schizophrenic and schizoaffective hospitalized patients. Acta Psychiatr Scand 1991;84:221–4.

[71] Shamir E, Laudon M, Barak Y, et al. Melatonin improves sleep quality of patients with chronic schizophrenia. J Clin Psychiatry 2000;61:373–7.

[72] Burke M, Sebastian CS. Treatment of clozapine sedation. Am J Psychiatry 1993;150:1900–1.

[73] Makela EH, Miller K, Cutlip WD. Three case reports of modafinil use in treating sedation induced by antipsychotic medications. J Clin Psychiatry 2003;64:485–6.

[74] Rosenthal MH, Bryant SL. Benefits of adjunct modafinil in an open-label, pilot study in patients with schizophrenia. Clin Neuropharmacol 2004;27:38–43.

[75] Narendran R, Young CM, Valenti AM, et al. Is psychosis exacerbated by modafinil? Arch Gen Psychiatry 2002;59:292–3.
[76] Spence SA, Green RD, Wilkinson ID, et al. Modafinil modulates anterior cingulate function in chronic schizophrenia. Br J Psychiatry 2005;187:55–61.
[77] Charney DS, Kales A, Soldatos CR, et al. Somnambulistic-like episodes secondary to combined lithium-neuroleptic treatment. Br J Psychiatry 1979;135:418–24.
[78] Kolivakis TT, Margolese HC, Beauclair L, et al. Olanzapine-induced somnambulism. Am J Psychiatry 2001;158:1158.
[79] Allen RP, Earley CJ. Restless legs syndrome: a review of clinical and pathophysiologic features. J Clin Neurophysiol 2001;18:128–47.
[80] Benson KL, Zarcone VP. Sleep abnormalities in schizophrenia and other psychotic disorders. Rev Psychiatry 1994;13:677–705.
[81] Ancoli-Israel S, Martin J, Jones DW, et al. Sleep-disordered breathing and periodic limb movements in sleep in older patients with schizophrenia. Biol Psychiatry 1999;45: 1426–32.
[82] Kraus T, Schuld A, Pollmächer T. Periodic leg movements in sleep and restless legs syndrome probably caused by olanzapine. J Clin Psychopharmacol 1999;19:478–9.
[83] Wetter TC, Brunner J, Bronisch T. Restless legs syndrome probably induced by risperidone treatment. Pharmacopsychiatry 2002;35:109–11.
[84] Pinninti NR, Mago R, Townsend J, et al. Periodic restless legs syndrome associated with quetiapine use: a case report. J Clin Psychopharmacol 2005;25:617–8.
[85] Sharafkhaneh A, Giray N, Richardson P, et al. Association of psychiatric disorders and sleep apnea in a large cohort. Sleep 2005;28:1405–11.
[86] Takahashi KI, Shimizu T, Sugita T, et al. Prevalence of sleep-related respiratory disorders in 101 schizophrenic patients. Psychiatry Clin Neurosci 1998;52:229–31.
[87] Winkelman JW. Schizophrenia, obesity, and obstructive sleep apnea. J Clin Psychiatry 2001;62:8–11.
[88] Wirshing DA, Pierre JM, Wirshing WC. Sleep apnea associated with antipsychotic-induced obesity. J Clin Psychiatry 2002;63:369–70.
[89] Boufidis S, Kosmidis MH, Bozikas VP, et al. Treatment outcome of obstructive sleep apnea syndrome in a patient with schizophrenia: case report. Int J Psychiatry Med 2003;33: 305–10.

Sleep and Anxiety Disorders

Thomas A. Mellman, MD

Department of Psychiatry, Howard University Mental Health Clinic, 530 College Street, Washington, DC, 20059, USA

S leep disturbances frequently are associated with and can comprise core features of anxiety disorders. Two anxiety disorders feature sleep disturbances among their diagnostic criteria in the *Diagnostic and Statistical Manual of Mental Disorders, Fourth Edition (DSM-IV)* [1]. Posttraumatic stress disorder (PTSD) criteria include nightmares with trauma-related content and difficulty initiating and maintaining sleep, which is a common definition of insomnia. Insomnia also is a symptom criterion for generalized anxiety disorder (GAD). Panic disorder, with and without agoraphobia, also is associated with complaints of difficulty initiating and maintaining sleep in many studies. There also is interest in the phenomenon of panic attacks that arise from sleep, which are not an uncommon occurrence with panic disorder. Sleep disturbances can occur with, but seem to be less salient features of, obsessive-compulsive disorder (OCD) and specific and social phobic disorders. In addition to comprising prominent features, insomnia, as with depression, is a risk factor for the subsequent onset of anxiety disorders There is overlap between interventions that target insomnia and other sleep disturbances and those that are used in treating anxiety disorders. Overlapping approaches include medications and cognitive behavioral strategies that target worry, tension, and maladaptive cognitions. Optimal sequencing or integration of treatments targeting anxiety and sleep disturbance is not well investigated, however.

Finally, links between anxiety and sleep disturbances may be relevant to understanding mechanisms and dysfunctions of arousal regulation that underlie both types of problems. Whereas sleep is a necessary and restorative state of diminished cortical arousal, anxiety and fear states manifest with heightened cortical and peripheral arousal. Increased arousal also is implicated when sleep initiation or maintenance is disturbed.

Polysomnographic (PSG) studies provide objective information regarding disturbances in sleep initiation and maintenance. This tool and other laboratory methods applied to sleep can offer unique perspectives on the function of the neurobiologic systems involved in arousal, sleep, and anxiety phenomena.

E-mail address: TMellman@Howard.edu

0193-953X/06/$ – see front matter
doi:10.1016/j.psc.2006.08.005

In the following sections, clinical issues and laboratory information when available regarding sleep aspects of specific anxiety disorders are discussed, followed by a discussion of treatment issues that interface sleep and anxiety disorders.

SLEEP IN SPECIFIC AND SOCIAL PHOBIAS
Fear and avoidance of situations are the key features of phobic disorders. Because these situations occur during interactions with the environment during wakefulness, sleep disturbances typically are not regarded as central to or commonly associated with these conditions. Nonetheless, persons who have phobic disorders may experience anticipatory anxiety that affects their sleep and dreams. Investigations relating sleep to phobias are limited. In one study, persons who had social phobia subjectively reported poorer sleep quality, longer sleep latency, more frequent sleep disturbance, and increased daytime dysfunction compared with controls [2]. However, the one pilot study of social phobia identified that used PSG, reported normal findings [3]. Clark and colleagues [4] noted that sleep architecture was similar in depressed persons who did and did not have simple phobias (the term that predated the *DSM-IV*). A study on parasomnias, including sleep terrors and sleepwalking, among adolescents found an increased comorbidity with simple phobias and other anxiety disorders [5].

SLEEP IN OBSESSIVE-COMPULSIVE DISORDER
Sleep disturbances also are not included in either the core syndromal manifestations or prominent associated features of OCD. An early PSG study noted impaired sleep maintenance and a reduced latency to rapid eye movement (REM) sleep in a group with persons who had OCD, which suggests a possible linkage between OCD and affective illness [6]. Two more recent PSG studies, however, of persons who had OCD failed to replicate these results, reporting instead that the sleep patterns of persons who had OCD essentially were normal [7,8].

SLEEP IN GENERALIZED ANXIETY DISORDER
There is a high degree of overlap between GAD and insomnia. *DSM-IV* criteria for GAD are chronic worry and three of six additional criteria that include difficulty initiating or maintaining sleep or restless and unsatisfying sleep. Two of the other symptom criteria, fatigue and irritability, can be consequences of sleep loss. In addition, the principal attribute of GAD, excessive worry or apprehensive expectation, commonly is implicated in the genesis and maintenance of insomnia problems.

Ohayon and coworkers [9] find that the comorbidity of GAD and insomnia is greater than for all of the other psychiatric disorders surveyed. Studies using objective sleep recordings corroborate the reported associations of GAD and insomnia by demonstrating impaired sleep initiation and maintenance in persons who have GAD [10–12]. High comorbidity with major depression has generated interest in comparing biologic markers of the disorders. Latency to

REM sleep was normal in these studies, in contrast to findings from major depression where REM sleep latency is reduced [10–12].

Consistent with their high degree of overlap and comorbidity, there also is substantial overlap of treatment approaches for GAD and insomnia. Overlapping approaches include the use of medications that target benzodiazepine receptors and psychotherapeutic interventions that target excessive worry. Application of these approaches in treating co-occurring generalized anxiety and sleep disturbances is discussed later.

SLEEP IN PANIC DISORDER

The core feature of panic disorder is recurring panic attacks that occur in a sudden, crescendo-like, and, at times unpredictable, manner. Panic attacks can emerge from sleep. Panic disorder also typically features chronic anxiety related to anticipating subsequent attacks and phobic avoidance (agoraphobia). Panic attacks arising from sleep (sleep panic attacks) are suggested to condition fear and apprehension of sleep resulting in secondary insomnia [13]. Insomnia conditioned by sleep panic and theories that panic disorder represents an endogenous type of dysregulation of arousal lead to the prediction that panic disorder is associated with impairment in initiating and maintaining sleep. Surveys document that insomnia is more frequent in patients who have panic disorder than in control populations [14,15]. Most [16–19] but not all [20,21] published studies of panic disorder that use objective methods of sleep recording (PSG) find evidence of impaired sleep initiation and maintenance. One of these studies finds increased motor activity during sleep [21]. Although there seems to be an association between excess body movement during sleep and panic disorder, two studies indicate the paradox that overall movement during sleep is reduced on nights when patients experience sleep panic attacks [16,22].

Survey data note associations between sleep complaints and comorbid depression in persons who have panic disorder [20]. There are several possible explanations for the relationship between sleep disturbance and the presence of depression in persons who have panic disorder. First, much of the associated sleep disturbance may be the result of depressive illness that commonly coexists with panic disorder. The two studies that failed to identify any impairment in sleep duration and maintenance specifically excluded depression. One of the studies documenting sleep disturbance in panic disorder, however, excluded depressive illness and it is uncertain whether or not depression accounted for the entire sleep disturbance documented in the remaining positive studies. A second consideration is that comorbid depression may be more common with a more severe variant of panic disorder that also features sleep disturbance. Because insomnia is a risk factor for the subsequent onset of depression [23,24], a third possibility is that depression is more likely to evolve as a comorbid condition when panic disorder features disturbed sleep.

Sleep panic attacks are a not uncommon occurrence in persons who have panic disorder. In a study that monitored panic attacks prospectively, 18%

occurred during sleep hours [25]. In surveys and clinical evaluations, 33% to 71% of panic disorder populations reported having experienced sleep panic attacks [14,26–28]. As many as a third of panic disorder patients experience sleep panic as or more frequently than wake panic attacks [13,14]. It is not known how common it is for patients to have only sleep panic; however, in the author's experience, patients who exclusively panic from sleep are rare. These episodes are described as being awakened with a jolt and feature apprehension and somatic symptoms, similar to panic attacks that are triggered during wake states. Studies that capture sleep panic attacks during PSG recordings find that the episodes were preceded by either stage 2 or stage 3 of non-REM sleep [16,29]. Mellman and Uhde [16] note more specifically that the sleep panic attacks originated during the transition from stage 2 into early slow wave sleep, which is a period of diminishing arousal. Slow wave sleep also is a state where cognitive activity is at a relative nadir [30]. The phenomenon of sleep panic during sleep indicates that in addition to the more intuitively explainable circumstance of panic attacks evolving from states of heightening arousal where apprehension is building, panic can be precipitated during states of diminishing arousal. The paradox of panic attacks arising during states of diminishing arousal seems consistent with theories of endogenous, physiologic mechanisms for triggering anxiety. Specific mechanisms postulated to underlie sleep panic include increased sensitivity to increased carbon dioxide blood levels [31], irregular breathing during slow wave sleep [32], and rebound noradrenergic surges [16,17]. A cognitive mechanism of sensitivity to and catastrophic interpretation of interoceptive stimuli also is suggested to underlie sleep panic [27].

The greater sensitivity of panic disorder patients to pharmacologic challenges that induce panic has provided an important research paradigm for investigating the psychobiology of panic attacks. Sodium lactate and pentagastrin challenges, which trigger panic attacks from wake states, are demonstrated also to trigger panic attacks from sleep [33,34]. Greater cardiac and respiratory responses to lactate infusion during sleep absent panic awakenings also are noted [17,35]. Findings that panicogenic triggers can elicit attacks from sleep states indicate that elevated basal arousal is not required for experimentally inducing panic.

The significance of sleep panic also is explored by comparing patients who experience sleep panic attacks with patients who experience panic attacks only from wake states. Associations of sleep panic with early illness onset, higher symptom load, depression, and suicidal ideation suggest a relationship to a more severe variant of the illness [26,36]. Patients who have sleep panic also are noted to experience anxiety from relaxation and hypnosis and to have less agoraphobic avoidance and fewer catastrophic cognitions compared with panic patients who do not experience sleep panic [14,27,37,38]. Thus, having sleep panic seems to mark a propensity to having panic attacks triggered by lower arousal and for attacks to occur relatively independently of situational and cognitive stimuli that are associated with nonsleep panic. The association with markers of severity may reflect a stronger disease diathesis.

Sleep panic attacks can present in a manner that mimics medical conditions. Holter cardiac monitoring or overnight poysomnography may be indicated when associated symptomatology suggests cardiac arrhythmias or sleep breathing disorders. Patient education and informed reassurance are helpful to patients who have these frequently upsetting occurrences. Sleep panic attacks are observed anecdotally to respond to the antidepressant types of antipanic medications but not necessarily benzodiazepine anxiolytics [13].

SLEEP IN POSTTRAUMATIC STRESS DISORDER

Sleep disturbances, including trauma-related nightmares and difficulty initiating and maintaining sleep, are *DSM-IV* criteria and prominent symptoms of PTSD, which is an anxiety disorder that develops in some but not all people who are exposed to severely threatening events [39,40]. Nightmares and insomnia also seem to be common in the early aftermath of trauma, especially among those who are developing PTSD [41–44]. Furthermore, sleep disruption leads to fatigue and irritability, which are daytime symptoms of PTSD. Sleep disruption also may interfere with healthy emotional adaptation and regulation and, thereby, contribute to the early development of the disorder.

Findings from sleep laboratory studies have not yielded a consensus regarding the fundamental nature of sleep disturbances in PTSD. All but a few of the studies are focused on the chronic phase of the disorder and many include only male war veterans. These studies are mixed in terms of finding objective indices of impaired sleep initiation and maintenance (reviewed in Mellman [45] and Lavie [46]). There also is controversy as to whether or not PTSD is associated with sleep breathing abnormalities. Krakow and colleagues [47] find evidence for sleep-disordered breathing in all but 4 of 44 subjects seeking treatment who were referred for PSG. There was no increase in sleep-disordered breathing with PTSD, however, in a study of community-recruited participants [48].

Evidence for abnormalities related to REM sleep in PTSD is more consistent. Increased phasic motor activity and eye movement density during REM sleep is reported in combat veterans who have PTSD [49–51]. Nightmares and other symptomatic awakenings arise disproportionately from REM sleep [52,53]. Breslau and coworkers recently reported more frequent transitions from REM sleep to stage 1 or wake in a community sample with either lifetime only (ie, remitted) or current PTSD compared with trauma-exposed and trauma-unexposed controls [48]. Thus, there is converging evidence for disruptions of REM sleep continuity (symptomatic awakenings, increased awakening/arousals, and motor activity) and increased REM activation (eye movement density) with chronic PTSD.

When PTSD exists for many years, a variety of secondary factors can influence sleep patterns and complicate their investigation. In addition to providing data that is less confounded than studies of chronic PTSD, an understanding of sleep alterations during the early aftermath of trauma and their relationship to

PTSD could have implications for understanding the pathogenesis of the disorder and rationales for preventive interventions.

Trauma-related nightmares are among the *DSM-IV* criteria for PTSD. Mellman and colleagues evaluated relationships of recalled dream content elicited within a month of traumatic injuries with the development of PTSD. Reports of dreams rated as "highly similar" to the traumatic experience and distressing were associated with concurrent and subsequent PTSD severity. The trauma-exposed group who did not develop PTSD subsequently either did not recall dreaming or reported dreams that did not depict actual memories, although some represented threatening scenarios. The investigators theorized that dreams with highly replicative content represent a failure of adaptive emotional memory processing that is a normal function of REM sleep and dreaming [44].

Insomnia also is a common feature of acute posttraumatic reactions. Green finds insomnia the most frequent symptom endorsed by survivors in the aftermath of a natural disaster [41]. Koren and colleagues find that complaints of insomnia and excessive daytime sleepiness 1 month after motor vehicle accidents predicted being diagnosed with PTSD at 3 months [43].

There is a limited number of studies that used objective recordings of sleep after trauma. An early report of three cases of "acute combat fatigue" described "markedly disrupted sleep" and "rare or absent REM episodes" [54]. In contrast, whereas Koren and colleagues [43] find an association of early subjective reports of sleep disturbance with the development of PTSD, these investigators did not find differences in early actigraphic measurements of sleep initiation or maintenance in their prospective study of traffic accident victims or in PSG measures in a subgroup recorded 1 year later [55]. Mellman and coworkers [56] report PSG findings from PSG recordings conducted within a month of trauma in 21 recently injured patients and 10 healthy controls. Sleep duration was reduced and REM eye movement density was elevated in the recently trauma exposed, injured patients compared with healthy controls but were similar among those who did and did not develop PTSD. The patients who were developing PTSD had shorter continuous periods of REM sleep before stage shifts or arousals. This finding suggests a relationship between fragmented patterns of REM sleep with the early development of PTSD.

A role for noradrenergic functioning in sleep disturbances during the early development of PTSD is suggested by previously established relationships of noradrenergic activity with PTSD [57] and PTSD sleep disturbances [58] and the noradrenergic signal terminating REM sleep [59]. Mellman and coworkers [60] also evaluated heart rate variability during sleep after trauma, which indexes autonomic regulation of heart rate, including sympathetic nervous system activity [61], which is a peripheral manifestation of noradrenergic function. The index of sympathetic nervous system activity, the low-frequency–to–high-frequency ratio, was greater in the subgroup that developed PTSD during their initial REM sleep periods.

In summary, subjective sleep complaints are common in the aftermath of trauma, especially among those developing PTSD. Nightmares that are similar to trauma memories seem to be relatively specific to developing PTSD. More recent studies do not indicate that sleep initiation and maintenance is markedly more impaired among those developing PTSD. Findings of Mellman and coworkers [56,60] preliminarily implicate fragmented patterns of and increased sympathetic nervous system activity during REM sleep. Thus, in both studies of chronic PTSD and the more limited data from acute trauma, objective sleep recordings do not indicate consistently the degree of impairment of sleep initiation and maintenance that might be expected from subjective reports of those developing or who have established PTSD. There is somewhat converging data from studies of chronic and acute PTSD implicating disruption of REM sleep. How this phenomenon relates to the prominent role of nightmares in the disorder and their divergence with normal REM sleep associated dreaming [62] is an important question.

TREATMENT AND PREVENTION

Sleep disturbances are are associated with anxiety disorders, in particular GAD, panic disorder, and PTSD. In contrast to melancholic subtypes of depression where mood paradoxically can improve, anxiety disorders do not benefit and can worsen from sleep deprivation [63–65]. Insomnia also is found a prospective risk factor for psychiatric disorders, including anxiety disorders [23,24]. Therefore, in addition to alleviating distress from insomnia, amelioration of sleep disturbances possibly can have therapeutic impact on other symptoms and serve to prevent relapse and exacerbation.

Therapies for anxiety disorders and sleep disturbances overlap. Cognitive behavioral treatments developed for insomnia have well-established efficacy [66]. One intervention component is providing instruction on sleep hygiene, including maintaining consistent bedtimes and wake times, avoiding maladaptive use of substances, and not spending excessive time awake in bed. Additional components sometimes include relaxation techniques and identifying and challenging dysfunctional beliefs that perpetuate insomnia. Anxiety management, exposure, and cognitive restructuring are key components of effective cognitive behavioral treatments for anxiety disorders [67]. Thus, it seems that behavioral interventions designed for insomnia and anxiety disorders can be applied synergistically. One study documents improvement in insomnia symptoms in association with cognitive behavioral treatment of GAD [68]. In contrast, De-Viva and colleagues [69] identified a group of patients who had significant residual insomnia who had otherwise benefited from cognitive behavioral treatment for PTSD. They further describe a series of these cases where the residual insomnia was reduced by a subsequently administered cognitive behavioral intervention focused specifically on the insomnia. These observations notwithstanding, development and evaluation of sequential or integrated treatments for insomnia and anxiety disorders are limited.

Various benzodiazepine receptor agonist medications are approved and marketed for hypnotic indications or treatment of anxiety disorders, particularly for GAD. One study finds agents that are marketed and approved as hypnotics had benefits toward daytime anxiety in treating insomnia associated with GAD [70]. The novel agents, pregabalin and tiagebine, that also target benzodiazepine receptors or related γ-aminobutyric acid (GABA)-ergic neurotransmission are reported to benefit insomnia symptoms associated with GAD, although neither have FDA approval for GAD or insomnia [71,72].

The newer antidepressant medications, in particular those in the selective serotonin reuptake inhibitor (SSRI) and selective serotonin and norepinephrine inhibitor (SNRI) categories, have become established as effective for a range of anxiety disorders. They also have advantages with respect to tolerance and dependence concerns relative to benzodiazepines and now are considered first-line treatments for panic disorder, social phobia, GAD, OCD, and PTSD. The effects on sleep of these agents vary between agents and to a greater degree between individuals and some are noted to stimulate insomnia [73]. Among the novel antidepressants, mirtazipine, which is neither an SSRI nor an SNRI, tends to have sedating/sleep effects. Mirtazapine recently was reported to have been beneficial to patients who have GAD in a preliminary open label trial [74], although it is not FDA approved for this indication. A study using the SSRI, citalopram, for late-life anxiety disorders indicates improved sleep with treatment in this subpopulation [75].

Currently, SSRIs, specifically sertraline and paroxetine, are the only agents approved by the FDA for the treatment of PTSD. Benefits of these treatments tend to be modest and typically do not include reductions in sleep disturbance. Therefore, adjunctive interventions often are used, often with the intent of targeting nightmare and insomnia symptoms [76]. Among these, there is support from controlled trials for adjunctive prescription of olanzapine [77] and prazosin [78], which are not FDA approved for PTSD. A behavioral intervention that involves exposure and restructuring of dream content, referred to as imagery rehearsal, also is found to benefit sleep disturbances of PTSD [79].

The model presented in the previous section regarding compromised REM sleep functions related to emotional memory processing and disinhibited noradrenerigic signaling provides a framework for conceptualizing the benefits of these treatments. Imagery rehearsal seems to facilitate habituation to and further processing of trauma memories expressed in dreams that are disruptive to sleep. The apparent benefits of prazosin and possibly olanzapine may relate to interfering with the response to noradrenergic signaling hypothesized to disrupt REM sleep. Applying these and related strategies holds promise for ameliorating disturbed sleep during the early aftermath of trauma and perhaps contributing to the prevention of PTSD.

SUMMARY

Sleep disturbances commonly are associated with anxiety disorders, in particular GAD, panic disorder, and PTSD. Sleep loss may exacerbate and contribute to relapse of these conditions. Core features of panic disorder and PTSD occur in relation to sleep (sleep panic attacks and re-experiencing nightmares). Investigation of sleep in anxiety disorders provides clues to mechanisms of arousal regulation relevant to insomnia and pathologic anxiety. Established treatments for anxiety disorders and insomnia have many overlapping components; however, optimal sequencing and integration of the approaches remain underinvestigated.

Acknowledgment

The author wishes to acknowledge Denver Brown for her assistance in preparing this article.

References

[1] American Psychiatric Association. Diagnostic and statistical manual of mental disorders. 4th edition. Washington, DC: American Psychiatric Press; 1994.

[2] Stein M, Kroft C, Walker J. Sleep impairment in patients with social phobia. Psychiatry Res 1993;49(Suppl 3):251–6.

[3] Brown T, Black B, Uhde T. The sleep architecture of social phobia. Biol Psychiatry 1994;35(Suppl 6):420–1.

[4] Clark C, Gillin J, Golshan S. Do differences in sleep architecture exist between depressives with comorbid simple phobia as compared with pure depressives? J Affect Disord 1995;33: 251–5.

[5] Gau S, Soong W. Psychiatric comorbidity of adolescents with sleep terrors or sleepwalking: a case-control study. Aust N Z J Psychiatry 1999;33:734–9.

[6] Insel T, Gillin J, Moore A, et al. The sleep of patients with obsessive-compulsive disorder. Arch Gen Psychiatry 1982;39:1372–7.

[7] Robinson D, Walsleben J, Pollack S, et al. Nocturnal polysomnography in obsessive-compulsive disorder. Psychiatry Res 1998;80:257–63.

[8] Hohagan F, Lis S, Krieger S, et al. Sleep EEG of patients with obsessive-compulsive disorder. Eur Arch Psychiatry Clin Neurosci 1994;243:273–8.

[9] Oyahan M, Caulet M, Lemoine P. Comorbidity of mental and insomnia disorders in the general population. Compr Psychiatry 1998;39:185–97.

[10] Saletu-Zyhlarz G, Saletu B, Anderer P, et al. Nonorganic insomnia in generalized anxiety disorder. Controlled studies on sleep, awakening and daytime vigilance utilizing polysomnography and EEG mapping. Neuropsychobiology 1997;36:117–29.

[11] Arriaga F, Paiva T. Clinical and EEG sleep changes in primary dysthymia and generalized anxiety: a comparison with normal controls. Neuropsychobiology 1990–1991;24:109–14.

[12] Papdimitriou G, Kerkhofs M, Kempenaers C, et al. EEG sleep studies in patients with generalized anxiety disorder. Psychiatry Res 1988;26:183–90.

[13] Mellman T, Uhde T. Patients with frequent sleep panic: clinical findings and response to medication treatment. J Clin Psychiatry 1990;51:513–6.

[14] Mellman T, Uhde T. Sleep panic attacks: new clinical findings and theoretical implications. Am J Psychiatry 1989;146:1204–7.

[15] Stein M, Chartier M, Walker J. Sleep in nondepressed patients with panic disorder: I. Systematic assessment of subjective sleep quality and sleep disturbance. Sleep 1993;16: 724–6.

[16] Mellman T, Uhde T. Electroencephalographic sleep in panic disorder. A focus on sleep-related panic attacks. Arch Gen Psychiatry 1989;46:178–84.

[17] Sloan E, Natarajan M, Baker B, et al. Nocturnal and daytime panic attacks- comparison of sleep architecture, heart rate variablity, and response to sodium lactate challenge. SociBiol Psychiatry 1999;45:1313–20.

[18] Lydiard R, Zealberg J, Laraia M, et al. Electroencephalography during sleep of patients with panic disorder. J Neuropsychiatry Clin Neurosci 1989;1:372–6.

[19] Arriaga F, Paiva T, Matos-Pires A, et al. The sleep of non-depressed patients with panic disorder: a comparison with normal controls. Acta Psychiatr Scand 1996;93:191–4.

[20] Stein M, Enns M, Kryger M. Sleep in nondepressed patients with panic disorder. II. Polysom-nographic assessment of sleep architecture and sleep continuity. J Affect Disord 1993;28: 1–6.

[21] Uhde T, Roy-Byrne P, Gillin J, et al. The sleep of patients with panic disorder. Psychiatry Res 1984;12:251–9.

[22] Brown T, Uhde TW. Sleep panic attacks: a micro-movement analysis. Depress Anxiety 2003;18:214–20.

[23] Ford D, Kamerow D. Epidemiologic study of sleep disturbances and psychiatric disorders. An opportunity for prevention? JAMA 1989;262:1479–84.

[24] Breslau N, Roth T, Rosenthal L, et al. Sleep disturbance and psychiatric disorders: a longitu-dinal epidemiological study of young adults. Biol Psychiatry 1996;39:411–8.

[25] Taylor C, Skeikh J, Agras S, et al. Ambulatory heart rate changes in patients with panic attacks. Am J Psychiatry 1986;143:478–82.

[26] Krystal J, Woods S, Hill C, et al. Characteristics of panic attack subtypes: assessment of spontaneous panic, situational panic, sleep panic, and limited symptom attacks. Compr Psychiatry 1991;32:474–80.

[27] Craske M, Lang A, Rowe M, et al. Presleep attributions about arousal during sleep: noctur-nal panic. J Abnorm Psychol 2002;111:53–62.

[28] Shapiro C, Sloan E. Nocturnal panic: an underrecognized entity. J Psychosom Res 1998;44:21–3.

[29] Hauri P, Freidman M, Ravaris C, et al. Sleep in patients with spontaneous panic attacks. Sleep 1989 12:323–37.

[30] Hobson JA, Pace-Schott E, Stickgold R. Dreaming and the brain: towards a cognitive neuro-science of conscious states. Behav Brain Sci 2000;23:793–842.

[31] Klein D. False suffocation alarms, spontaneous panics, and related conditions: an integra-tive hypothesis. Arch Gen Psychiatry 1993;50:306–17.

[32] Stein M, Millar T, Larsen D, et al. Irregular breathing during sleep in patients with panic dis-order. Am J Psychiatry 1995;152:1168–73.

[33] Koenigsberg H, Pollack C, Ferro D. Can panic be induced in deep sleep? Examining the necessity of cognitive processing for panic. Depress Anxiety 1998;8:126–30.

[34] Geraci M, Anderson T, Slate-Cothren S, et al. Pentagastrin-induced sleep panic attacks: panic in the absence of elevated baseline arousal. Biol Psychiatry 2002;52:1183–9.

[35] Koenigsberg H, Pollack C, Fine J, et al. Cardiac and respiratory activity in panic disorder: effects of sleep and sleep lactate infustions. Am J Psychiatry 1994;151:1148–52.

[36] Labbate L, Pollack M, Otto M, et al. Sleep panic attacks: an association with childhood anxiety and adult psychopathology. Biol Psychiatry 1994;36:57–60.

[37] Tsao J, Craske M. Fear of loss of vigilance: development and preliminary validation of a self-report instrument. Depress Anxiety 2003;18:177–86.

[38] Craske M, Lang A, Mystkowski J, et al. Does nocturnal panic represent a more severe form of panic disorder? J Nerv Ment Dis 2002;190:611–8.

[39] American Psychiatric Association. Diagnostic and statistical manual of mental disorders. 4th ed. Washington, DC: American Psychiatric Press; 1994.

[40] Neylan T, Marmar C, Metzler T, et al. Sleep disturbances in the Vietnam generation: findings from a nationally representative sample of male Vietnam veterans. Am J Psychiatry 1998;155:929–33.

[41] Green BL. Disasters and posttraumatic stress disorder. In: Davidson JRT, Foa EB, editors. Post-traumatic stress disorder DSM-IV and beyond. Washington, DC: American Psychiatric Press; 1993. p. 75–97.

[42] Mellman T, David D, Kulick-Bell R, et al. sleep disturbance and its relationship to psychiatric morbidity following Hurricane Andrew. Am J Psychiatry 1995;152:1659–63.

[43] Koren D, Arnon I, Lavie P, et al. Sleep complaints as early predictors of posttraumatic stress disorder: a 1-year prospective study of injured survivors of motor vehicle accidents. Am J Psychiatry 2002;159:855–7.

[44] Mellman T, David D, Bustamante V, et al. Dreams in the acute aftermath of trauma and their relationship to PTSD. J Trauma Stress 2001;14:241–7.

[45] Mellman TA. Sleep and the pathogenesis of PTSD. In: Shalev A, Yehuda R, McFarlane AC, editors. International handbook of human response to trauma. New York: Plenum Publishing; 2000. p. 299–306.

[46] Lavie P. Current concepts: sleep disturbances in the wake of traumatic events. N Engl J Med 2001;345:1825–32.

[47] Krakow B, Melendrez D, Pederson B, et al. Complex insomnia: insomnia and sleep-disordered breathing in a consecutive series of crime victims with nightmares and PTSD. Biol Psychiatry 2001;49:948–53.

[48] Breslau N, Roth T, Burduvali E, et al. Sleep in lifetime posttraumatic stress disorder: a community-based polysomnographic study. Arch Gen Psychiatry 2004;61:508–16.

[49] Ross R, Ball W, Dinges D, et al. Rapid eye movement sleep disturbance in posttraumatic stress disorder. Biol Psychiatry 1994;35:195–202.

[50] Ross R, Ball W, Dinges D, et al. Motor dysfunction during sleep in posttraumatic stress disorder. Sleep 1994;17:723–32.

[51] Mellman T, Nolan B, Hebding J, et al. A polysomnographic comparison of veterans with combat-related PTSD, depressed men, and non-ill controls. Sleep 1996;20:46–51.

[52] Mellman T, Kulick-Bell R, Ashlock L, et al. Sleep events among veterans with combat-related posttraumatic stress disorder. Am J Psychiatry 1995;152:110–5.

[53] Woodward S, Arsenault N, Santerre C, et al. Polysomnographic characteristics of trauma-related nightmares. Presented at annual meeting of Association of Professional Sleep Societies. Las Vegas, Nevada, June, 2000.

[54] Schlosberg A, Benjamin M. Sleep patterns in three acute combat fatigue cases. J Clin Psychiatry 1978;39:546–9.

[55] Klein E, Koren D, Arnon I, et al. Sleep complaints are not corroborated by objective sleep measures in post-traumatic stress disorder: a 1-year prospective study in survivors of motor vehicle crashes. J Sleep Res 2003;12:35–41.

[56] Mellman T, Bustamante V, Fins A, et al. REM sleep and the early development of posttraumatic stress disorder. Am J Psychiatry 2002;159:1696–701.

[57] Southwick S, Bremner J, Rasmusson A, et al. Role of norepinephrine in the pathophysiology and treatment of posttraumatic stress disorder. Biol Psychiatry 1999;46:1192–204.

[58] Mellman T, Kumar A, Kulick-Bell R, et al. Noradrenergic and sleep measures in combat-related PTSD. Biol Psychiatry 1995;38:174–9.

[59] Hobson J, McCarley R, Wyzinski P. Sleep cycle oscillation: reciprocal discharge by two brainstem neuronal groups. Science 1975;189:55–8.

[60] Mellman T, Knorr B, Pigeon W, et al. Heart rate variability during sleep and the early development of PTSD. Biol Psychiatry 2004;55:953–6.

[61] Task Force of the European Society of Cardiology and the North American Society of Pacing and Electrophysiology. Heart rate variability: standards of measurement, physiological interpretation, and clinical use. Circulation 1996;93:1043–65.

[62] Ross R, Ball W, Sullivan K, et al. Sleep disturbance as the hallmark of post-traumatic stress disorder. Am J Psychiatry 1989;146:697–707.

[63] Labbate L, Johnson M, Lydiard R, et al. Sleep deprivation in panic disorder and obsessive-compulsive disorder. Can J Psychiatry 1997;42:982–3.

[64] Labbate L, Johnson M, Lydiard R, et al. Sleep deprivation in social phobia and generalized anxiety disorder. Biol Psychiatry 1998;43:840–2.

[65] Roy-Byrne P, Uhde T, Post R. Effects of one night's sleep deprivation on mood and behavior in panic disorder. Patients with panic disorder compared with depressed patients and normal controls. Arch Gen Psychiatry 1986;43:895–9.

[66] Morin C, Culbert J, Schwartz S. Nonpharmacological interventions for insomnia: a meta-analysis of treatment efficacy. Am J Psychiatry 1994;151:1172–80.

[67] Falsetti SA, Combs-Lane A, Davis JL. Cognitive behavioral treatment of anxiety disorders. In: Nutt DJ, Ballenger JC, editors. Anxiety disorders. Oxford (UK): Blackwell Science; 2003. p. 425–44.

[68] Belanger L, Morin CM, Langlois F, et al. Insomnia and generalized anxiety disorder: effects of cognitive behavior therapy for gad on insomnia symptoms. J Anxiety Disord 2004;18: 561–71.

[69] DeViva J, Zayfert C, Pigeon W, et al. Treatment of residual insomnia after CBT for PTSD: case studies. J Trauma Stress 2005;18:155–9.

[70] Fontaine R, Beaudry P, Le Morvan P, et al. Zopiclone and triazolam in insomnia associated with generalized anxiety disorder: a placebo-controlled evaluation of efficacy and daytime anxiety. Int Clin Psychopharmacol 1990;5:173–83.

[71] Rickels K, Pollack M, Feltner D, et al. Pregabalin for treatment of generalized anxiety disorder: a 4-week, multicenter, double-blind, placebo-controlled trial of pregabalin and alprazolam. Arch Gen Psychiatry 2005;62:1022–30.

[72] Rosenthal M. Tiagabine for the treatment of generalized anxiety disorder: a randomized, open-label, clinical trial with paroxetine as a positive control. J Clin Psychiatry 2003;64: 1245–9.

[73] Winokur A, Gary KA, Rodner S, et al. Depression, sleep physiology, and antidepressant drugs. Depress Anxiety 2001;14:19–28.

[74] Gambi F, De Berardis D, Campanella D, et al. Mirtazapine treatment of generalized anxiety disorder: a fixed dose, open label study. J Psychopharmacol 2005;19:483–7.

[75] Blank S, Lenze E, Mulsant B, et al. Outcomes of late-life anxiety disorders during 32 weeks of citalopram treatment. J Clin Psychiatry 2006;67:468–72.

[76] Freidman M, Davidson J, Mellman T, et al. Guidelines for treatment of PTSD: pharmacotherapy. J Trauma Stress 2000;13:563–6.

[77] Stein M, Kline N, Matloff J. Adjunctive olanzapine for SSRI-resistant combat-related PTSD: a double-blind, placebo-controlled study. Am J Psychiatry 2003;160:1189–90.

[78] Raskind M, Peskind E, Kanter E, et al. Reduction of nightmares and other PTSD symptoms in combat veterans by prazosin: a placebo-controlled study. Am J Psychiatry 2003;160: 371–3.

[79] Krakow B, Hollifield M, Johnston L, et al. Imagery rehearsal therapy for chronic nightmares in sexual assault survivors with posttraumatic stress disorder: a randomized controlled trial. JAMA 2001;286:537–45.

Psychiatr Clin N Am 29 (2006) 1059–1076

PSYCHIATRIC CLINICS
OF NORTH AMERICA

ELSEVIER
SAUNDERS

Sleep and Sleep Disorders in Children and Adolescents

Lisa J. Meltzer, PhD[a],*, Jodi A. Mindell, PhD[b,c]

[a]Division of Pulmonary Medicine, The Children's Hospital of Philadelphia and University of Pennsylvania School of Medicine, Philadelphia, PA, USA
[b]Saint Joseph's University, Philadelphia, PA, USA
[c]The Sleep Center at The Children's Hospital of Philadelphia, Philadelphia, PA, USA

Pediatric sleep disorders are common, affecting approximately 25% to 40% of children and adolescents [1]. Although there are several different types of sleep disorders that affect youth, each disorder can have a significant impact on daytime functioning and development, including learning, growth, behavior, and emotion regulation [2]. Although the relationship between sleep and psychiatric disorders has been established in adults, researchers are only beginning to uncover the interaction between sleep and psychiatric disorders in children and adolescents, including depression, attention-deficit/hyperactivity disorder (ADHD), and autism. The purpose of this article is to review normal sleep and sleep disorders in children and adolescents, the assessment of sleep in pediatric populations, common pediatric sleep disorders, and sleep in children who have common psychiatric disorders.

SLEEP IN CHILDREN

Parents often ask practitioners how much sleep their child needs. This can be a difficult question to answer as sleep needs not only change with developmental stages, but recent studies and surveys show that there is a large variability in both children's sleep need, especially in the first few years of life [3], as well as the actual amount of sleep that youth in America are getting [4,5]. Table 1 describes what typically is seen in terms of sleep patterns in children across development.

Newborns (0 to 3 Months)

There is no clear sleep pattern in the first few weeks of life; however, most newborns sleep between 10 and 18 hours per day, although this may be longer if infants are premature. This total sleep time is divided into many short sleep periods across the 24-hour clock, with no differentiation between day and night. This polyphasic sleep schedule (multiple sleep periods), although age appropriate, often is difficult for new parents. The discrepancy between newborn sleep

*Corresponding author. The Children's Hospital of Philadelphia, 3535 Market Street, 14th Floor, Philadelphia, PA 19104. E-mail address: meltzerL@email.chop.edu (L.J. Meltzer).

0193-953X/06/$ – see front matter
doi:10.1016/j.psc.2006.08.004

Table 1
Typical sleep need for children and adolescents by developmental stage

Age group	Years	Total sleep need
Infants	3 to 12 months	14 to 15 hours
Toddlers	1 to 3 years	12 to 14 hours
Preschoolers	3 to 5 years	11 to 13 hours
School-aged	6 to 12 years	10 to 11 hours
Adolescents	12 to 18 years	8.5 to 9.5 hours

patterns and parental expectations and need for prolonged nighttime sleep may result in parents stating that their baby "never sleeps."

Infants (3 to 12 Months)

Sleep patterns begin to consolidate by 3 months of age, with babies beginning to show a diurnal cycle of sleep at night and wakefulness during the day. Infants typically sleep approximately 10 to 12 hours at night and up to 3 or 4 hours during the day (divided into two or three daytime naps). At approximately 6 months of age, 90% of infants take only two naps, with their nighttime sleep progressively lengthening. It is important to keep in mind that with the onset of each developmental milestone (eg, pulling to standing or walking), children's sleep can become disrupted for several nights to weeks before and after the milestone occurs [6].

All children wake for brief periods during the night, with many infants able to return to sleep independently (self-soothers). Parents should be encouraged from an early age to put their babies to bed drowsy, but still awake, at bedtime in order for babies to learn how to fall asleep independently. In contrast, infants who are nursed or rocked to sleep are more likely to develop behavioral insomnia of childhood, sleep-onset association type, which presents as frequent night wakings (see later discussion for further description) [2]. Other common sleep disorders in infants include confusional arousals, bedtime problems, and rhythmic movement disorders (RMD).

Toddlers (12 Months to 3 Years)

By 18 months of age, the majority of toddlers transition from two daytime naps to one and continue to sleep approximately 10 to 12 hours at night. Approximately 25% to 30% of toddlers have sleep problems [1], with bedtime resistance (behavioral insomnia of childhood, limit-setting type) and frequent night wakings (behavioral insomnia of childhood, sleep-onset association type) the two primary disorders in this age group. In addition, daytime behavior is markedly worse in children who are poor sleepers.

Preschool-Aged Children (3 to 5 Years)

Sleep amounts in preschool-aged children decrease, mostly the result of the discontinuation of daytime naps. By the age of 5 years, 75% of children have given up their nap and sleep a total of 11 to 12 hours at night. As children develop language, cognitive reasoning, and imagination, they also can develop

effectiveness and potential side effects of melatonin for children and adolescents are sparse and inconclusive.

Sleep-Disordered Breathing

Sleep-disordered breathing (SDB) in children can range from primary snoring to obstructive sleep apnea syndrome (OSAS) and is related to significant cognitive and behavioral sequelae, including learning, attention, concentration, hyperactivity, and aggressive behavior. The incidence of habitual snoring has been reported at 3% to 12% of the general pediatric population, with OSAS seen in 1% to 3% of children [2,27]. Although recent evidence suggests that snoring itself is related to negative neurobehavioral functioning [28,29], OSAS is a more serious disorder that poses significant risk for the developing brain [27].

The clinical presentation of OSAS differs from that in adults, where the typical presentation is obese individuals who snore and are excessively sleepy during the day. In contrast, children who have OSAS may or may not be obese; the typical cause of this disorder in children is enlarged tonsils and adenoids. Although snoring alone is not indicative of OSAS in children, the American Academy of Pediatrics recommends that all children who have habitual snoring should be evaluated for OSAS [30]. Additional symptoms of OSAS in children include restless sleep, sleeping in an upright position or with the neck hyperextended (to keep the airway open), noisy breathing, and frequent infections of the tonsils or inner ear [27]. Although children may present typical symptoms of daytime sleepiness (eg, difficulty waking in the morning, falling asleep in school, or frequent naps that are not age appropriate), some children actually may be hyperactive, especially as they get more tired. Neurobehavioral problems also may be present in children with OSAS, including mood lability, aggression or other acting out behaviors, ADHD-like symptoms (eg, inattention or hyperactivity), and learning problems [31–33]. Studies find that academic functioning improves in children who have OSAS who have been treated with adenotonsillectomy compared with children who were not treated [32,34].

OSAS occurs in children of all ages and both genders, although the peak prevalence of this disorder is seen in preschool-aged children (3 to 5 years). Children who have craniofacial abnormalities, Down syndrome, or micrognathia are at increased risk for OSAS. In addition, with the rise in childhood obesity, increasingly more children are at risk for OSAS because of their weight, similar to adults.

For 70% of children, symptoms of OSAS are alleviated with a tonsillectomy and/or adenoidectomy [27,35]. A follow-up overnight sleep study post surgery is recommended. For children who are overweight, weight loss is the recommended treatment. Pharmacologic approaches may be indicated for children who have chronic nasal congestion that interferes with the quality of their breathing during sleep. Finally, in children in whom a tonsillectomy or adenoidectomy is contraindicated or unsuccessful, nasal continuous positive airway pressure (CPAP) may be appropriate. CPAP can be a successful treatment for children and adolescents; however, young children and children who have developmental delays may have greater difficulty tolerating this treatment and may need to participate in systematic desensitization to improve compliance with wearing the CPAP during sleep [36].

Narcolepsy

Narcolepsy is a chronic neurologic disorder that involves excessive daytime sleepiness, cataplexy (sudden loss of muscle control in response to strong emotional stimuli), hypnagogic hallucinations (vivid dreams at sleep onset), sleep paralysis, and fragmented nighttime sleep [17]. Although the onset of narcolepsy previously was believed to be in late adolescence or adulthood, it now seems that the symptoms of narcolepsy, most notably excessive daytime sleepiness, may begin to manifest in some individuals during childhood [37]. The prevalence of narcolepsy in children is difficult to establish, with retrospective studies reporting that approximately 34% of adults who have narcolepsy experienced the onset of symptoms before age 15 [38].

As sleepiness may be the only symptom present in children, the diagnosis of narcolepsy is more difficult in children and adolescents than in adults [39]. The symptoms of cataplexy and hypnagogic hallucinations may not be present or may be difficult to elicit in clinic from a child or the parent's history. Further, in young children, a diagnosis of narcolepsy may be confounded by a child's developmental need for regular naps. Polysomnography (PSG) with a multiple sleep latency test (MSLT) may provide clear evidence of narcolepsy, but in children, results are not always conclusive, and repeat studies may be necessary for a final diagnosis.

The current treatment recommendations for narcolepsy in children are similar to that of adults, and include education, sleep hygiene, and pharmacologic interventions. Education must be conducted not only with the family but also the other systems within which the child functions, including school and peer networks. Appropriate sleep scheduling is essential, with a consistent bedtime, wake time, and good sleep hygiene (eg, no TV in the bedroom and sleeping in a cool, dark environment). In addition, children and adolescents who have narcolepsy may benefit from a scheduled daily nap in the early afternoon. Medications commonly are used to target the primary symptoms of narcolepsy: daytime sleepiness and cataplexy. Stimulants are the class of drugs prescribed most commonly to counteract daytime sleepiness [37,40]. Modafinil (Provigil) also is reported to be effective in improving alertness and improved performance; however, most studies have been conducted with adults, with few pediatric trials completed [41,42]. Cholinergic pathways mediate cataplexy; thus, medications with anticholinergic properties are used to treat cataplexy, including clomipramine and imipramine. Currently, there are no Food and Drug Administration (FDA)–approved medications for the treatment of narcolepsy (either the symptoms of daytime sleepiness or cataplexy).

Disorders of Arousal

Disorders of arousal, more commonly referred to as partial arousal parasomnias, are common pediatric sleep disorders that tend to cease with development. These events occur during the transition from slow wave sleep (stages 3 and 4) to lighter sleep, rapid eye movement (REM) sleep, or a brief arousal, with transitions most common during the first few hours after sleep onset (at bedtime and during naps). Partial arousal parasomnias include confusional arousals, sleep terrors, sleep talking, and sleepwalking [17,43]. Events generally last a few minutes but can last much longer for some children. During an event, although children are asleep, they may appear awake (eyes open), talk, or seem frightened or confused (eg, screaming in the case of sleep terrors). During a partial arousal parasomnia, children may not recognize their parents and resist attempts to be comforted or soothed, with attempts to wake the child often prolonging the event. Typical parasomnias resolve spontaneously with children rapidly returning to a deep sleep.

A common feature of these disorders is retrograde amnesia, with children having no recollection of the event in the morning. In addition to the amnesia, partial arousal parasomnias are distinguishable from nightmares by the timing of the events, with sleep terrors occurring in the first part of the evening and nightmares in the early hours of the morning (during REM sleep). Clinically, practitioners often say that when parents are more upset by the episode, it usually is a sleep terror. Alternatively, when a child can recount vividly why he/she was terrified after waking, the child likely is experiencing nightmares.

There is a strong genetic component to partial arousal parasomnias, with a family history typically reported [44]. In addition, studies find little evidence that these events are related to anxiety, depression, or other psychological problem, although there is an increased rate of psychiatric issues in adolescents who have sleep terrors [45]. Partial arousals are more likely to be triggered by insufficient sleep, a disruption to the sleep environment or sleep schedule, stress, illness, or certain medications (eg, chloral hydrate or lithium). In addition, SDB is found in approximately 60% of school-aged children who have sleep terrors [44].

Treatment for partial arousal parasomnias includes providing families with information about creating a safe sleep environment (eg, preventing windows from opening or putting alarms or bells on doors to alert if a sleep walker is up), education about the events, and how to interact with children appropriately during an event. Finally, as some children may develop a fear of going to sleep (because they are afraid of having a partial arousal event) and a prolonged sleep onset in turn increases the likelihood of an event occurring, parents should be encouraged to not discuss these events in the morning with the child or other children in the home. Medications rarely are used to treat this sleep disorder but may be indicated if partial arousal events are very frequent, highly disruptive to the family, or when the child or others in the home are in danger because of the behavior. Additional information about parasomnias in general are provided elsewhere in this issue.

Restless Legs Syndrome and Periodic Limb Movement Disorder

Although the prevalence of RLS and periodic limb movement disorder (PLMD) is not well defined in the general pediatric population, it is worthy of discussion because of the strong relationship between these disorders and ADHD (discussed later). RLS manifests as uncomfortable sensations in the legs that worsen in the evening and with long periods of inactivity (eg, long car ride or movie) [17]. Sensations often are described as creepy-crawly or tingling feelings, most commonly in the legs, which can be alleviated temporarily with movement. In children, this can include running and jumping around. Symptoms also sometimes can be improved if the affected area is rubbed or stretched. PLMD commonly co-occurs with RLS but also may appear independently. PLMS are brief repetitive movements or jerks, lasting on average 2 seconds and occurring every 5 to 90 seconds during stages 1 and 2 of sleep [17,46]. PLMD occurs when PLMS are associated with frequent, but brief, arousals from sleep.

Pharmacologic treatment for RLS and PLMD in children and adolescents may include benzodiazepine and dopaminergic medications, although these medications have not been studied adequately in these age groups. In addition, some children who have RLS or PLMD have low iron/ferritin and many of these children and adolescents respond favorably to iron therapy [47]. At this time, there are no FDA-approved medications available to treat RLS and PLMD in children.

Sleep-Related Rhythmic Movement Disorders

Sleep-related RMD include head banging and body rocking and are considered to be a sleep-wake transition disorder, occurring as children attempt to fall asleep at bedtime, naptime, or after a normal nighttime arousal [17,48]. The etiology for RMD is unknown and, although they are common in infants (60% of 9 month olds), the behaviors tend to resolve spontaneously with development (only 8% of 4 year olds demonstrate these behaviors), but they can continue into adolescence and adulthood [49]. Events typically last 5 to 15 minutes, but prolonged events can go for several hours. The rhythmic behaviors generally are benign and self-limiting in normal children, with children rocking side to side, rocking back and forth while elevated on all four limbs, or banging their head against the pillow.

It is important to ensure that children are safe and protected from injury when they engage in these behaviors, and although treatments for this disorder are suggested, most are supported only anecdotally. In cases that result in injury, or when the behavior may be highly disruptive to others for a short duration (eg, family vacation or overnight sleepover), benzodiazepines may be indicated. For more severe cases or when the behavior persists past the age of 3 years, however, a thorough psychiatric and neurologic evaluation is recommended to rule out other disorders, such as autism, pervasive developmental disorder, or hypnogenic dystonia.

EVALUATION OF SLEEP PATTERNS AND SLEEP DISORDERS IN CHILDREN AND ADOLESCENTS

Unlike the evaluation of sleep problems in adults, information about a child's sleep and functioning most likely is presented by a parent or other primary caregiver. Although in general the sleep history is similar to that of adults (eg, sleep patterns and daytime functioning), the social and environmental context of a child's daily life also needs to be considered. This context includes the impact of the child's sleep problems on the family, including parent sleep and functioning, and the effects on other siblings in the home. The psychosocial history needs to include questions about parental marital status and living arrangements, as children's sleep patterns are influenced greatly by their environment and inconsistencies in parenting practices or sleeping environments also can disrupt sleep. Finally, daytime sleepiness can present differently across the lifespan, with young children getting more active and seemingly energetic when they get sleepy, while older children and adolescents become moody and more fatigued.

A thorough sleep history should cover all areas of a child's sleep habits, keeping in mind that sleep patterns can differ significantly from weekdays to weekends and from school days to summer vacation and holidays. Starting with bedtime behavior, it is important to assess children's evening routine, bedtime, sleep environment (eg, cosleeping, shared room or bed, or television in the bedroom), behavior at bedtime (eg, bedtime stalling, bedtime refusal, or difficulties falling asleep independently), and sleep-onset latency. Nocturnal behaviors should be discussed, including night wakings, symptoms of SDB (eg, snoring or pauses in breathing), sleep terrors or sleepwalking, seizures, and enuresis. Daytime behaviors also should be reviewed, including children's morning wake time (and difficulty waking in the morning), daytime sleepiness, fatigue, naps, meals, and caffeine or energy drink consumption.

Additional information about daytime functioning also is needed, including mood, school performance, social interactions, and significant life events. Children and adolescents are greatly affected by their day-to-day environment, including home and school, and changes or stressors in either area may affect children's sleep quality and sleep quantity. Events that may have an impact on children's sleep include the death of a family member, social and peer pressure, the birth of a new sibling, a recent move, or marital discord between the parents. In particular, children who "worry" more than their peers are at risk for difficulties with sleep onset and prolonged night wakings because of rumination over social interactions, academic expectations, family problems, or even current events (eg, September 11th, Hurricane Katrina, or the war in Iraq).

Along with a detailed sleep history, sleep diaries provide a wealth of information about children's sleep patterns. If completed on a daily basis, diaries can provide information about the consistency of a child's bedtime, duration of sleep onset, occurrence of night wakings, and whether or not the child oversleeps on weekends and holiday mornings. In addition, the timing, frequency, and duration of naps can provide additional information about why a child may have difficulty falling asleep at a given bedtime.

Objective measures of sleep include actigraphy and PSG. An actigraph is a small device the size of a watch worn on a child's wrist or ankle that measures sleep-wake patterns for extended periods of time (eg, 3 days to 2 weeks). By measuring children's movements and activity levels, a clearer picture of their bedtime, wake time, night wakings, and naps can be provided (Figs. 1 and 2). The strength of actigraphy is that it can be collected easily for an extended period of time in children's natural sleeping environment. The two primary clinical limitations for using actigraphy are the need for an accurate sleep diary to interpret actigraphy patterns and the inability of actigraphy to provide information on sleep architecture or underlying sleep disruptors (eg, SDB or periodic movements during sleep).

PSG is considered the gold standard for assessing sleep stages and underlying sleep disruptors, such as OSA and PLMD. As with adults, the MSLT is used in combination with an overnight PSG for the diagnosis of narcolepsy, although normative values for children and adolescents differ by Tanner stage [37]. Although PSG can be conducted in the home, it is done more commonly in a laboratory where the child stays overnight. Many physiologic measures are recorded (eg, electroencephalogram [EEG], electromyogram, electro-oculogram, EKG, and oxygen saturation), providing information about the quantity and quality of children's sleep. PSG has several drawbacks, including cost and availability. In addition, PSG is only a single night measure, which does not provide information about sleep patterns over time. In addition, there is some concern about children's ability to sleep comfortably in a strange environment (in particular young children). Finally, as discussed, PSG is expensive, and laboratories that are child friendly, with appropriately trained technicians, are limited.

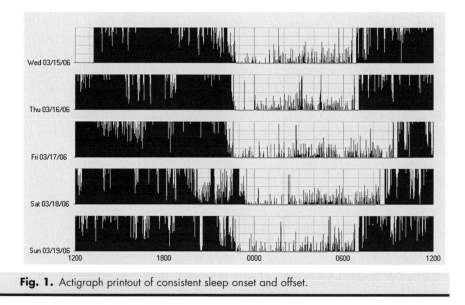

Fig. 1. Actigraph printout of consistent sleep onset and offset.

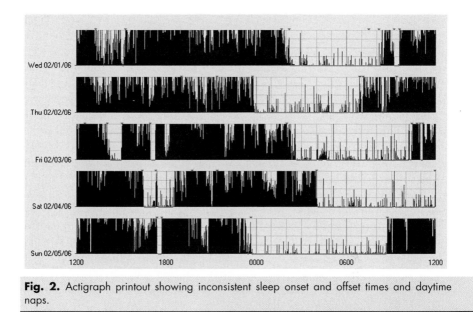

Fig. 2. Actigraph printout showing inconsistent sleep onset and offset times and daytime naps.

SLEEP AND PSYCHIATRIC DISORDERS IN CHILDREN

Sleep difficulties are common in many different populations of children, including children and adolescents who have developmental disabilities, chronic health conditions, and psychiatric disorders. The three groups of children who have persistent sleep problems seen most commonly in psychiatric practice are children who have ADHD, autism, and mood/anxiety disorders [50]. The following is a brief review of the complex relationship between sleep and these disorders in children and adolescents.

Attention-Deficit/Hyperactivity Disorder

Sleep problems are common in children who have ADHD, affecting approximately 25% to 50% of children who have this diagnosis [51]. Sleep clearly has been shown to differ between children who have and who do not have ADHD. Using parent report, actigraphy, and PSG, children who have ADHD have been found to have greater variability in their sleep patterns, greater difficulty with sleep onset, more activity during sleep, restless sleep and poor sleep quality, shortened sleep duration, and daytime sleepiness. Further, medications used to treat ADHD (eg, stimulants) can prolong sleep-onset latency and result in poorer sleep quality. These studies suggest that ADHD disrupts a child's sleep significantly.

The relationship between sleep problems and ADHD, however, is complex and bidirectional [52]. Although children who have ADHD have greater difficulties with sleep, children who have SDB display an increase in daytime behavior symptoms that mimic ADHD or exacerbate underlying ADHD symptoms. In studies of children who have SDB, including snoring and OSAS, an increase in hyperactivity, inattentive behaviors, poor emotion regulation, and peer problems is found [28,33,53]. When these sleep disorders were treated, many of the ADHD symptoms also resolved [54,55]. Finally, higher rates of RLS/PLMD are found in children who have ADHD compared with children who do not have ADHD [56,57]. When the PLMD was treated with dopamine agonists, sleep quality, sleep quantity, and ADHD symptoms that previously were resistant to psychostimulants improved [58]. More research is needed to help elucidate the relationship between sleep and ADHD in children and adolescents, but this population is at risk for increased sleep difficulties that should be evaluated and treated when appropriate.

Autism Spectrum Disorders

Sleep problems commonly are reported in children who have autism spectrum disorders (ASDs), affecting 44% to 83% of children who have ASDs [59–61]. The sleep problems reported most commonly include prolonged sleep onset, frequent and prolonged night wakings, early morning wakings, and shorter total sleep time, with differences reported by parent questionnaires and actigraphy [61–64]. The etiology of sleep problems in children who have ASDs is unclear, although suggested causes include alterations in the timing of melatonin production, anxiety, abnormal sleep EEG, or brain pathology.

Although knowledge is limited by the few studies conducted, sleep problems in children who have ASDs seem to be related to daytime functioning. In particular, sleep problems have been shown to be related to more energetic, excited, and problematic daytime behaviors [59]. In addition, shorter total sleep time is related to social skills deficits and increased stereotypic behaviors in children who have ASDs [65]. Behavioral interventions have been used, although with limited to moderate success. Pediatric sleep specialists agree that children who have ASDs have a lower response rate to behavioral interventions for sleep problems, and this population recently was identified as the highest priority in terms of clinical trials for the pharmacologic management of pediatric sleep problems [66].

Depression and Anxiety

As with ADHD, the relationship between mood/anxiety disorders and sleep is complex and bidirectional. Sleep disturbances (eg, hypersomnia or insomnia) are a symptom of anxiety and depression; at the same time, the consequences of disrupted or insufficient sleep often exacerbate these disorders. Ninety percent of children who have major depressive disorder report sleep disturbances, with insomnia or difficulty initiating sleep the most common complaint [67,68]. Hypersomnolence, or sleeping too much, also is a common complaint in depressed adolescents [69]. These typically are subjective reports, however, as objective measures of sleep do not always capture these sleep disturbances. Sleep complaints also are common in children who have anxiety disorders. Along with generalized anxiety, children who experience severe stress reactions, adjustment disorders, fears and phobias, or separation anxiety also experience increased difficulties with sleep.

As sleep disturbances and mood/anxiety disorders often are comorbid complaints, the most effective treatment is a multimodal integrated approach that addresses both the sleep difficulties and the mood/anxiety problems [68]. When treating mood/anxiety disorders pharmacologically, it is important to consider the impact of the medication on a child or adolescent's sleep, especially as some antidepressants may exacerbate sleep problems. Having a clear and consistent sleep routine and schedule helps ensure that children or adolescent's are getting sufficient sleep. Relaxation strategies (eg, diaphragmatic breathing or imagery) also may be used to improve sleep-onset latency and decrease bedtime fears and worries. Finally, the inclusion of a cognitive component (eg, positive self-statements or restructuring sleep-onset expectations) also can be highly effective in addressing sleep disturbances and mood/anxiety disorder.

SUMMARY

Sleep disturbances are common in children and range from behaviorally based sleep disorders, including behavioral insomnia of childhood and DSPS, to physiologically based sleep disorders, including OSAS, narcolepsy, RLS, and PLMD. Given that children and adolescents who have psychiatric issues commonly experience sleep disorders, it is critical that child psychiatrists conduct a thorough sleep assessment on all patients. Furthermore, not only are sleep disorders frequently comorbid with psychiatric illness but, in many cases, contribute significantly to daytime symptoms and daytime functioning.

References

[1] Owens JA. Epidemiology of sleep disorders during childhood. In: Sheldon SH, Ferber R, Kryger MH, editors. Principles and practices of pediatric sleep medicine. Philadelphia: Elsevier Saunders; 2005. p. 27–33.

[2] Mindell JA, Owens JA. A clinical guide to pediatric sleep: diagnosis and management of sleep problems. Philadelphia: Lippincott, Williams & Wilkins; 2003.

[3] Iglowstein I, Jenni OG, Molinari L, et al. Sleep duration from infancy to adolescence: reference values and generational trends. Pediatrics 2003;111:302–7.

[4] National Sleep Foundation. Sleep in America poll. 2004.

[5] National Sleep Foundation. Sleep in America poll. Washington, DC. 2006. Available at: www.sleepfoundation.org.

[6] Scher A, Cohen D. Locomotion and nightwaking. Child Care Health Dev 2005;31: 685–91.

[7] Kataria S, Swanson MS, Trevathan GE. Persistence of sleep disturbances in preschool children. Behav Pediatr 1987;110:642–6.

[8] Owens JA, Spirito A, McGuinn M, et al. Sleep habits and sleep disturbance in elementary school-aged children. J Dev Behav Pediatr 2000;21:27–36.

[9] Sadeh A, Raviv A, Gruber R. Sleep patterns and sleep disruptions in school-age children. J Dev Psychol 2000;36:291–301.

[10] Sadeh A, Gruber R, Raviv A. The effects of sleep restriction and extension on school-age children: what a difference an hour makes. Child Dev 2003;74:444–55.

[11] Sadeh A, Gruber R, Raviv A. Sleep, neurobehavioral functioning, and behavior problems in school-age children. Child Dev 2002;73:405–17.

[12] Fallone G, Acebo C, Seifer R, et al. Experimental restriction of sleep opportunity in children: effects on teacher ratings. Sleep 2005;28:1279–85.

[13] Carskadon MA, Acebo C. Regulation of sleepiness in adolescents: update, insights, and speculation. Sleep 2002;25:606–14.

[14] Wolfson AR, Carskadon MA. Sleep schedules and daytime functioning in adolescents. Child Dev 1998;69:875–87.

[15] Carskadon MA, Wolfson AR, Acebo C, et al. Adolescent sleep patterns, circadian timing, and sleepiness at a transition to early school days. Sleep 1998;21:871–81.

[16] Dahl RE, Lewin DS. Pathways to adolescent health sleep regulation and behavior. J Adolesc Health 2002;31:175–84.

[17] American Academy of Sleep Medicine. International classification of sleep disorders. 2nd ed. Diagnostic and coding manual. Westchester (IL): American Academy of Sleep Medicine; 2005.

[18] Mindell JA, Kuhn BR, Lewin DS, et al. Behavioral treatment of bedtime problems and night wakings in infants and young children. Sleep 2006;29(10):in press.

[19] Sadeh A. Assessment of intervention for infant night waking: parental reports and activity-based home monitoring. J Consult Clin Psychol 1994;62:63–8.

[20] Goodlin-Jones BL, Burnham MM, Gaylor EE, et al. Night waking, sleep-wake organization, and self-soothing in the first year of life. J Dev Behav Pediatr 2001;22:226–33.

[21] Morgenthaler TI, Owens J, Alessi C, et al. Practice parameters for behavioral treatment of bedtime problems and night wakings in infants and young children: an American Academy of Sleep Medicine report. Sleep, in press.

[22] Wyatt JK. Delayed sleep phase syndrome: pathophysiology and treatment options. Sleep 2004;27:1195–203.

[23] Herman JH. Circadian rhythm disorders: diagnosis and treatment. In: Sheldon SH, Ferber R, Kryger MH, editors. Principles and practice of pediatric sleep medicine. Philadelphia: Elsevier Saunders; 2005. p. 101–11.

[24] Mundey K, Benloucif S, Harsanyi K, et al. Phase-dependent treatment of delayed sleep phase syndrome with melatonin. Sleep 2005;28:1271–8.

[25] Smits MG, Nagtegaal EE, van der HJ, et al. Melatonin for chronic sleep onset insomnia in children: a randomized placebo-controlled trial. J Child Neurol 2001;16:86–92.

[26] Scheer FA, Cajochen C, Turek FW, et al. Melatonin in the regulation of sleep and circadian rhythms. In: Kryger MH, Roth C, Dement WC, editors. Principles and practices of sleep medicine. 4th ed. Philadelphia: Elsevier Saunders; 2005. p. 395–404.

[27] Katz ES, Marcus CL. Diagnosis of obstructive sleep apnea syndrome in infants and children. In: Sheldon SH, Ferber R, Kryger MH, editors. Principles and practice of pediatric sleep medicine. Philadelphia: Elsevier Saunders; 2005. p. 197–210.

[28] Urschitz MS, Eitner S, Guenther A, et al. Habitual snoring, intermittent hypoxia, and impaired behavior in primary school children. Pediatrics 2004;114:1041–8.

[29] O'Brien LM, Mervis CB, Holbrook CR, et al. Neurobehavioral implications of habitual snoring in children. Pediatrics 2004;114:44–9.

[30] American Academy of Pediatrics. Clinical practice guideline: diagnosis and management of childhood obstructive sleep apnea syndrome. Pediatrics 2002;109:704–12.

[31] Chervin RD, Archbold KH, Dillon JE, et al. Inattention, hyperactivity, and symptoms of sleep-disordered breathing. Pediatrics 2002;109:449–56.

[32] Chervin RD, Ruzicka DL, Giordani BJ, et al. Sleep-disordered breathing, behavior, and cognition in children before and after adenotonsillectomy. Pediatrics 2006;117:e769–78.

[33] O'Brien LM, Holbrook CR, Mervis CB, et al. Sleep and neurobehavioral characteristics of 5- to 7-year-old children with parentally reported symptoms of attention-deficit/hyperactivity disorder. Pediatrics 2003;111:554–63.

[34] Ray RM, Bower CM. Pediatric obstructive sleep apnea: the year in review. Curr Opin Otolaryngol Head Neck Surg 2005;13:360–5.

[35] Marcus CL. Sleep-disordered breathing in children. Am J Resp Crit Care 2001;164:16–30.

[36] Marcus CL, Rosen G, Ward SL, et al. Adherence to and effectiveness of positive airway pressure therapy in children with obstructive sleep apnea. Pediatrics 2006;117:e442–51.
[37] Kotagal S. Narcolepsy in children. In: Sheldon SH, Ferber R, Kryger MH, editors. Principles and practice of pediatric sleep medicine. Philadelphia: Elsevier Saunders; 2005. p. 171–82.
[38] Challamel MJ, Mazzola ME, Nevsimalova S, et al. Narcolepsy in children. Sleep 1994;17: S17–20.
[39] Ohayon MM, Ferini-Strambi L, Plazzi G, et al. How age influences the expression of narcolepsy. J Psychosom Res 2005;59:399–405.
[40] Greenhill LL, Pliszka S, Dulcan MK, et al. Practice parameter for the use of stimulant medications in the treatment of children, adolescents, and adults. J Am Acad Child Adolesc Psychiatry 2002;41:26S–49S.
[41] Ballon JS, Feifel D. A systematic review of modafinil: potential clinical uses and mechanisms of action. J Clin Psychiatry 2006;67:554–66.
[42] Ivanenko A, Tauman R, Gozal D. Modafinil in the treatment of excessive daytime sleepiness in children. Sleep Med 2003;4:579–82.
[43] Mason TB, Pack AL. Sleep terrors in childhood. J Pediatr 2005;147:388–92.
[44] Guilleminault C, Palombini L, Pelayo R, et al. Sleepwalking and sleep terrors in prepubertal children: what triggers them? Pediatrics 2003;111:e17–25.
[45] Gau SF, Soong WT. Psychiatric comorbidity of adolescents with sleep terrors or sleepwalking: a case-control study. Aust N Z J Psychiatry 1999;33:734–9.
[46] Simakajornboon N. Periodic limb movement disorder in children. Paediatr Respir Rev 2006;7(Suppl 1):S55–7.
[47] Mahowald MW. Restless legs syndrome: the CNS/iron connection. J Lab Clin Med 2006;147:56–7.
[48] Hoban TF. Rhythmic movement disorder in children. CNS Spectr 2003;8:135–8.
[49] Sheldon SH, Glaze D. Sleep in neurologic disorders. In: Sheldon SH, Ferber R, Kryger MH, editors. Principles and Practice of Pediatric Sleep Medicine. Philadelphia: Elsevier Saunders; 2005. p. 269–92.
[50] Ivanenko A, Crabtree VM, Gozal D. Sleep in children with psychiatric disorders. Pediatr Clin North Am 2004;51:51–68.
[51] Corkum P, Tannock R, Moldofsky H. Sleep disturbances in children with attention-deficit/hyperactivity disorder. J Am Acad Child Psy 1998;37:637–46.
[52] Owens JA. The ADHD and sleep conundrum: a review. J Dev Behav Pediatr 2005;26: 312–22.
[53] Melendres MCS, Lutz JM, Rubin ED, et al. Daytime sleepiness and hyperactivity in children with suspected sleep-disordered breathing. Pediatrics 2004;114:768–75.
[54] Gozal D. Sleep-disordered breathing and school performance in children. Pediatrics 1998;102:616–20.
[55] Ali NJ, Pitson D, Stradlin JR. Sleep disordered breathing: effects of adenotonsillectomy on behavior and psychological function. Eur J Pediatr 1996;155:156.
[56] Cortese S, Konofal E, Lecendreux M, et al. Restless legs syndrome and attention-deficit/hyperactivity disorder: a review of the literature. Sleep 2005;28:1007–13.
[57] Picchietti DL, England SJ, Walters AS, et al. Periodic limb movement disorder and restless legs syndromme in children with attention-deficit hyperactivity disorder. J Child Neurol 1998;1998:588–94.
[58] Walters AS, Mandelbaum DE, Lewin DS, et al. Dopaminergic therapy in children with restless legs/periodic limb movements in sleep and ADHD. Dopaminergic Therapy Study Group. Pediatr Neurol 2000;22:182–6.
[59] Richdale AL, Prior MR. The sleep/wake rhythm in children with autism. Eur Child Adolesc Psychiatry 1995;4:175–86.
[60] Richdale AL. Sleep problems in autism: prevalence, cause, and intervention. Dev Med Child Neurol 1999;41:60–6.

[61] Wiggs L, Stores G. Sleep patterns and sleep disorders in children with autistic spectrum disorders: insights using parent report and actigraphy. Dev Med Child Neurol 2004;46: 372–80.

[62] Patzold LM, Richdale AL, Tonge BJ. An investigation into sleep characteristics of children with autism and Asperger's Disorder. J Pediatr Child Hlth 1998;h34:528–33.

[63] Honomichl RD, Goodlin-Jones BL, Burnham M, et al. sleep patterns of children with pervasive developmental disorders. J Autism Dev Disord 2002;32:553–61.

[64] Williams GP, Sears LL, Allard A. Sleep problems in children with autism. J Sleep Res 2004;13:265–8.

[65] Schreck KA, Mulick JA, Smith AF. Sleep problems as possible predictors of intensified symptoms of autism. Res Dev Disabil 2004;25:57–66.

[66] Mindell JA, Emslie G, Blumer J, et al. Pharmacologic management of insomnia in children and adolescents: consensus statement. Pediatrics 2006;117:e1223–32.

[67] Roberts RE, Lewinsohn PM, Seeley JR. Symptoms of DSM-III-R major depression in adolescence: evidence from an epidemiological survey. J Am Acad Child Adolesc Psychiatry 1995;34:1608–17.

[68] Ivanenko A, Crabtree VM, Gozal D. Sleep and depression in children and adolescents. Sleep Med Rev 2005;9:115–29.

[69] Ryan ND, Puig-Antich J, Ambrosini P, et al. The clinical picture of major depression in children and adolescents. Arch Gen Psychiatry 1987;44:854–61.

Sleep and Its Disorders in Older Adults

Jana R. Cooke, MD[a], Sonia Ancoli-Israel, PhD[b],*

[a]Division of Pulmonary and Critical Care Medicine,
University of California San Diego School of Medicine, San Diego, California
[b]Department of Psychiatry, University of California San Diego School of Medicine,
San Diego, California

O ver the past few decades, research has shown that with age, several normal, age-related changes occur in sleep architecture and sleep patterns. Along with these expected changes, however, aging is often accompanied by a variety of sleep complaints, with up to 50% of older Americans reporting chronic difficulties with their sleep [1]. Furthermore, studies find that those older adults who have sleep complaints have a higher use of health services [2]. Problems with sleep are not an inevitable part of aging, however, as many of these complaints are comorbid with medical or psychiatric illnesses, medications, or primary sleep disorders. This article reviews sleep and its disorders in older adults.

SLEEP AND AGING

Subjectively, older adults report spending more time in bed but sleeping less, waking more often during the night, waking up earlier in the morning, taking more naps, and taking longer to fall asleep than younger adults [1]. Polysomnography (PSG) has provided objective evidence for these complaints, showing that older people do indeed spend more time in bed, sleep less, have more awakenings at night, and take longer to fall asleep [3]. As Vitiello and colleagues report, even healthy adults who do not complain about their sleep display PSG evidence of impaired sleep [4].

A recent meta-analysis of approximately 65 studies, representing 3577 subjects across the entire age spectrum, finds that with age, percentages of stage 1 and stage 2 sleep increased whereas the percentage of rapid eye movement (REM) sleep decreased [5]. When studies that included only elderly participants were reviewed, the amount of slow wave sleep remained constant and

Supported by NIA AG08415, NIA AG15301, NCI CA112035, CBCRP 11IB-0034, NIH M01 RR00827, the Department of Veterans Affairs VISN-22 Mental Illness Research, Education and Clinical Center (MIRECC), and the Research Service of the Veterans Affairs San Diego Healthcare System.

*Corresponding author. Department of Psychiatry 0603, UCSD, 9500 Gilman Drive, La Jolla, CA 92093-0603. E-mail address: sancoliisrael@ucsd.edu (S. Ancoli-Israel).

0193-953X/06/$ – see front matter
doi:10.1016/j.psc.2006.08.003

did not change with increasing age. Rather, the percentage of slow wave sleep actually began decreasing linearly at a rate of 2% per decade in young and middle-aged adults [5]. Sleep does become more fragmented in older adults, with an increase in the number of sleep stage shifts, arousals, and awakenings, resulting in a decrease in sleep efficiency (amount of time spent in bed asleep). Additionally, the total sleep time during the night may decrease despite an increase in the amount of time spent in bed. Van Cauter and colleagues find that in men ages 16 to 83, total sleep time decreased on average by 27 minutes per decade from midlife until the eighth decade [6].

It is believed that the absolute need for sleep does not decrease with age but rather the ability to sleep does [3,7]. Results of objective tests of daytime sleepiness show that the elderly are sleepier than younger adults [8], and because daytime sleepiness is suggestive of insufficient nighttime sleep, the conclusion is that older adults simply are not able to obtain an adequate amount of sleep at night.

This insufficient sleep is associated with significant morbidity and mortality. Studies show that patients who have difficulty sleeping report decreased quality of life and increased symptoms of depression and anxiety compared with those who do not have sleep difficulties [9]. In older adults, sleep problems are associated with an increased risk for falls, difficulty ambulating, difficulty with balance, and difficulty seeing—even after controlling for medication use [10]. The risk for falls is especially concerning, as this is found to be a strong predictor of nursing home placement for the community-dwelling, independent-living older adult [11]. In addition, when compared with matched controls, aged patients who have sleep difficulties are found to have slower reaction times and cognitive dysfunction, including impaired memory [12]. This is not surprising, as chronic sleep difficulties at any age can lead to deficits in attention, response times, short-term memory, and performance level [13].

In addition to increased morbidity, there also is increased mortality associated with sleeping problems. In a longitudinal study of healthy older adults, reduced amounts of REM sleep and sleep efficiency are reported to increase the risk for all-cause mortality, even after controlling for a variety of related covariates [14]. In addition, as discussed previously, the elderly often spend more time in bed, which is associated with an increased risk for death.

There are a variety of reasons that explain older adults' sleep difficulties, including the presence of specific sleep disorders, circadian rhythm disturbances, and medical and psychiatric illness or medication use. Each potential etiology is described in more detail later.

INSOMNIA

Insomnia, defined as the inability to initiate or maintain sleep resulting in daytime consequences, is the most common sleep disturbance reported in older adults. Complaints may range from difficulty falling asleep to difficulty with sleep maintenance to frequent nighttime awakenings and early morning awakenings. In a study of more than 9000 adults over age 65, 42% of participants had difficulty falling asleep and staying asleep [1]. On follow-up 3 years later, insomnia complaints had resolved in 15% of the study's population, but the incidence of new sleep complaints was 5% [15]. Studies also find that older women are more likely to complain about insomnia than older men [16].

Causes of Insomnia

Although insomnia may be a primary sleep disorder, sleep complaints in the older adult increasingly are recognized as being comorbid with chronic medical and psychiatric conditions [17]. Comorbid conditions associated with the development of insomnia in the elderly include depression, chronic pain, cancer, chronic obstructive pulmonary disease, and cardiovascular disease. Foley and colleagues report that although 28% of older adults suffered from complaints of chronic insomnia, only 7% of the incident cases of insomnia in the elderly occur in the absence of one of these related conditions [15]. Foley and colleagues conclude that it was not, therefore, aging, per se that caused insomnia in older adults, rather, all the conditions that occur with aging.

Medical and psychiatric illnesses

Reports of trouble with sleep are correlated strongly with complaints about health and depression [1]. In the 2003 National Sleep Foundation survey of adults ages 65 years and over, those who had more medical conditions, including cardiac and pulmonary disease and depression, reported significantly more sleep complaints [17]. Furthermore, as the number of medical conditions increased, the likelihood of having sleep difficulties increased (Fig. 1). Studies examining the prevalence of sleep disturbances in patients who had chronic medical diseases report that 31% of arthritis and 66% of chronic pain patients report difficulty falling asleep, whereas 81% of arthritis, 85% of chronic pain, and 33% of diabetes patients report difficulty staying asleep [18–20]. Shortness of breath resulting from chronic obstructive pulmonary disease or congestive heart failure, nocturia resulting from an enlarged prostate, and neurologic

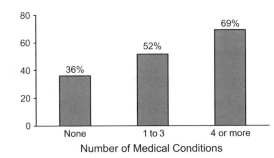

Fig. 1. The prevalence of one or more sleep problems by the number of medical conditions in adults ages 65 years or older. (*From* Foley D, Ancoli-Israel S, Britz P, et al. Sleep disturbances and chronic disease in older adults: results of the 2003 National Sleep Foundation Sleep in America survey. J Psychosom Res 2004;56:497–502; with permission.)

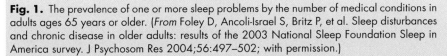

deficits related to cerebrovascular accidents or Parkinson's disease all are associated with sleep complaints and insomnia [21–23].

It long has been known that depression and insomnia are associated with each other [24], as the presence of depressed mood may predict insomnia and untreated insomnia may result in depression [25,26]. In a large cross-sectional survey, Ohayon and Roth find that insomnia was present in 65% of respondents who had major depression, 61% of those who had panic disorder, and 44% who had generalized anxiety disorder [27]. Anxiety and stress during the day are common causes of transient insomnia. Depression related to serious life events, such as divorce or death, however, can trigger long-lasting, chronic insomnia. Additionally, patients who have insomnia are more likely to have a psychiatric disorder. Buysee and colleagues report that insomnia at baseline significantly predicts an increased risk for developing depression 1 to 3 years later [26]. A recent study by Perlis and colleagues also finds that elderly subjects, in particular women, who have persistent insomnia are at greater risk for the development of depression [28]. Studies in younger adults suggest that treating the insomnia also might improve depression [29], but these types of studies have not been conducted in the elderly.

Medications
The medications used to treat these various underlying chronic medical and psychiatric conditions also can contribute to or cause sleep disruptions. Polypharmacy increasingly is common among older adults, often without consideration of its effect on patient sleep. Several medications are known to disturb sleep, including β-blockers, bronchodilators, corticosteroids, decongestants, diuretics, and other cardiovascular, neurologic, psychiatric, and gastrointestinal medications. Whenever feasible, sedating medications should be administered before bedtime, whereas stimulating medications and diuretics should be taken earlier in the day.

Treatment of Insomnia
Although insomnia traditionally has been treated with medications, research finds that behavioral therapy may be more effective than medications and, therefore, should be the first treatment option considered, although a combined approach may be required initially [30,31].

Behavioral
Behavioral treatments are shown to be highly effective in the treatment of insomnia [32]. A set of guidelines for the maintenance of healthy sleep and wake habits (called sleep hygiene) should be introduced (Box 1). Patients should be educated on how to modify poor sleep hygiene practices that may be interfering with their sleep. Cognitive behavioral therapy (CBT), which combines stimulus control or sleep restriction with cognitive restructuring, good sleep hygiene, and relaxation, is the most effective behavioral therapy [30]. Stimulus control is based on the belief that insomnia may be the result of maladaptive classical conditioning [33]. Patients are instructed to eliminate

Box 1: Sleep hygiene rules

1. Do not spend too much time in bed.
2. Maintain consistent sleep and wake times.
3. Get out of bed if unable to fall asleep.
4. Restrict naps to 30 minutes in the late morning or early afternoon.
5. Exercise regularly.
6. Spend more time outside, without sunglasses, especially late in the day.
7. Increase overall light exposure.
8. Eat a light snack (ie, milk or bread) before bed.
9. Avoid caffeine, tobacco, and alcohol after lunch.
10. Limit liquids in the evening

all in-bed activities other than sleep, such as reading and television watching. If they are not able to fall asleep within 20 minutes, they are instructed to get out of bed until they feel sufficiently sleepy, when they can return to bed and attempt to again fall asleep. If they are not able to fall asleep within 20 minutes, the pattern of getting out of bed until sleepy repeats itself. This therapy tries to break the association between the bed and wakefulness. Sleep restriction therapy limits the time spent in bed to approximately 15 minutes beyond the duration of time spent asleep at night [34]. As sleep efficiency improves, the amount of time spent in bed gradually increases.

In a study of insomnia in older adults, CBT was compared with temazepam, with a combination of CBT plus temazepam, and with placebo for 8 weeks [30]. All three active treatments were better than placebo in reducing wake time during the night immediately post treatment but only those treated with CBT maintained clinical gains during the 3-, 12-, and 24-month follow-up period. Even abbreviated sessions of CBT (two 25 minute sessions) are found effective in reducing wake time during the night and insomnia symptoms. The 2005 National Institutes of Health (NIH) State-of-the-Science Conference on Insomnia [31] concludes that CBT is as effective as prescription medications for the treatment of chronic insomnia. One disadvantage of CBT, however, is that the clinical effect may take up to 2 weeks or longer to appear [32,35].

Pharmacologic

Several different classes of medications have been used to treat insomnia in the elderly, including sedative-hypnotics, antihistamines, antidepressants, antipsychotics, and anticonvulsants. The 2005 NIH State-of-the-Science Conference on Insomnia concludes that there is no systematic evidence for the effectiveness of the antihistamines, antidepressants, antipsychotics, or anticonvulsants in the treatment of insomnia [31]. The panel also recognized and expressed significant concerns about the risks associated with the use of these medications in the elderly, stating that the risks outweighed the benefits.

Sedative-hypnotic medications are appropriate at times for the management of insomnia although studies show that it should be accompanied by behavioral therapy for the most effective treatment [30,31]. Choosing the sedative-hypnotic that best fits the specific complaint related to insomnia is the key to using this class of medications successfully. For example, agents with a long onset of action do not benefit patients who have difficulty falling asleep. Furthermore, the potentially harmful effects of this type of medication, especially the benzodiazepines, must be considered, as long-acting hypnotics can cause excessive daytime sleepiness (EDS) and poor motor coordination, which may lead to injuries. Chronic use of benzodiazepines can lead to tolerance and withdrawal symptoms if discontinued abruptly, and the benefits of these agents for long-term use have not been studied in randomized clinical trials.

Several medications with different and novel mechanisms of action are now available and should be considered first-line agents in the pharmacologic treatment of insomnia in older adults. The selective short-acting nonbenzodiazepines (type-1 γ-aminobutyric acid [GABA] benzodiazepines receptor agonists), such as eszopiclone, zaleplon, zolpidem, and zolpidem CR, are shown to be safe and effective in the management of insomnia in the elderly, with a low propensity for causing clinical residual effects, withdrawal, dependence, or tolerance [36–39]. Ramelteon, a melatonin agonist, and the only sleeping agent not controlled by the Drug Enforcement Agency, recently has been approved for the treatment of sleep-onset insomnia and is shown to be effective in the elderly [40]. Table 1 lists the five newest agents approved for sleep.

By combining the two types of therapies, pharmacologic and behavioral, patients may gain relief from insomnia in the short-term with medications while

Table 1
Newest Food and Drug Administration–approved nonbenzodiazepines for insomnia

Name	Trade name	Indication	Dose	Half-life (h)	Time required to stay in bed (h)
Zaleplon	Sonata	Short-term treatment of sleep-onset insomnia	5 mg 10 mg 20 mg	1	4
Zolpidem	Ambien	Short-term treatment of sleep-onset insomnia	5 mg 10 mg	2.5	7–8
Zolpidem CR	Ambien CR	Long-term treatment of sleep-onset or maintenance insomnia	6.25 mg 12.5 mg	2.8	7–8
Eszopiclone	Lunesta	Long-term treatment of sleep-onset or maintenance insomnia	1 mg 2 mg 3 mg	6	≥8
Ramelteon	Rozerem	Long-term treatment of sleep-onset insomnia	8 mg	1–2.6	≥8

learning the techniques of CBT, which may allow long-term treatment of insomnia.

CIRCADIAN RHYTHM DISTURBANCES

In humans, many physiologic variables, including the sleep-wake cycle, are regulated by a biologic clock that operates over a 24-hour period, termed the circadian rhythm. This rhythm entrains to the 24-hour day by external time cues or zeitgebers, with the light-dark cycle the most important in addition to other internal rhythms. Circadian rhythm sleep disturbances may develop if dysynchrony between the internal circadian pacemaker, located in the suprachiasmatic nucleus of the anterior hypothalamus, and external environment cues occur.

With aging, there are several factors that may contribute to a desynchronized circadian rhythm, which may lead to sleep disturbances. The suprachiasmatic nucleus deteriorates with age, resulting in weaker or more disrupted rhythms [41]. Other circadian rhythm disturbances known to be involved in the entrainment of the circadian rhythm of sleep also may develop. For example, the nocturnal secretion of endogenous melatonin, known to play an important role in the sleep-wake cycle, gradually decreases with age, which may result in reduced sleep efficiency and an increased incidence of circadian rhythm sleep disturbances [42]. In addition, external cues that are necessary to entrain the circadian rhythm of sleep-wake may be missing or weak in elderly patients. This point is exemplified by the fact that the elderly, especially those institutionalized, spend little time being exposed to bright light, one of the most powerful zeitgebers. Daily bright light exposure averages 60 minutes for healthy elderly, 30 minutes for Alzheimer's disease patients living at home, and 0 minutes for nursing home patients [43–45]. This reduced level of bright light exposure is associated with nighttime sleep fragmentation and circadian rhythm sleep disorders [45]. Finally, the amplitude of the circadian rhythm also may decrease with age. Reductions in rhythm amplitude can increase the frequency of nighttime awakenings and the severity of daytime sleepiness [46].

Older adults can develop changes in the phasing of the circadian rhythm, thereby causing changes in the timing of the sleep period. Many older patients experience a phase advance in their sleep-wake cycle, causing them to feel sleepy early in the evening and to awaken very early in the morning. Individuals who have advanced sleep rhythms typically fall asleep between 7:00 PM and 9:00 PM, correlating with the drop in body temperature, and wake up some 8 hours later, at 3:00 AM to 5:00 AM (Fig. 2). Because of societal norms, many older individuals who have an advanced sleep-wake cycle opt to stay up late, in spite of their sleepiness, yet awaken early in the morning because of this advancement, resulting in restricted time in bed and daytime sleepiness.

Like insomnia, circadian rhythm changes are considered to be common with older age, and presenting symptoms may mimic those of insomnia. Making a distinction between the two disturbances is important as the treatment approaches differ. A careful and detailed sleep history, sleep diaries, and activity

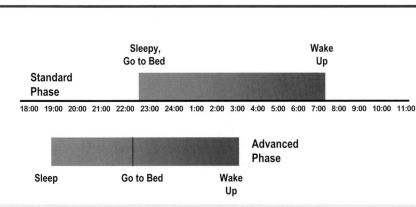

Fig. 2. Standard of sleep versus advanced phase of sleep. (*From* Ancoli-Israel S. All I want is a good night's sleep. St. Louis: Mosby; 1996; with permission.)

monitoring with wrist actigraphy all can be useful in distinguishing between the two conditions.

Treatments known to strengthen and entrain the sleep-wake cycle are the most appropriate therapies for shifts in the circadian rhythm. As bright light is the strongest cue for circadian entrainment, the most common and effective treatment for circadian rhythm shifts is bright light therapy. For patients who have advanced sleep-wake cycle, evening light exposure is found to delay circadian rhythms and strengthen the sleep-wake cycle in healthy, community-living older subjects and in nursing home patients [47]. In addition, these patients should avoid bright light in the morning hours and adhere to a regular sleep schedule. If patients are unable to spend enough time outdoors, studies show that exposure to artificial light via a bright light box in the early evening can improve sleep continuity in healthy and institutionalized elderly patients [47].

Endogenous secretion of melatonin tends to be reduced in older adults, and some studies suggest that melatonin replacement therapy may improve sleep efficiency in this population [48]. The NIH State-of-the-Science Insomnia Conference concludes that melatonin seems to be safe and effective for the treatment of circadian rhythm disorders, but that there is little evidence for efficacy in the treatment of insomnia. In general, clinicians should exercise caution when considering a trial of melatonin replacement therapy in elderly patients.

PRIMARY SLEEP DISORDERS
There are three primary sleep disorders commonly found in the elderly: sleep-disordered breathing (SDB), periodic limb movements in sleep/restless legs syndrome (PLMS/RLS), and REM sleep behavior disorder (RBD).

Sleep-Disordered Breathing
SDB (details of which are discussed elsewhere in this publication) is more common in older adults than younger adults and more common in elderly nursing home patients, in particular those who have dementia, than those who live

independently. In a large series of randomly selected, community-dwelling elderly, 65 to 95 years of age, Ancoli-Israel and colleagues [49] report that 81% of the study subjects had an apnea hypopnea index (AHI) greater than or equal to 5, with prevalence rates of 62% for an AHI greater than or equal to 10, 44% for an AHI greater than or equal to 20, and 24% for an AHI greater than or equal to 40. Studying a large cohort of patients with a mean age of 63.5 years, the Sleep Heart Health Study [50] reports prevalence rates of SDB by 10-year age groups. For those subjects ages 60 to 69, 32% had an AHI 5–14 and 19% had an AHI greater than or equal to 15. For those ages 70 to 79, 33% had an AHI 5–14 and 21% had an AHI greater than or equal to 15. For those ages 80 to 98, 36% had an AHI 5–14 and 20% had an AHI greater than or equal to 15. This is in contrast to the prevalence of SDB among middle-aged adults, estimated at 4% of men and 2% of women as defined by an AHI greater than or equal to 5 and the presence of EDS [51].

Most longitudinal and cross-sectional studies show that the prevalence of SDB increases or stabilizes with increasing age [52–54]. Hoch and colleagues [53] find that the prevalence of SDB increases from ages 60 to 90 years. The Sleep Heart Health Study [50] also reports an increase in SDB prevalence with age, although this was found only in those subjects who had an AHI greater than or equal to 15. In a longitudinal study that followed older adults for 18 years, Ancoli-Israel and colleagues [54] find that the AHI remained stable and changed only with associated changes in body mass index.

Patients who have certain progressive dementias that involve degeneration in areas of the brainstem responsible for regulating respiration and other autonomic functions relevant to sleep maintenance may be at higher risk for developing SDB. Ancoli-Israel and colleagues [55] find that those institutionalized elderly who had more severe dementia had more severe SDB compared with those who had mild-moderate or no dementia. Furthermore, those who had more severe SDB performed worse on the dementia rating scales, suggesting that more severe SDB was associated with more severe dementia.

Risk factors for SDB in older adults include increasing age, gender, and obesity [56]. Other conditions that increase the risk for developing SDB include the use of sedating medications, alcohol consumption, family history, race, smoking, and upper airway configuration [56].

Snoring and EDS are the two main symptoms of SDB in the elderly. Other less common presentations in older adults include insomnia, nocturnal confusion, and daytime cognitive impairment, including trouble concentrating or paying attention and short-term memory loss. Approximately 50% of patients who have habitual snoring have some degree of SDB, and snoring is identified as an early predictor of SDB [57]. EDS is a major feature of SDB in the elderly and results from recurrent nighttime arousals and sleep fragmentation. Unintentional napping and falling asleep at inappropriate times during the day are common manifestations of the daytime sleepiness experienced by patients who have EDS secondary to untreated SDB. This excessive sleepiness can cause social and occupational difficulties and reduced vigilance and cognitive deficits, which may be relevant particularly in those patients who have baseline cognitive impairment [58].

The presence of SDB is associated with significant morbidity, including cardiovascular disease and cognitive dysfunction. In older adults, severe SDB (AHI $\geq$ 30) is consistently reported to cause impairments in attention, immediate and delayed recall, executive tasks, planning and sequential thinking, and manual dexterity, whereas milder SDB (AHI 10–20) may cause only cognitive dysfunction in the presence of excessive sleepiness [59].

The exact relationship between SDB and cardiovascular disease, including myocardial infarction, stroke, congesting heart failure, and hypertension, in older adults remains relatively unknown, although results from a few recent studies provide some insight. The Sleep Heart Health Study [60] finds a positive association between the severity of SDB (based on overnight PSG) and the risk for developing cardiovascular disease, including coronary artery disease, congestive heart failure, and stroke [61]. A recent study of patients who had acute ischemic stroke reports that SDB was common, particularly in older male patients who had diabetes and a nighttime stroke onset [62].

To assess the presence of SDB accurately in the elderly, practitioners should use a step-wise approach. A complete sleep history should be obtained, preferably in the presence of a bed partner or caregiver, focusing on symptoms of SDB, specifically EDS, unintentional napping, and snoring, symptoms of other sleep disorders (ie, RLS), and sleep-related habits and routines. Patients' medical history should be reviewed thoroughly, with particular attention paid to SDB-associated medical conditions, medications, the use of alcohol, and evidence of cognitive impairment. Lastly, if any of these is suggestive of SDB, an overnight sleep recording should be obtained.

Continuous positive airway pressure (CPAP) is the gold standard for treatment of SDB. CPAP treatment is shown to improve cognition functioning in older adults [59]. As with any adults who have SDB, CPAP compliance can be an issue, although clinicians should not assume that elderly patients will be noncompliant simply because of age. The authors' laboratory finds that patients who have Alzheimer's disease tolerate CPAP treatment [63], and the only factor associated with poor CPAP compliance is the presence of depression—not age, severity of dementia, or severity of SDB [63].

Alternatives to CPAP include oral appliances and surgery, although neither is as effective as CPAP. All patients should be counseled on weight loss, smoking cessation, and abstinence from alcohol consumption, if indicated. Medications known to cause respiratory depression, including long-acting benzodiazepines and narcotics, generally should be avoided in the elderly who have SDB, as these agents may increase the number and duration of apneas.

As the body of literature exploring SDB in the elderly grows, discussions about the significance of its presence in this population and who should be treated continue. Whether or not SDB is an age-dependent condition, in which aging causes the pathology, or an age-related condition, in which the disease occurs only during a particular age period, remains unknown. As the prevalence seems to increase with age, it could be argued that SDB is an age-dependent condition, and the same condition with the same outcomes as seen in younger adults and therefore, warrants the same aggressive treatment [52–54]. Although prevalence in the elderly may be age-dependent, the severity of SDB and its clinical significance in the elderly may be age-related. Studies aimed at answering these questions and those related to mortality and SDB in the elderly are ongoing.

Currently, most experts in the field agree that in general, treatment of SDB in the elderly should be guided by the significance of patient symptoms and the severity of the SDB [64]. If older adults have other comorbid conditions, such has hypertension, cognitive dysfunction, and cardiac disease, or if the SDB is severe, treatment should be considered. Age alone never should be a reason to withhold treatment

Periodic Limb Movements in Sleep/Restless Legs Syndrome

PLMS and RLS also are common in older adults. Details of these disorders are discussed elsewhere in this publication. The prevalence of PLMS increases dramatically with age, with an estimated prevalence of 45% in older adults [65]. It is equally prevalent in older men and women. Despite its high prevalence in older adults, the severity of PLMS does not worsen progressively with increasing age [66]. Like PLMS, the prevalence of RLS increases significantly with age, with older women affected twice as often as older men [67].

Medications that target the leg movements or the associated arousals are the treatments currently recommended for PLMS/RLS in older adults. Dopamine agonists are considered the preferred therapy for PLMS/RLS in the elderly, as this class of medications is found effective in reducing the number of kicks and associated arousals [68,69]. The only drug currently Food and Drug Administration approved for the treatment of RLS is ropinirole, although the off-label use of other dopamine agonists (eg, pergolide, pramipexole, and carbidopa-levodopa) also is shown to be effective [69].

Rapid Eye Movement Sleep Behavior Disorder

RBD is more common in the elderly, specifically elderly men [70], although the exact prevalence is unknown. Details of this disorder are discussed elsewhere in this publication.

SLEEP IN DEMENTIA

Patients who have dementia commonly experience disturbed sleep, with reports that 19% to 44% of patients who are community dwelling and demented complain of sleep disturbances [71]. This may be a consequence of the dementing process itself, causing irreversible damage to areas in the brain responsible for regulating sleep. This theory is supported by the finding that those patients who have more severe dementia have more severe sleep disruptions [72]. Daytime napping resulting from EDS is a common feature of sleep in demented patients along with abnormal nighttime behavior, including wandering, confusion, and agitation (sundowning). These sleep disturbances cause significant caregiver distress and are related to patient institutionalization [73].

Although the dementing process itself may be responsible for the disturbed sleep experienced by patients who have dementia, it is important to evaluate each patient for other potential causes of sleep disturbances. Like older adults who are not demented, patients who have dementia may have disturbed sleep related to pain from medical illnesses, medications, circadian rhythm changes, depression, and primary sleep disorders, such as SDB, PLMS/RLS, or RBD.

Treatment of specific sleep disturbances in the elderly who have dementia should be guided by that specific sleep disorder. Patients who have SBD should be treated with CPAP if appropriate; those who have PLMS/RLS should be treated with a dopamine agonist; and those who have circadian rhythm disturbances should be treated with bright light therapy. In general, nonpharmacologic interventions, such as regular physical activity, social interactions, restricting time in bed, and so forth, are preferred to pharmacologic interventions. Medications, including sedative-hypnotics, antihistamines, and antipsychotics, all have significant side effects, including drug interactions and residual daytime sleepiness (hang-over effect), which may result in impaired motor and cognitive function. Furthermore, the 2005 NIH State-of-the-Science Conference on Insomnia concludes that there is no evidence to support the use of antihistamines, antidepressants, antipsychotics, or anticonvulsants in the treatment of sleep difficulties [31].

Institutionalized older adults experience even more fragmented and disturbed sleep than those elderly who are demented and living in the community [74]. Middelkoop and colleagues [75] report that when compared with elderly patients living in the community or in assisted living facilities, patients residing in nursing homes had poorer sleep quality, more disturbed sleep onset, more advanced sleep-wake cycles, and higher use of sedative-hypnotics. In a 24-hour day, institutionalized, severely demented older adults may not spend a single hour completely awake or asleep [72,74].

A variety of environmental factors may be responsible for the poor sleep quality experienced by most institutionalized elderly patients. Nighttime noise and ambient light exposure may contribute significantly to sleep disruption in nursing home patients [76]. Ancoli-Israel and Kripke [74] report that these patients were exposed to less than 10 minutes of bright light per day and those who had more light exposure had fewer sleep disruptions [45]. Nursing home patients typically spend large amounts of each day in bed and chronic bed rest is known to disrupt circadian rhythms [74]. Interventions aimed at reducing nighttime noise and light exposure and at changing sleep hygiene and the sleep environment may improve the sleep quality of nursing home residents greatly [77]. Increased bright light exposure also is shown to consolidate sleep and strengthen circadian rhythms in this population of patients [78,79]. Strategies to reduce nighttime disturbances and to promote stronger sleep-wake cycles are listed in Box 2.

Box 2: Tips for improving sleep in the nursing home

1. Determine cause of sleep problem and initiate specific treatment.
2. Limit naps to 1 hour in the early afternoon.
3. Adjust medications.
4. Avoid all caffeine.
5. Improve environment.
a. Keep the environment dark at night.
b. Keep the environment bright during the day.
c. Keep the environment quiet at night.
d. Match roommates.

Adapted from Ancoli-Israel S. Sleep disorders. In: Morris JN, Lipsitz LA, Murphy K, et al, editors. Quality care for the nursing home. St. Louis: Mosby; 1997. p. 64–73.

SUMMARY

For many older adults, aging is associated with significant changes in sleep. There is a variety of potential causes, including primary sleep disorders, circadian rhythm disturbances, insomnia, depression, medical illness, and medications. As with younger adults, the diagnosis requires a thorough sleep history and an overnight sleep recording when appropriate. Treatment should address the primary sleep problem and can result in significant improvement in quality of life and daytime functioning in older adults.

References
   [1] Foley DJ, Monjan AA, Brown SL, et al. Sleep complaints among elderly persons: an epidemiologic study of three communities. Sleep 1995;18425–32.
   [2] Novak M, Mucsi I, Shapiro CM, et al. Increased utilization of health services by insomniacs—an epidemiological perspective. J Psychosom Res 2004;56:527–36.
   [3] Bliwise DL. Review: sleep in normal aging and dementia. Sleep 1993;16:40–81.
   [4] Vitiello MV, Larsen LH, Moe KE. Age-related sleep change gender and estrogen effects on the subjective–objective sleep quality relationships of healthy, noncomplaining older men and women. J Psychosom Res 2004;56:503–10.
   [5] Ohayon MM, Carskadon MA, Guilleminault C, et al. Meta-analysis of quantitative sleep parameters from childhood to old age in healthy individuals: Developing normative sleep values across the human lifespan. Sleep 2004;27:1255–73.
   [6] Van Cauter EV, Leproult R, Plat L. Age-related changes in slow wave sleep and REM sleep and relationship with growth hormone and cortisol levels in healthy men. JAMA 2000;284:861–8.
   [7] Ancoli-Israel S. Sleep problems in older adults: putting myths to bed. Geriatrics 1997;52: 20–30.
   [8] Carskadon MA, van den Hoed J, Dement WC. Sleep and daytime sleepiness in the elderly. J Geriatr Psychiatry 1980;13:135–51.
   [9] Barbar SI, Enright PL, Boyle P, et al. Sleep disturbances and their correlates in elderly Japanese American men residing in Hawaii. J Gerontol A Biol Sci Med Sci 2000;55: M406–11.

[10] Brassington GS, King AC, Bliwise DL. Sleep problems as a risk factor for falls in a sample of-community- dwelling adults aged 64–99 years. J Am Geriatr Soc 2000;48:1234–40.

[11] Tinetti ME, Williams CS. Falls, injuries due to falls and the risk of admission to a nursing home. N Engl J Med 1997;337:1279–84.

[12] Crenshaw MC, Edinger JD. Slow-wave sleep and waking cognitive performance among older adults with and without insomnia complaints. Physiol Behav 1999;66:485–92.

[13] Walsh JK, Benca RM, Bonnet M, et al. Insomnia: assessment and management in primary care: National Heart, Lung, and Blood Institute Working Group on Insomnia. Am Fam Physician 1999;59:3029–37.

[14] Dew MA, Hoch CC, Buysse DJ, et al. Healthy older adults' sleep predicts all-cause mortality at 4 to 19 years of follow-up. Psychosom Med 2003;65:63–73.

[15] Foley DJ, Monjan A, Simonsick EM, et al. Incidence and remission of insomnia among elderly adults: an epidemiologic study of 6,800 persons over three years. Sleep 1999;22(Suppl 2):S366–72.

[16] Rediehs MH, Reis JS, Creason NS. Sleep in old age: focus on gender differences. Sleep 1990;13:410–24.

[17] Foley D, Ancoli-Israel S, Britz P, et al. Sleep disturbances and chronic disease in older adults: results of the 2003 National Sleep Foundation Sleep in America Survey. J Psychosom Res 2004;56:497–502.

[18] Wilcox S, Brenes GA, Levine D, et al. Factors related to sleep disturbance in older adults experiencing knee pain or knee pain with radiographic evidence of knee osteoarthritis. J Am Geriatr Soc 2000;48:1241–51.

[19] Sridhar GR, Madhu K. Prevalence of sleep disturbance in diabetes mellitus. Diabetes Res Clin Pract 1994;23:183–6.

[20] Ancoli-Israel S, Moore P, Jones V. The relationship between fatigue and sleep in cancer patients: a review. Eur J Cancer Care (Engl) 2001;10:245–55.

[21] Klink ME, Quan SF, Kaltenborn WT, et al. Risk factors associated with complaints of insomnia in a general adult population. Influence of previous complaints of insomnia. Arch Intern Med 1992;152:1634–7.

[22] Quan SF, Katz R, Olson J, et al. Factors associated with incidence and persistence of symptoms of disturbed sleep in an elderly cohort: the cardiovascular health study. Am J Med Sci 2005;329:163–72.

[23] Garcia-Borreguero D, Larrosa O, Bravo M. Parkinson's disease and sleep. Sleep Med Rev 2003;7:115–29.

[24] Ford DE, Kamerow DB. Epidemiologic study of sleep disturbances and psychiatric disorders: an opportunity for prevention? JAMA 1989;262:1479–84.

[25] Cole MG, Dendukuri N. Risk factors for depression among elderly community subjects: a systematic review and meta-analysis. Am J Psychiatry 2003;160:1147–56.

[26] Buysse DJ, Reynolds CF, Kupfer DJ, et al. Clinical diagnoses in 216 insomnia patients using the international classification of sleep disorders (ICSD), DSM-IV and ICD-10 categories: a report from the APA/NIMH DSM-IV field trial. Sleep 1994;17:630–7.

[27] Ohayon MM, Roth T. What are the contributing factors for insomnia in the general population? J Psychosom Res 2001;51:745–55.

[28] Perlis ML, Smith LJ, Lyness JM, et al. Insomnia as a risk factor for onset of depression in the elderly. Behav Sleep Med 2006;4:104–13.

[29] Nowell PD, Buysse DJ. Treatment of insomnia in patients with mood disorders. Depress Anxiety 2006;14:7–18.

[30] Morin CM, Colecchi C, Stone J, et al. Behavioral and pharmacological therapies for late life insomnia. JAMA 1999;281:991–9.

[31] NIH State of the Science Conference Statement on Insomnia. manifestations and management of chronic insomnia in adults June 13–15, 2005. Sleep 2005;28:1049–58.

[32] Morin CM, Hauri PJ, Espie CA, et al. Nonpharmacologic treatment of chronic insomnia. An American Academy of Sleep Medicine review. Sleep 1999;22:1134–56.

[33] Bootzin RR, Nicassio PM. Behavioral treatments for insomnia. In: Hersen M, Eisler RM, Miller PM, editors. Progress in behavior modification, vol. 6. New York: Academic Press; 1978. p. 1–45.
[34] Spielman AJ, Saskin P, Thorpy MJ. Treatment of chronic insomnia by restriction of time in bed. Sleep 1987;10:45–56.
[35] Sateia MJ. Insomnia. Lancet 2004;364:1959–73.
[36] Roger M, Attali P, Coquelin JP. Multicenter, double-blind, controlled comparison of zolpidem and triazolam in elderly patients with insomnia. Clin Ther 1993;15:127–36.
[37] Ancoli-Israel S, Walsh JK, Mangano RM, et al. Zaleplon Clinical Study Group. Zaleplon, a novel nonbenzodiazepine hypnotic, effectively treats insomnia in elderly patients without causing rebound effects. Primary Care Companion to J Clin Psychiatry 1999;1: 114–20.
[38] Ancoli-Israel S, Richardson GS, Mangano R, et al. Long-term use of sedative hypnotics in older patients with insomnia. Sleep Med 2005;6:107–13.
[39] Scharf MB, Erman M, Rosenberg R, et al. A 2-week efficacy and safety study of eszopiclone in elderly patients with primary insomnia. Sleep 2005;28:720–7.
[40] Roth T, Stubbs CD, Walsh JK. Ramelteon (TAK-375). A selective MT1/MT2 receptor agonist reduces latency to persistant sleep in a model of transient insomnia related to a novel sleep environment. Sleep 2005;28303–7.
[41] Swaab DF, Fliers E, Partiman TS. The suprachiasmatic nucleus of the human brain in relation to sex, age and senile dementia. Brain Res 1985;342:37–44.
[42] Touitou Y. Human aging and melatonin. Clinical relevance. Exp Gerontol 2001;36: 1083–100.
[43] Espiritu RC, Kripke DF, Ancoli-Israel S, et al. Low illumination by San Diego adults: association with atypical depressive symptoms. Biol Psychiatry 1994;35:403–7.
[44] Ancoli-Israel S, Klauber MR, Jones DW, et al. Variations in circadian rhythms of activity, sleep and light exposure related to dementia in nursing home patients. Sleep 1997;20: 18–23.
[45] Shochat T, Martin J, Marler M, et al. Illumination levels in nursing home patients: effects on sleep and activity rhythms. J Sleep Res 2000;9:373–80.
[46] Vitiello MV. Sleep disorders and aging. Curr Opin Psychiatry 1996;9:284–9.
[47] Campbell SS, Terman M, Lewy AJ, et al. light treatment for sleep disorders: consensus report. V. Age-related disturbances. J Biol Rhythms 1995;10:151–4.
[48] Haimov I, Lavie P. Potential of melatonin replacement therapy in older patients with sleep disorders. Drugs Aging 1995;7:75–8.
[49] Ancoli-Israel S, Kripke DF, Klauber MR, et al. Sleep disordered breathing in community-dwelling elderly. Sleep 1991;14:486–95.
[50] Young T, Shahar E, Nieto FJ, et al. Predictors of sleep-disordered breathing in community-dwelling adults: the Sleep Heart Health Study. Arch Intern Med 2002;162:893–900.
[51] Young T, Palta M, Dempsey J, et al. The occurrence of sleep disordered breathing among middle-aged adults. N Engl J Med 1993;328:1230–5.
[52] Bliwise DL, Carskadon MA, Carey E, et al. Longitudinal development of sleep-related respiratory disturbance in adult humans. J Gerontol 1984;39:290–3.
[53] Hoch CC, Reynolds CFI, Monk TH, et al. Comparison of sleep-disordered breathing among healthy elderly in the seventh, eighth, and ninth decades of life. Sleep 1990;13: 502–11.
[54] Ancoli-Israel S, Gehrman P, Kripke DF, et al. Long-term follow-up of sleep disordered breathing in older adults. Sleep Med 2001;2:511–6.
[55] Ancoli-Israel S, Klauber MR, Butters N, et al. Dementia in institutionalized elderly: relation to sleep apnea. J Am Geriatr Soc 1991;39:258–63.
[56] Phillips B, Ancoli-Israel S. Sleep disorders in the elderly. Sleep Med 2001;2:99–114.
[57] Collop NA, Cassell DK. Snoring and sleep-disordered breathing. In: Lee-Chiong TL, Sateia MJ, Carskadon MA, editors. Sleep medicine. Philadelphia: Hanley & Belfus; 2002. p. 349–55.

[58] Martin J, Stepnowsky C, Ancoli-Israel S. Sleep apnea in the elderly. In: McNicholas WT, Phillipson EA, editors. Breathing disorders during sleep. London: W.B. Saunders Company; 2002. p. 278–87.

[59] Aloia MS, Ilniczky N, Di Dio P, et al. Neuropsychological changes and treatment compliance in older adults with sleep apnea. J Psychosom Res 2003;54:71–6.

[60] Haas DC, Foster GL, Nieto FJ, et al. Age-dependent associations between sleep-disordered breathing and hypertension: importance of discriminating between systolic/diastolic hypertension and isolated systolic hypertension in the Sleep Heart Health Study. Circulation 2005;111:614–21.

[61] Shahar E, Whitney CW, Redline S, et al. Sleep-disordered breathing and cardiovascular disease: cross sectional results of the Sleep Heart Health Study. Am J Respir Crit Care Med 2001;163:19–25.

[62] Bassetti CL, Milanova M, Gugger M. Sleep-disordered breathing and acute ischemic stroke: diagnosis, risk factors, treatment, evolution, and long-term clinical outcome. Stroke 2006;37:967–72.

[63] Ayalon L, Ancoli-Israel S, Stepnowsky C, et al. Adherence to continuous positive airway pressure treatment in patients with Alzheimer's disease and obstructive sleep apnea. Am J Geriatr Psychiatry 2006;14:176–80.

[64] Ancoli-Israel S, Coy TV. Are breathing disturbances in elderly equivalent to sleep apnea syndrome? Sleep 1994;17:77–83.

[65] Ancoli-Israel S, Kripke DF, Klauber MR, et al. Periodic limb movements in sleep in community-dwelling elderly. Sleep 1991;14:496–500.

[66] Gehrman PR, Stepnowsky C, Cohen-Zion M, et al. Long-term follow-up of periodic limb movements in sleep in older adults. Sleep 2002;25:340–6.

[67] Hornyak M, Trenkwalder C. Restless legs syndrome and periodic limb movement disorder in the elderly. J Psychosom Res 2004;56:543–8.

[68] Hening W, Allen RP, Picchietti DL, et al. Restless Legs Syndrome Task Force of the Standards of Practice Committee of the American Academy of Sleep Medicine. An update on the dopaminergic treatment of restless legs syndrome and periodic limb movement disorder. Sleep 2004;27:560–83.

[69] Littner M, Kushida C, Anderson WM, et al. Practice parameters for the dopaminergic treatment of restless legs syndrome and periodic limb movement disorder. Sleep 2004;27:557–9.

[70] Olson EJ, Boeve BF, Silber MH. Rapid eye movement sleep behaviour disorder: demographic, clinical and laboratory findings in 93 cases. Brain 2000;123:331–9.

[71] McCurry SM, Reynolds CF, Ancoli-Israel S, et al. Treatment of sleep disturbances in Alzheimer's disease. Sleep Med Rev 2000;4:603–28.

[72] Pat-Horenczyk R, Klauber MR, Shochat T, et al. Hourly profiles of sleep and wakefulness in severely versus mild-moderately demented nursing home patients. Aging Clin Exp Res 1998;10:308–15.

[73] Gaugler JE, Edwards AB, Femia EE, et al. Predictors of institutionalization of cognitively impaired elders: family help and the timing of placement. J Gerontol B Psychol Sci Soc Sci 2000;55:247–55.

[74] Ancoli-Israel S, Kripke DF. Now I lay me down to sleep: the problem of sleep fragmentation in elderly and demented residents of nursing homes. Bull Clin Neurosci 1989;54:127–32.

[75] Middelkoop HA, Kerkhof GA, Smilde-van den Doel DA, et al. Sleep and ageing: the effect of institutionalization on subjective and objective characteristics of sleep. Age Ageing 1994;23:411–7.

[76] Schnelle JF, Cruise PA, Alessi CA, et al. Sleep hygiene in physically dependent nursing home residents. Sleep 1998;21:515–23.

[77] Alessi CA, Schnelle JF. Approach to sleep disorders in the nursing home setting. Sleep Med Rev 2000;4:45–56.

[78] Ancoli-Israel S, Gehrman PR, Martin JL, et al. Increased light exposure consolidates sleep and strengthens circadian rhythms in severe Alzheimer's disease patients. Behav Sleep Med 2003;1:22–36.
[79] Ancoli-Israel S, Martin JL, Kripke DF, et al. Effect of light treatment on sleep and circadian rhythms in demented nursing home patients. J Am Geriatr Soc 2002;50:282–9.

Psychiatr Clin N Am 29 (2006) 1095–1113

PSYCHIATRIC CLINICS
OF NORTH AMERICA

ELSEVIER
SAUNDERS

Sleep Disorders in Women: Clinical Evidence and Treatment Strategies

Claudio N. Soares, MD, PhD[a,b,*], Brian J. Murray, MD[c,d,e]

[a]Department of Psychiatry and Behavioural Neurosciences, McMaster University, Hamilton, ON, Canada
[b]Women's Health Concerns Clinic, St. Joseph's Healthcare Hamilton, Hamilton, ON, Canada
[c]Division of Neurology, Department of Medicine, University of Toronto, Toronto, ON, Canada
[d]Sunnybrook Health Sciences Centre, Toronto, ON, Canada
[e]Women's College Hospital, Toronto, ON, Canada

Several epidemiologic surveys suggest that insomnia occurs more frequently in women than men [1–3]. Overall, women have a 1.3- to 1.8-fold greater risk for developing insomnia [4]. Insomnia and other sleep disturbances are reported during specific situations associated with the female reproductive cycle, such as symptomatic premenstrual periods [5], pregnancy [6,7], and menopause [8].

Sleep patterns may change in older women, and sleep disorders become more frequent. These changes possibly are influenced by the emergence of co-existing medical conditions and the presence of other hormonal, physiologic, and even psychosocial factors [9–11]. Some reports suggest that women are more likely to experience insomnia during peri- and early postmenopausal years [12]. Insomnia is a common complaint during the menopausal transition, affecting up to 60% of women [13–15]. Putative causes of insomnia associated with the menopausal transition and postmenopausal years include the occurrence or severity of nocturnal hot flashes, mood disorders, and sleep-disordered breathing [8,16–18].

This article reviews what currently is known about sleep problems in women, with emphasis on common sleep disorders of particular relevance to various lifespan stages throughout the female reproductive lifecycle. Existing evidence on the clinical characteristics, risk factors, and treatment options for insomnia and sleep-disordered breathing in women and the potential implications of hormonal changes for their clinical management are discussed. This review focuses primarily on disorders of initiation and maintenance of sleep, which are some of the most common presenting complaints to physician practices.

*Corresponding author. Women's Health Concerns Clinic, St. Joseph's Healthcare Hamilton, 301 James Street South, FB #638, Hamilton, ON L8P 3B6, Canada. E-mail address: csoares@mcmaster.ca (C.N. Soares).

0193-953X/06/$ – see front matter
doi:10.1016/j.psc.2006.09.002

Virtually all sleep disorders can be affected by hormonal factors, however, and that there are many aspects of management that are specific to women.

PREVALENCE, RISK FACTORS, AND CLINICAL CHARACTERISTICS OF INSOMNIA IN WOMEN

Adult women are affected significantly by insomnia and other sleep complaints. The National Sleep Foundation's Women and Sleep Poll, involving 1012 women, ages 30 to 60, finds that 53% of women experienced one or more symptoms of insomnia during the month before the assessment; the most common symptom reported was related to poor sleep quality, or "feeling tired upon awakening," endorsed by 35% of the women. Other characteristics of insomnia (difficulty falling asleep, several awakenings during the night followed by difficulties getting back to sleep, and waking too early in the morning) were reported by approximately 20% of the women surveyed [19].

Various studies identify female gender as a risk factor for insomnia [2,20]; community-based studies that examine gender differences in insomnia complaints consistently show a higher prevalence of insomnia among women than among men [3,21–23]. A community survey including 9000 participants (ages 65 and older, men and women), demonstrates that women, compared with men, had more trouble falling asleep (36% versus 29%), woke up too early (31% versus 21%), or were unable to fall asleep again (25% versus 20%) [22]. Gender differences also seem to exist in younger populations; in another survey of 529 participants, ages 20 to 45, there is a significantly higher percentage of women reporting difficulties maintaining sleep (20% versus 10%, female versus male) [24]. The gender difference remains significant after adjustments for age, smoking, and psychologic status. In this study, female gender is an independent predictor of excessive daytime sleepiness and difficulty maintaining sleep almost every night. Female gender also is related significantly to increased number of awakenings per night after controlling for age, anxiety, depression, and smoking. These findings are consistent with other reports of difficulty initiating or maintaining sleep in a significant percentage of women, particularly among the elderly [25], subjects who have depression [26,27], or those who are medically ill [28–30], especially those who have pain or dyspnea [31,32].

Various factors might contribute to a heightened risk for insomnia in women compared with men. Although psychiatric disorder is a strong risk factor for insomnia in men and women, [2,33] depression [34] and anxiety [35] affect women more commonly, which may contribute to the higher prevalence of insomnia. Lindberg and colleagues examined differences in psychologic status as a possible explanation for gender differences in sleep disturbances in 529 young adults (ages 20–45 years) [24]. There was a higher percentage of women suffering from anxiety symptoms (33% versus 19%, women compared with men, respectively); women who had anxiety showed an increased prevalence of difficulty initiating sleep (9% versus 3%), difficulty maintaining sleep (32%

versus 15%), and early morning awakening (10% versus 3%) compared with those who did not have anxiety. In contrast, no significant difference was observed between anxious and nonanxious men with respect to sleep disturbances. This relationship is likely to become bidirectional (ie, altered sleep may be a perpetuating factor in various mood and anxiety disorders). For example, sleep deprivation is known to affect mood negatively [36]; in addition, conditions, such as sleep apnea, are associated with a higher prevalence of psychiatric disorders, including depression and anxiety [37]. Li and colleagues identified some female-specific risk factors in a study of gender differences in insomnia in a Chinese population (N = 9851), ages 18 to 65 [1]. Women who were divorced or widowed were more susceptible to insomnia than men under the same circumstances. Exposure to environmental noise at night was a stronger risk factor for insomnia in women than men. Frequent alcohol intake also contributed more significantly to the occurrence of insomnia in women. In a Japanese study of 650 women selected from the general population, depressive states, major life events, and "poor self-rated health" were identified as risk factors for insomnia [38]. In Finland, in a community survey of 1600 individuals, the presence of worries, human relationship problems, and regrets were the top-ranked risk factors affecting sleep, more significantly among women (19%) than men (13%) [39]. Conversely, work-related stress was the most important risk factor for insomnia among men.

The relative contribution of sex steroids for the occurrence of gender differences in insomnia is complex, understudied [40], and a point of controversy in the literature. For some women during reproductive years, sleep problems may emerge secondary to menstrual symptoms (eg, cramping, bloating, headaches, and tender breasts) or dysmenorrhea [41,42]. Polysomnographic (PSG) data indicate that women who have dysmenorrhea experience less efficient sleep (ratio of the time spent asleep to the time in bed) and more wakefulness than women who do not have painful menstrual cycles [43]. Also, sex hormone receptors are present in the suprachiasmatic nucleus, the key biologic clock in the brain, and gender differences in its stimulation do exist [44]. Similarly, female-specific conditions, such as polycystic ovarian syndrome, can be associated with endocrine changes and result in a significant increase in sleep-disordered breathing, which can contribute to sleep fragmentation and daytime sleepiness [45].

PERIMENSTRUAL SLEEP AND MOOD PROBLEMS

Studies examining a putative association between phases of the menstrual cycle and sleep problems have produced mixed results. Although clinically intuitive, some [46] but not all [47] studies corroborated the existence of significant sleep disruption associated with premenstrual complaints, premenstrual syndrome, or diagnosis of premenstrual dysphoric disorder [48–50]. There are reports of hypersomnia [51] and insomnia [46] temporally linked to the premenstrual phase of the menstrual cycle. Consistent evidence of changes in sleep architecture (eg, PSG measures) associated with symptomatic premenstrual periods is lacking, however, despite patients' subjective reports of sleep being disrupted during this period. The inconsistency in the literature likely is related to small sample sizes studied and significant heterogeneity of underlying sleep or endocrine characteristics assessed [12].

SLEEP, PREGNANCY, AND POSTPARTUM PERIOD

Pregnancy is a time of significant physiologic changes, and it is not surprising that sleep is altered. Sleep seems to be disrupted substantially during pregnancy and the postpartum period; prevalence rates for altered sleep during pregnancy range from 15% to 80%, depending on the population studied and the time of assessment (eg, higher rates during the third trimester of pregnancy compared with first trimester) [52]. Sleep in the postpartum period is disrupted markedly by care of the infant and can be assessed objectively with tools, such as actigraphy [53]. Even in the absence of infant care, the sleep that follows pregnancy is disrupted and often does not return to the prepregnancy state [54]. This may reflect the outcome of some of the physiologic changes that occurred during the course of pregnancy or even the emergence of anxiety and hypervigilance behaviors toward the newborn. In summary, existing literature suggests that the peripartum sleep disruption and the emergence of anxiety symptoms may affect mood during this period; further studies are needed to explore more objective measures of sleep in the postpartum period [55].

Survey studies indicate that women attribute many different reasons to justify their altered sleep during pregnancy; during the first trimester, nausea and vomiting frequently are associated with sleep problems [56]; psychosocial stressors also are reported, particularly in cases involving first-time pregnancies, unplanned pregnancies, or the absence of solid psychosocial support or networks [57].

As pregnancy progresses into the second and third trimesters, there are more reports of increased number of awakenings, fatigue, leg cramps, and shortness of breath. One of the authors of this article has observed that leg cramps noted in overnight PSG sometimes follow a series of periodic limb movements of which patients often are unaware (Brian J. Murray, MD, unpublished observations, 2006). Overall, women are more likely to go to bed earlier and nap frequently during the day as they try to compensate for the disruption of the nighttime sleep pattern [58].

When assessing altered sleep during pregnancy, consider changes in sex steroids that may occur during this process and the relative contribution of these hormonal changes for the occurrence of sleep-disordered breathing in this population. Snoring tends to increase during pregnancy, possibly resulting from changes in upper airway resistance, which is sensitive to hormonal factors, in particular progesterone levels [59]. In addition, pregnant women, particularly during the final trimester, seem to have a heightened risk for developing sleep apnea and restless legs syndrome (RLS) [6,60]. Studies suggest that RLS might be more associated with lower ferritin and folate levels. Thus, nutritional supplements should be considered for symptomatic individuals or subpopulations at risk [61].

Objective assessments of sleep during pregnancy produce inconsistent results, again likely because of limited sample sizes and differing research methodology [62]. A well-designed study assessed 33 women from prepregnancy throughout pregnancy and post partum and included in-home PSG and measures of fatigue. This study revealed changes in sleep during the first trimester, with a significant increase in total sleep time and decrease in slow wave sleep (restorative sleep) compared with prepregnancy assessments [7]. Subjective fatigue increased during the first trimester and was correlated with prepregnancy levels of iron, ferritin (a better marker of iron stores in the brain) [63], and younger age. Total sleep time tends to return to normal levels at the end of the third trimester, as women report more frequent awakenings and a decline in sleep efficiency. The same study shows that experienced mothers (multiparous) are more likely to increase their time in bed compared with first-time mothers, in a possible attempt to improve their sleep time in the context of reduced sleep efficiency.

RLS is surprisingly common in pregnancy and affects approximately 25% of mothers [60,64]. This may be related at least partially to iron deficiency, as progressive iron depletion occurs with fetal development and standard iron supplementation in pregnancy often is insufficient to replace the need; in addition, iron deficiency remains common in women of childbearing age [65]. One third of pregnant patients in one study had iron stores that were in the range where RLS was particularly prominent [61]. Depletion of iron can be noted in basal ganglia structures in the brain of patients who have RLS [66], which is even more interesting, given the roles of these structures for mood regulation [67]. Furthermore, iron is the rate-limiting step in the synthesis of dopamine in the brain [68]. Therefore, the relationship between iron loss, RLS, and peripartum mood disorders warrants further investigation.

Similarly, sleep-disordered breathing increases over the course of pregnancy because of many factors, including weight gain, mucosal edema, and changes in respiratory mechanics. Although frank obstructive sleep apnea generally is not common in this population, it can occur and its treatment is important given potential implications for maternal health; there also are data suggesting intrauterine growth retardation may be more common in children of these mothers [69]. More commonly, upper airway resistance increases throughout pregnancy [70] and may contribute to frequent arousals and, therefore, sleep maintenance insomnia with subsequent daytime sleepiness.

Disrupted sleep during pregnancy is associated with poor obstetric outcomes, in particular length of labor and type of delivery. In a prospective, longitudinal follow-up of 131 pregnant women, Lee and Gay demonstrate that women who slept less than 6 hours at night had longer labors and were 4.5 times more likely to have cesarean deliveries. The researchers, therefore, highlight the importance of monitoring sleep quantity and quality during prenatal assessments, as they are potential predictors of labor duration and delivery type [71].

The assessment of changes in sleep architecture and sleep efficiency during the postpartum period constitutes a challenging task given the various components of this equation (eg, hormonal changes inherent to the postpartum period, sleep deprivation resulting from frequent awakenings associated with breastfeeding, and the presence or severity of postnatal mood and behavior changes). Objective assessments (PSG) of women immediately after delivery indicate an increase in wake time after sleep onset and awakenings even in the absence of nocturnal activities involving infant care and nursing [54]. Women in the postpartum period seem to develop a lower sleep efficiency, with shorter latency to rapid eye movement (REM) sleep (characteristic of depression) and reduction in total sleep time. Although the majority of studies suggest that most awakenings and changes in sleep/wake ratios are related directly to newborns' direct nursing care, it is hypothesized that other factors could contribute to this disruption, including an abrupt decline in progesterone (a hormone with known sedative properties) immediately after delivery and changes in melatonin levels—the latter possibly affecting the normal circadian rhythm [12,47]. Moreover, the occurrence of increased irritability and mood swings post partum (postnatal blues) could lead to a disruption of new mothers' sleep efficiency and increase the risk for subsequent development of postpartum depression [55,72]. Another possibility is that the sleep disruption itself contributes directly to many of these mood changes. Preliminary, but intriguing, evidence suggests that some strategies to promote protected sleep time immediately after delivery (eg, prolonged hospital stay, "rooming out" infants under a partner's or nurse's care, and use of sedatives as needed) may reduce the risk of clinically significant depression or anxiety in the first few months of the postpartum period (Meir Steiner, MD, PhD, personal communication, 2005).

MENOPAUSE
Menopausal Transition, Hot Flashes, and Insomnia
Menopause is a natural event that occurs typically when a woman is in her early 50s and is associated most commonly with the aging process and ovarian failure [73]. The menopausal transition, however, usually begins several years earlier [74] and is characterized by the occurrence of vasomotor symptoms (eg, hot flashes and night sweats), sleep disturbances, and changes in sexual function that can affect quality of life adversely [75–78]. Women approaching menopause also may present with increased risk for developing osteoporosis, cardiovascular disease, and cognitive deficits [79–81]. More recently, several studies revealed that women entering perimenopause are at higher risk for developing depression, even in the absence of prior episodes of depression [82–86].

Approximately 45% to 75% of women in menopausal transition experience hot flashes [87,88]. Hot flashes are transient sensations of heat dissipation and may be accompanied by palpitations, nausea, dizziness, headache, and ultimately insomnia [89]. The presence of nocturnal hot flashes commonly is associated with sleep disturbances [12,90].

The pathophysiology of hot flashes is not understood fully, but it is believed to be mediated through the anterior hypothalamus, an area that regulates temperature and sleep [91–94]. Despite more recent evidence [16], a direct association between hot flashes and insomnia is considered controversial, because most studies using objective sleep measures (ie, PSG) or subjective measures (ie, sleep questionnaires) show inconsistent findings. Early PSG studies in menopausal women suggested a significant correlation between hot flashes and sleep disturbances [95]. Additionally, the use of estrogen therapy resulted in a significant reduction of sleep latency, frequency of awakenings, and improvement of REM sleep [96,97]. More recent studies, however, fail to show positive effects of hormone therapy (HT) on sleep architecture in menopausal women [98,99]. Some of the confusion in this literature may be related to different formulations of HTs.

Subjective sleep studies provide more consistent, but perhaps less rigorous, evidence of the association between hot flashes and insomnia; there seems to be a positive impact of hormonal interventions on sleep complaints and vasomotor symptoms [100–102]. Subjective sleep quality measures in women who have hot flashes and insomnia not always are corroborated by PSG characteristics, however [98].

Menopause-Related Depression and Insomnia

The extent to which mood and behavior are affected during the menopausal transition is unknown [103,104]. Many women who develop depressive symptoms during this period also experience hot flashes and insomnia [86], suggesting a potential association between sleep disruption and the occurrence or severity of vasomotor symptoms, leading to an adverse impact on mood and well-being [105,106]. Depression is found in some menopausal women, however, even in the absence of clinically significant hot flashes [107].

Evidence that depression and insomnia may share similar mediators through the hypothalamic-pituitary-adrenal (HPA) axis comes from profound changes in sleep patterns and mood observed in patients who are medically ill and receiving synthetic corticosteroids [108]. Fluctuating estrogen (E2) levels during the perimenopause also could exacerbate the HPA axis activity in response to stress, resulting in mood and sleep disorders [109].

Estrogen modulates the synthesis, release, and metabolism of monoamines that affect mood, behavior, and sleep [110]. Estrogen exerts an agonist effect on serotonergic activity by increasing the number of serotonin receptors, increasing transport and uptake of the neurotransmitter, increasing synthesis of serotonin, up-regulating serotonin 1 receptors, down-regulating serotonin 2 receptors, and decreasing monoamine oxidase activity [111]. Gonadal hormones also regulate γ-aminobutyric acid (GABA), which plays a central role in sleep initiation and maintenance. Preclinical studies show that gonadal hormones have a barbiturate-like action on the GABA receptor complex [112]. Estrogen seems to reduce the number of GABA-A receptors, but progesterone is shown to counter that effect [112]. Therefore, consideration of particular hormone formulations is critical when interpreting conflicting data on the effects of hormones on sleep. Fluctuations in estrogen and progesterone may alter GABA function and play a role in menopause-related insomnia [113].

Sleep-Disordered Breathing in Menopause

Sleep-disordered breathing is most prevalent in men but often under-recognized in women [114,115]. Very conservatively, the prevalence of obstructive sleep apnea syndrome (OSAS) in women is 1.2% compared with 3.9% in men [23]. The prevalence of milder forms of sleep-disordered breathing in women is higher and seems to increase with age, however [115]. Studies show that OSAS has a different clinical pattern in women than in men. Women have fewer respiratory events per hour of sleep and episodes are of shorter duration compared with those in men [116].

OSAS in women can be hormonally related. Diminishing progesterone levels during menopause may be a cause of OSAS, as progesterone is a known respiratory stimulant and upper airway dilator [117]. Increased body weight associated with menopause also may be a cause. Menopause is associated significantly with increased risk of OSAS, independently of body weight [115]. Some of this effect may be mediated by testosterone, which may decrease the threshold for the occurrence of apnea [118]. Sleep-disordered breathing in various studies is confounded by different methodologies for measuring airway resistance [119] and different definitions for what constitutes a hypopnea. Definitions that include more severe frank apneic events or oxygen desaturation are more likely to identify events in men, whereas definitions that include arousal may be more likely to identify the sleep fragmentation and daytime sleepiness in women, as women are less likely to manifest complete cessation of airflow or oxygen desaturation. Differences in the definition of respiratory events, therefore, may contribute to bias and underdetection of clinically relevant sleep-disordered breathing in women, leading not only to missed treatment opportunities but also to misinterpretation or misdiagnosis of daytime sleepiness [120].

ESTABLISHING A DIAGNOSIS

The first step in management is to establish a clear diagnosis. A careful interview of patients (and more importantly bed partners, who are objective observers for behaviors of which patients may be unaware) is essential. To address women's sleep problems fully, a routine history and physical examination is required, with particular attention to medical and psychiatric contributors to a patient's problem. Hormonal status must be considered. A typical day's sleep behavior can be obtained chronologically and should include details of sleep onset, sleep maintenance, and daytime alertness.

Often a sleep problem has medical and behavioral components. Both factors need to be addressed to ensure clinical improvement. To that end, ensure that medical causes of insomnia (RLS, in particular, for sleep initiation difficulties and sleep-disordered breathing for sleep maintenance problems) are treated adequately before embarking on behavioral management. Some intrinsic sleep disorders, such as poor sleep hygiene or RLS, can be established based purely on history, whereas others, such as obstructive sleep apnea, require formal PSG assessment.

INSOMNIA TREATMENTS

A wide range of nonpharmacologic and pharmacologic therapies is available for the treatment of insomnia and is reviewed in detail in articles elsewhere in this issue; studies focused on female-specific conditions, however, are scarce. In general, insomnia therapies should improve daytime functioning by improving sleep continuity (reducing interrupted sleep) and increasing total sleep time [121]. Establishing an appropriate diagnosis is the first step, and ensuring elimination of medical contributors is paramount. Specific treatment for RLS is reviewed elsewhere, but first-line therapy includes dopaminergic agents [122]. Sleep apnea often is treated with weight loss, positional therapy, dental appliances, continuous positive airway pressure, or surgery, in more severe cases [123]. Once these factors are addressed, symptomatic therapy often is pursued. In pregnancy and breast-feeding scenarios, special attention must be made to the safety of medications that may be considered for treatment. Unfortunately, many medications are not tested formally in these populations, leaving significant knowledge gaps. Nonpharmacologic therapies, therefore, become critically important for these patients.

Nonpharmacologic Therapies

Nonpharmacologic approaches to insomnia could be seen as the mainstay of insomnia treatment. Some patients are reluctant to use medications for insomnia, particularly because of the possibility of habituation, withdrawal, and rebound insomnia with the use of pharmacologic therapies [124]. Few clinicians know, however, how to use nonpharmacologic interventions, such as behavioral therapies; other negative aspects of nonpharmacologic strategies include limited number of controlled studies for specific interventions (particularly for herbal preparations), cost or lack of insurance reimbursement, and slower speed of onset [122,125–128].

Behavioral Therapies

Behavioral approaches provide similar short-term clinical benefits for the management of insomnia compared with pharmacologic therapies but have better long-term benefits, especially in older adults [125,126,129]. Overall, stimulus control and sleep restriction therapies are the most effective behavioral approaches [122,130]. Details of these therapies are reviewed elsewhere in this issue. Developing good sleep hygiene habits is important but shows limited efficacy when used alone [130,131]. Other behavioral techniques include meditation, biofeedback, and hypnotherapy. Hypnotherapy shows some efficacy in small trials [132]. In one of these studies, hypnotherapy was used in women treated for breast cancer and had a positive impact on hot flashes and improved quality of sleep [133].

Data on the efficacy of behavioral therapies for the treatment of insomnia in menopausal women are limited. Given many unique factors contributing to insomnia in this population (ie, the higher incidence of hot flashes and sleep-disordered breathing), it is difficult to predict the extent to which these treatments would be efficacious when used alone.

Herbal and Dietary Supplements for the Management of Insomnia: Focus on Menopause

Several herbal preparations have putative therapeutic benefits for the treatment of menopause-related symptoms, including vasomotor symptoms and insomnia. *Cimicifuga racemosa* (black cohosh) shows more positive results than placebo for the treatment of menopause-related physical and psychologic complaints [134–137], although no objective studies for the treatment of insomnia are published to date.

Valerian (*Valerian officinalis*) seems to have sedative and muscle-relaxant effects and its use has become increasingly popular among women [138,139]. The evidence for its efficacy as a treatment for insomnia is inconclusive, based on a systematic review of nine clinical trials [140]. In addition, sleep benefit may be delayed for 2 weeks and some patients experience residual daytime effects [141].

Chamomile (*Matricaria recutita*) and passionflower (*Passiflora incarnata*) seem to have sedative properties resulting from their flavinoid components. No clinical studies have been conducted in female-specific subpopulations, however [141].

Hormone Therapy

For several decades, HT has been the gold standard treatment for many menopausal complaints, including hot flashes and insomnia [96,98,142,143]. There also is evidence for its efficacy for the treatment of depression during perimenopause and, to a lesser extent, for OSAS [144–148]. The long-term safety of HT is questioned, however, particularly in light of the results from the Women's Health Initiative study [149]. Consequently, many physicians and patients are seeking nonHTs for the relief of menopausal symptoms. In addition, the use of HT for the management of menopause-related insomnia shows limited results when objective parameters of sleep are used [99]. HT is not uniform, however, and consists of various estrogen and progesterone formulations and doses that may lead to differential effects on sleep [150].

Antidepressants

The past 20 years have seen an increase in the off-label use of antidepressants for insomnia, with little or no evidence of their efficacy for the treatment of sleep complaints [151]. When used in women who are perimenopausal or postmenopausal, some antidepressants (eg, paroxetine, citalopram, and mirtazapine) may have an indirect effect on sleep and quality of life by improving other menopause-related symptoms (eg, vasomotor symptoms, pain, and mood swings); thus, these agents might constitute a treatment option for symptomatic women who are unable or unwilling to receive HTs [101,152–154].

Benzodiazepines

Pharmacologic therapies indicated for insomnia modulate primarily GABA-A receptors and exert their effect on the benzodiazepine site of the receptors, thereby potentiating the inhibitory effect of GABA on neurotransmission

[155]. To date, no studies have examined the efficacy of benzodiazepines for the treatment of insomnia related to more female-specific conditions.

Nonbenzodiazepines

Replacing benzodiazepines as first-line agents for insomnia are the nonbenzo-diazepine receptor agonists (non-BZRAs), commonly known as Z compounds, such as zolpidem, zaleplon, and eszopiclone [155–158]. Currently, most non-BZRAs are recommended for short-term treatment of insomnia. Both zolpidem and eszopiclone demonstrate sustained efficacy and safety without the development of tolerance or rebound insomnia over 6 months to 1 year [157,159].

A 4-week, placebo-controlled trial (N = 141) with zolpidem shows statistically significant improvement in some parameters of insomnia (increased total sleep time, decreased wake time after sleep onset, and number of awakenings) in women who are perimenopausal or postmenopausal; however, the study does not assess if zolpidem affected positively or negatively other menopause-related complaints.

In a larger study (N = 410), eszopiclone shows superior efficacy compared with placebo for the treatment of insomnia in perimenopause and early menopause subjects who had developed insomnia in the context of transitioning to menopause and reported other menopause-related symptoms (eg, hot flashes or night sweats) without comorbid depression or anxiety [160]. Subjects receiving eszopiclone reported significantly greater improvement in sleep induction, sleep maintenance (total awakenings, awakenings because of hot flashes, and time awake after sleep onset), sleep duration, sleep quality, and next-day functioning. The use of eszopiclone resulted in improvement of quality of life and other menopause-specific symptoms, assessed by the Greene Climacteric Scale, the Menopause-Specific Quality of Life questionnaire, and changes in family life or home disability domains of the Sheehan Disability Scale.

SUMMARY

Women commonly report sleep disorders that may predispose or contribute to the occurrence of other psychiatric problems. Many phases of the life cycle are associated with unique features of sleep disruption that are modulated at least partially by hormonal factors. Pregnancy and peripartum and perimenopausal states are associated particularly with sleep disruption and have the clearest published evidence base. Many factors contribute to a heightened incidence of insomnia in women, including the occurrence or severity of somatic symptoms (eg, hot flashes and dysmenorrhea); psychiatric symptoms, such as depression or anxiety; and intrinsic sleep disorders. The presence of insomnia is associated with poorer quality of life and impaired daytime functioning; its management, therefore, is imperative.

Significant physiologic changes in pregnancy lead to several sleep disorders. Sleep-disordered breathing and RLS are common in women but even more in this subpopulation. Given the strong possibility that sleep disorders are contributing to mood changes in pregnant women, careful attention must be paid to the development of treatment strategies that address medical and psychologic factors to assist this vulnerable population fully.

For symptomatic menopausal women, HT still is the treatment of choice for short-term management of menopause-related symptoms, in particular hot flashes; however, its safety as a long-term treatment option is questioned, and many physicians and their patients are seeking nonhormonal alternatives. An accurate diagnosis must be made in this population, and treatment of underlying sleep disorders is crucial. Most nonpharmacologic symptomatic treatments for insomnia (eg, stimulus control and sleep restriction) have not been studied systematically in patients who are menopausal, despite their proved efficacy for insomnia in general. The use of antidepressants and herbal preparations seem more helpful when sleep complaints result from the emergence of menopause-related symptoms, depression, or anxiety.

Women who suffer insomnia during the menopausal transition or post menopause may benefit from the therapeutic effects of newer agents, such as the non-BZRAs (zolpidem and eszopiclone) and melatonin receptor antagonists; more studies are needed to determine the extent to which these agents can offer a safe and efficacious long-term management of insomnia with a positive impact on daytime function and improvement of quality of life.

References

[1] Li RH, Wing YK, Ho SC, et al. Gender differences in insomnia—a study in the Hong Kong Chinese population. J Psychosom Res 2002;53:601–9.

[2] Klink ME, Quan SF, Kaltenborn WT, et al. Risk factors associated with complaints of insomnia in a general adult population. Influence of previous complaints of insomnia. Arch Intern Med 1992;152:1634–7.

[3] Rocha FL, Guerra HL, Lima-Costa MF. Prevalence of insomnia and associated socio-demographic factors in a Brazilian community: the Bambui study. Sleep Med 2002;3:121–6.

[4] Krystal AD. Insomnia in women. Clin Cornerstone 2003;5:41–50.

[5] Schenck CH, Mahowald MW. Two cases of premenstrual sleep terrors and injurious sleep-walking. J Psychosom Obstet Gynaecol 1995;16:79–84.

[6] Sahota PK, Jain SS, Dhand R. Sleep disorders in pregnancy. Curr Opin Pulm Med 2003;9:477–83.

[7] Lee KA, Zaffke ME. Longitudinal changes in fatigue and energy during pregnancy and the postpartum period. J Obstet Gynecol Neonatal Nurs 1999;28:183–91.

[8] Dennerstein L, Dudley EC, Hopper JL, et al. A prospective population-based study of menopausal symptoms. Obstet Gynecol 2000;96:351–8.

[9] Martin J, Shochat T, Ancoli-Israel S. Assessment and treatment of sleep disturbances in older adults. Clin Psychol Rev 2000;20:783–805.

[10] Ancoli-Israel S, Cooke JR. Prevalence and comorbidity of insomnia and effect on functioning in elderly populations. J Am Geriatr Soc 2005;53(7 Suppl):S264–71.

[11] McCrae CS, Rowe MA, Tierney CG, et al. Sleep complaints, subjective and objective sleep patterns, health, psychological adjustment, and daytime functioning in community-dwelling older adults. J Gerontol B Psychol Sci Soc Sci 2005;60:182–9.

[12] Moline ML, Broch L, Zak R, Gross V. Sleep in women across the life cycle from adulthood through menopause. Sleep Med Rev 2003;7:155–77.

[13] Owens JF, Matthews KA. Sleep disturbance in healthy middle-aged women. Maturitas 1998;30:41–50.

[14] Moline M, Broch L, Zak R. Sleep problems across the life cycle in women. Curr Treat Options Neurol 2004;6:319–30.
[15] Shin C, Lee S, Lee T, et al. Prevalence of insomnia and its relationship to menopausal status in middle-aged Korean women. Psychiatry Clin Neurosci 2005;59:395–402.
[16] Ohayon MM. Severe hot flashes are associated with chronic insomnia. Arch Intern Med 2006;166:1262–8.
[17] Shahar E, Redline S, Young T, et al. Hormone replacement therapy and sleep-disordered breathing. Am J Respir Crit Care Med 2003;167:1186–92.
[18] Krystal AD, Edinger J, Wohlgemuth W, et al. Sleep in peri-menopausal and post-menopausal women. Sleep Med Rev 1998;2:243–53.
[19] National Sleep Foundation. Sleep in America poll 2005. Washington (DC): National Sleep Foundation, 2005.
[20] Ford DE, Kamerow DB. Epidemiologic study of sleep disturbances and psychiatric disorders. An opportunity for prevention? JAMA 1989;262:1479–84.
[21] Radecki SE, Brunton SA. Management of insomnia in office-based practice. National prevalence and therapeutic patterns. Arch Fam Med 1993;2:1129–34.
[22] Foley DJ, Monjan AA, Brown SL, et al. Sleep complaints among elderly persons: an epidemiologic study of three communities. Sleep 1995;18:425–32.
[23] Bixler EO, Vgontzas AN, Lin HM, et al. Prevalence of sleep-disordered breathing in women: effects of gender. Am J Respir Crit Care Med 2001;163(3 Pt 1):608–13.
[24] Lindberg E, Janson C, Gislason T, et al. Sleep disturbances in a young adult population: can gender differences be explained by differences in psychological status? Sleep 1997;20:381–7.
[25] Liu X, Liu L. Sleep habits and insomnia in a sample of elderly persons in China. Sleep 2005;28:1579–87.
[26] McCall WV, Reboussin BA, Cohen W. Subjective measurement of insomnia and quality of life in depressed inpatients. J Sleep Res 2000;9:43–8.
[27] Breslau N, Roth T, Rosenthal L, et al. Sleep disturbance and psychiatric disorders: a longitudinal epidemiological study of young adults. Biol Psychiatry 1996;39:411–8.
[28] Gislason T, Almqvist M. Somatic diseases and sleep complaints. An epidemiological study of 3,201 Swedish men. Acta Med Scand 1987;221:475–81.
[29] Strang P. Emotional and social aspects of cancer pain. Acta Oncol 1992;31:323–6.
[30] Davison SN, Jhangri GS. The impact of chronic pain on depression, sleep, and the desire to withdraw from dialysis in hemodialysis patients. J Pain Symptom Manage 2005;30:465–73.
[31] Ohayon MM. Relationship between chronic painful physical condition and insomnia. J Psychiatr Res 2005;39:151–9.
[32] Meuser T, Pietruck C, Radbruch L, et al. Symptoms during cancer pain treatment following WHO-guidelines: a longitudinal follow-up study of symptom prevalence, severity and etiology. Pain 2001;93:247–57.
[33] Mallon L, Broman JE, Hetta J. Relationship between insomnia, depression, and mortality: a 12-year follow-up of older adults in the community. Int Psychogeriatr 2000;12:295–306.
[34] Piccinelli M, Wilkinson G. Gender differences in depression. Critical review. Br J Psychiatry 2000;177:486–92.
[35] Kohn L, Espie CA. Sensitivity and specificity of measures of the insomnia experience: a comparative study of psychophysiologic insomnia, insomnia associated with mental disorder and good sleepers. Sleep 2005;28:104–12.
[36] Durmer JS, Dinges DF. Neurocognitive consequences of sleep deprivation. Semin Neurol 2005;25:117–29.
[37] Sharafkhaneh A, Giray N, Richardson P, et al. Association of psychiatric disorders and sleep apnea in a large cohort. Sleep 2005;28:1405–11.
[38] Kawada T, Yosiaki S, Yasuo K, et al. Population study on the prevalence of insomnia and insomnia-related factors among Japanese women. Sleep Med 2003;4:563–7.

[39] Urponen H, Vuori I, Hasan J, et al. Self-evaluations of factors promoting and disturbing sleep: an epidemiological survey in Finland. Soc Sci Med 1988;26:443–50.

[40] Manber R, Armitage R. Sex, steroids, and sleep: a review. Sleep 1999;22:540–55.

[41] Baker FC, Driver HS. Self-reported sleep across the menstrual cycle in young, healthy women. J Psychosom Res 2004;56:239–43.

[42] Cluydts R, Visser P. Mood and sleep. I. Effects of the menstrual cycle. Waking Sleeping 1980;4:193–7.

[43] Baker FC, Driver HS, Rogers GG, et al. High nocturnal body temperatures and disturbed sleep in women with primary dysmenorrhea. Am J Physiol 1999;277(6 Pt 1):E1013–21.

[44] Kruijver FP, Swaab DF. Sex hormone receptors are present in the human suprachiasmatic nucleus. Neuroendocrinology 2002;75:296–305.

[45] Vgontzas AN, Legro RS, Bixler EO, et al. Polycystic ovary syndrome is associated with ob-structive sleep apnea and daytime sleepiness: role of insulin resistance. J Clin Endocrinol Metab 2001;86:517–20.

[46] Manber R, Bootzin RR. Sleep and the menstrual cycle. Health Psychol 1997;16:209–14.

[47] Lee KA, McEnany G, Zaffke ME. REM sleep and mood state in childbearing women: sleepy or weepy? Sleep 2000;23:877–85.

[48] Mauri M, Reid RL, MacLean AW. Sleep in the premenstrual phase: a self-report study of PMS patients and normal controls. Acta Psychiatr Scand 1988;78:82–6.

[49] Sheldrake P, Cormack M. Variations in menstrual cycle symptom reporting. J Psychosom Res 1976;20:169–77.

[50] Parry BL, Mostofi N, LeVeau B, et al. Sleep EEG studies during early and late partial sleep deprivation in premenstrual dysphoric disorder and normal control subjects. Psychiatry Res 1999;85:127–43.

[51] Sachs C, Persson HE, Hagenfeldt K. Menstruation-related periodic hypersomnia: a case study with successful treatment. Neurology 1982;32:1376–9.

[52] Hedman C, Pohjasvaara T, Tolonen U, et al. Effects of pregnancy on mothers' sleep. Sleep Med 2002;3:37–42.

[53] Shinkoda H, Matsumoto K, Park YM. Changes in sleep-wake cycle during the period from late pregnancy to puerperium identified through the wrist actigraph and sleep logs. Psychi-atry Clin Neurosci 1999;53:133–5.

[54] Karacan I, Williams RL, Hursch CJ, et al. Some implications of the sleep patterns of preg-nancy for postpartum emotional disturbances. Br J Psychiatry 1969;115:929–35.

[55] Ross LE, Murray BJ, Steiner M. Sleep and perinatal mood disorders: a critical review. J Psy-chiatry Neurosci 2005;30:247–56.

[56] Schweiger MS. Sleep disturbance in pregnancy. A subjective survey. Am J Obstet Gynecol 1972;114:879–82.

[57] Walker LO, Cooney AT, Riggs MW. Psychosocial and demographic factors related to health behaviors in the 1st trimester. J Obstet Gynecol Neonatal Nurs 1999;28:606–14.

[58] Mindell JA, Jacobson BJ. Sleep disturbances during pregnancy. J Obstet Gynecol Neona-tal Nurs 2000;29:590–7.

[59] Edwards N, Middleton PG, Blyton DM, et al. Sleep disordered breathing and pregnancy. Thorax 2002;57:555–8.

[60] Manconi M, Govoni V, De Vito A, et al. Restless legs syndrome and pregnancy. Neurology 2004;63:1065–9.

[61] Lee KA, Zaffke ME, Baratte-Beebe K. Restless legs syndrome and sleep disturbance during pregnancy: the role of folate and iron. J Womens Health Gend Based Med 2001;10:335–41.

[62] Santiago JR, Nolledo MS, Kinzler W, et al. Sleep and sleep disorders in pregnancy. Ann Intern Med 2001;134:396–408.

[63] Sorond FA, Ratan RR. Ironing-out mechanisms of neuronal injury under hypoxic-ischemic conditions and potential role of iron chelators as neuroprotective agents. Antioxid Redox Signal 2000;2:421–36.

[64] Goodman JD, Brodie C, Ayida GA. Restless leg syndrome in pregnancy. BMJ 1988;297: 1101–2.

[65] Looker AC, Dallman PR, Carroll MD, et al. Prevalence of iron deficiency in the United States. JAMA 1997;277:973–6.

[66] Earley CJ, B Parker P, Horska A, et al. MRI-determined regional brain iron concentrations in early- and late-onset restless legs syndrome. Sleep Med 2006;7:458–61.

[67] Bejjani BP, Damier P, Arnulf I, et al. Transient acute depression induced by high-frequency deep-brain stimulation. N Engl J Med 1999;340:1476–80.

[68] Sun ER, Chen CA, Ho G, et al. Iron and the restless legs syndrome. Sleep 1998;21:371–7.

[69] Franklin KA, Holmgren PA, Jonsson F, et al. Snoring, pregnancy-induced hypertension, and growth retardation of the fetus. Chest 2000;117:137–41.

[70] Edwards E, Whitaker-Azmitia PM, Harkins K. 5–HT1A and 5–HT1B agonists play a differential role on the respiratory frequency in rats. Neuropsychopharmacology 1990;3: 129–36.

[71] Lee KA, Gay CL. Sleep in late pregnancy predicts length of labor and type of delivery. Am J Obstet Gynecol 2004;191:2041–6.

[72] Soares CN. Insomnia in women: an overlooked epidemic? Arch Women Ment Health 2005;8:205–13.

[73] Shifren JL, Schiff I. The aging ovary. J Womens Health Gend Based Med 2000;9(Suppl 1): S3–7.

[74] Soules M, Sherman S, Parrott E, et al. Executive summary: Stages of Reproductive Aging Workshop (STRAW). Fertil Steril 2001;76:874–8.

[75] Barton D, Loprinzi C, Wahner-Roedler D. Hot flashes: aetiology and management. Drugs Aging 2001;18:597–606.

[76] Baker A, Simpson S, Dawson D. Sleep disruption and mood changes associated with menopause. J Psychosom Res 1997;43:359–69.

[77] Stone AB, Pearlstein TB. Evaluation and treatment of changes in mood, sleep, and sexual functioning associated with menopause. Obstet Gynecol Clin North Am 1994;21: 391–403.

[78] Soares CN, Joffe H, Steiner M. Menopause and mood. Clin Obstet Gynecol 2004;47: 576–91.

[79] Fiorano-Charlier C, Ostertag A, Aquino JP, et al. Reduced bone mineral density in postmenopausal women self-reporting premenopausal wrist fractures. Bone 2002;31:102–6.

[80] Hunter M, Battersby R, Whitehead M. Relationships between psychological symptoms, somatic complaints and menopausal status. Maturitas 1986;8:217–28.

[81] Grodstein F, Stampfer MJ, Colditz GA, et al. Postmenopausal hormone therapy and mortality. N Engl J Med 1997;336:1769–75.

[82] Maartens LW, Knottnerus JA, Pop VJ. Menopausal transition and increased depressive symptomatology: a community based prospective study. Maturitas 2002;42:195–200.

[83] Bromberger JT, Assmann SF, Avis NE, et al. Persistent mood symptoms in a multiethnic community cohort of pre- and perimenopausal women. Am J Epidemiol 2003;158:347–56.

[84] Schmidt PJ, Haq N, Rubinow DR. A longitudinal evaluation of the relationship between reproductive status and mood in perimenopausal women. Am J Psychiatry 2004;161: 2238–44.

[85] Freeman EW, Sammel MD, Lin H, et al. Associations of hormones and menopausal status with depressed mood in women with no history of depression. Arch Gen Psychiatry 2006;63:375–82.

[86] Cohen LS, Soares CN, Vitonis AF, et al. Risk for new onset of depression during the menopausal transition: the Harvard Study of Moods and Cycles. Arch Gen Psychiatry 2006;63:385–90.

[87] Freeman EW, Sammel MD, Grisso JA, et al. Hot flashes in the late reproductive years: risk factors for Africa American and Caucasian women. J Womens Health Gend Based Med 2001;10:67–76.

[88] Joffe H, Soares CN, Cohen LS. Assessment and treatment of hot flushes and menopausal mood disturbance. Psychiatr Clin North Am 2003;26:563–80.

[89] Freedman RR. Physiology of hot flashes. Am J Human Biol 2001;13:453–64.

[90] Bachmann GA. Vasomotor flushes in menopausal women. Am J Obstet Gynecol 1999;180(3 Pt 2):S312–6.

[91] Freedman RR. Biochemical, metabolic, and vascular mechanisms in menopausal hot flashes. Fertil Steril 1998;70:332–7.

[92] Steingold KA, Laufer L, Chetkowski RJ, et al. Treatment of hot flashes with transdermal estradiol administration. J Clin Endocrinol Metab 1985;61:627–32.

[93] Rebar RW, Spitzer IB. The physiology and measurement of hot flushes. Am J Obstet Gynecol 1987;156:1284–8.

[94] Berendsen HH. The role of serotonin in hot flushes. Maturitas 2000;36:155–64.

[95] Erlik Y, Tataryn IV, Meldrum DR, et al. Association of waking episodes with menopausal hot flushes. JAMA 1981;245:1741–4.

[96] Schiff I, Regestein Q, Tulchinsky D, et al. Effects of estrogens on sleep and psychological state of hypogonadal women. JAMA 1979;242:2405–14.

[97] Thompson J, Oswald I. Effect of oestrogen on the sleep, mood, and anxiety of menopausal women. BMJ 1977;2:1317–9.

[98] Polo-Kantola P, Erkkola R, Irjala K, et al. Effect of short-term transdermal estrogen replacement therapy on sleep: a randomized, double-blind crossover trial in postmenopausal women. Fertil Steril 1999;71:873–80.

[99] Purdie DW, Empson JA, Crichton C, et al. Hormone replacement therapy, sleep quality and psychological wellbeing. Br J Obstet Gynaecol 1995;102:735–9.

[100] Levine DW, Dailey ME, Rockhill B, et al. Validation of the Women's Health Initiative Insomnia Rating Scale in a multicenter controlled clinical trial. Psychosom Med 2005;67: 98–104.

[101] Soares CN, Arsenio HC, Joffe H, et al. Escitalopram versus ethinyl estradiol and norethindrone acetate for symptomatic peri- and postmenopausal women: impact on depression, vasomotor symptoms, sleep, and quality of life. Menopause 2006;13:780-6.

[102] Adler G, Young D, Galant R, et al. A multicenter, open-label study to evaluate satisfaction and menopausal quality of life in women using transdermal estradiol/norethindrone acetate therapy for the management of menopausal signs and symptoms. Gynecol Obstet Invest 2005;59:212–9.

[103] Anderson E, Hamburger S, Liu JH, et al. Characteristics of menopausal women seeking assistance. Am J Obstet Gynecol 1987;156:428–33.

[104] Hay AG, Bancroft J, Johnstone EC. Affective symptoms in women attending a menopause clinic. Br J Psychiatry 1994;164:513–6.

[105] Joffe H, Hennen J, Soares CN, et al. Hot flushes associated with depression in perimenopausal women seeking primary care. Menopause 2002;9:392–8.

[106] Avis NE, Stellato R, Crawford S, et al. Is there a menopausal syndrome? Menopausal status and symptoms across racial/ethnic groups. Soc Sci Med 2001;52:345–56.

[107] Freeman EW, Sammel MD, Liu L, et al. Hormones and menopausal status as predictors of depression in women in transition to menopause. Arch Gen Psychiatry 2004;61: 62–70.

[108] Wolkowitz OM, Reus VI. Treatment of depression with antiglucocorticoid drugs. Psychosom Med 1999;61:698–711.

[109] Puder JJ, Freda PU, Goland RS, et al. Estrogen modulates the hypothalamic-pituitary-adrenal and inflammatory cytokine responses to endotoxin in women. J Clin Endocrinol Metab 2001;86:2403–8.

[110] McEwen BS, Alves SE. Estrogen actions in the central nervous system. Endocr Rev 1999;20:279–307.

[111] Halbreich U, Kahn LS. Role of estrogen in the aetiology and treatment of mood disorders. CNS Drugs 2001;15:797–817.

[112] Harrison NL, Majewska MD, Harrington JW, et al. Structure-activity relationships for steroid interaction with the gamma-aminobutyric acidA receptor complex. J Pharmacol Exp Ther 1987;241:346–53.
[113] Krystal AD. Depression and insomnia in women. Clin Cornerstone 2004;6(Suppl 1B): S19–28.
[114] Resta O, Caratozzolo G, Pannacciulli N, et al. Gender, age and menopause effects on the prevalence and the characteristics of obstructive sleep apnea in obesity. Eur J Clin Invest 2003;33:1084–9.
[115] Young T, Rabago D, Zgierska A, et al. Objective and subjective sleep quality in premenopausal, perimenopausal, and postmenopausal women in the Wisconsin Sleep Cohort Study. Sleep 2003;26:667–72.
[116] Leech JA, Onal E, Dulberg C, et al. A comparison of men and women with occlusive sleep apnea syndrome. Chest 1988;94:983–8.
[117] Young T, Palta M, Dempsey J, et al. The occurrence of sleep-disordered breathing among middle-aged adults. N Engl J Med 1993;328:1230–5.
[118] Zhou XS, Rowley JA, Demirovic F, et al. Effect of testosterone on the apneic threshold in women during NREM sleep. J Appl Physiol 2003;94:101–7.
[119] Norman RG, Ahmed MM, Walsleben JA, et al. Detection of respiratory events during NPSG: nasal cannula/pressure sensor versus thermistor. Sleep 1997;20:1175–84.
[120] Kapsimalis F, Kryger MH. Gender and obstructive sleep apnea syndrome, part 1: clinical features. Sleep 2002;25:412–9.
[121] Roth T. Measuring treatment efficacy in insomnia. J Clin Psychiatry 2004;65(Suppl 8): 8–12.
[122] Chesson AL Jr, Anderson WM, Littner M, et al. Practice parameters for the nonpharmacologic treatment of chronic insomnia. An American Academy of Sleep Medicine report. Standards of Practice Committee of the American Academy of Sleep Medicine. Sleep 1999;22:1128–33.
[123] Strollo PJ Jr, Rogers RM. Obstructive sleep apnea. N Engl J Med 1996;334:99–104.
[124] Erman MK. Therapeutic options in the treatment of insomnia. J Clin Psychiatry 2005;66(Suppl. 9):18–23 [quiz 42–3].
[125] Wang MY, Wang SY, Tsai PS. Cognitive behavioural therapy for primary insomnia: a systematic review. J Adv Nurs 2005;50:553–64.
[126] Montgomery P, Dennis J. A systematic review of non-pharmacological therapies for sleep problems in later life. Sleep Med Rev 2004;8:47–62.
[127] Morin CM. Measuring outcomes in randomized clinical trials of insomnia treatments. Sleep Med Rev 2003;7:263–79.
[128] Vincent N, Lionberg C. Treatment preference and patient satisfaction in chronic insomnia. Sleep 2001;24:411–7.
[129] Espie CA, Inglis SJ, Tessier S, et al. The clinical effectiveness of cognitive behaviour therapy for chronic insomnia: implementation and evaluation of a sleep clinic in general medical practice. Behav Res Ther 2001;39:45–60.
[130] Morin CM. Cognitive-behavioral approaches to the treatment of insomnia. J Clin Psychiatry 2004;65(Suppl 16):33–40.
[131] Stepanski EJ, Wyatt JK. Use of sleep hygiene in the treatment of insomnia. Sleep Med Rev 2003;7:215–25.
[132] Stanton HE. Hypnotic relaxation and the reduction of sleep onset insomnia. Int J Psychosom 1989;36:64–8.
[133] Younus J, Simpson I, Collins A, et al. Mind control of menopause. Womens Health Issues 2003;13:74–8.
[134] Vermes G, Banhidy F, Acs N. The effects of remifemin on subjective symptoms of menopause. Adv Ther 2005;22:148–54.
[135] Pockaj BA, Loprinzi CL, Sloan JA, et al. Pilot evaluation of black cohosh for the treatment of hot flashes in women. Cancer Invest 2004;22:515–21.

[136] Osmers R, Friede M, Liske E, et al. Efficacy and safety of isopropanolic black cohosh extract for climacteric symptoms. Obstet Gynecol 2005;105(5 Pt 1):1074–83.

[137] Uebelhack R, Blohmer JU, Graubaum HJ, et al. Black cohosh and St. John's wort for climacteric complaints: a randomized trial. Obstet Gynecol 2006;107(2 Pt 1): 247–55.

[138] Krystal AD, Ressler I. The use of valerian in neuropsychiatry. CNS Spectr 2001;6: 841–7.

[139] Wheatley D. Kava and valerian in the treatment of stress-induced insomnia. Phytother Res 2001;15:549–51.

[140] Stevinson C, Ernst E. Valerian for insomnia: a systematic review of randomized clinical trials. Sleep Med 2000;1:91–9.

[141] Larzelere MM, Wiseman P. Anxiety, depression, and insomnia. Prim Care 2002;29: 339–60 [vii].

[142] Watts NB, Notelovitz M, Timmons MC, et al. Comparison of oral estrogens and estrogens plus androgen on bone mineral density, menopausal symptoms, and lipid-lipoprotein profiles in surgical menopause. Obstet Gynecol 1995;85:529–37.

[143] Boyle GJ, Murrihy R. A preliminary study of hormone replacement therapy and psychological mood states in perimenopausal women. Psychol Rep 2001;88:160–70.

[144] Schmidt PJ, Nieman L, Danaceau MA, et al. Estrogen replacement in perimenopause-related depression: a preliminary report. Am J Obstet Gynecol 2000;183: 414–20.

[145] Soares CN, Almeida OP, Joffe H, et al. Efficacy of estradiol for the treatment of depressive disorders in perimenopausal women: a double-blind, randomized, placebo-controlled trial. Arch Gen Psychiatry 2001;58:529–34.

[146] Cohen LS, Soares CN, Poitras JR, et al. Short-term use of estradiol for depression in perimenopausal and postmenopausal women: a preliminary report. Am J Psychiatry 2003;160:1519–22.

[147] Cistulli PA, Barnes DJ, Grunstein RR, et al. Effect of short-term hormone replacement in the treatment of obstructive sleep apnoea in postmenopausal women. Thorax 1994;49: 699–702.

[148] Keefe DL, Watson R, Naftolin F. Hormone replacement therapy may alleviate sleep apnea in menopausal women: a pilot study. Menopause 1999;6:196–200.

[149] Rossouw JE, Anderson GL, Prentice RL, et al. Risks and benefits of estrogen plus progestin in healthy postmenopausal women: principal results From the Women's Health Initiative randomized controlled trial. JAMA 2002;288:321–33.

[150] Montplaisir J, Lorrain J, Denesle R, et al. Sleep in menopause: differential effects of two forms of hormone replacement therapy. Menopause 2001;8:10–6.

[151] National Institutes of Health. NIH State-of-the-Science Conference Statement on Manifestations and Management of Chronic Insomnia in Adults. Washington (DC): National Institutes of Health 2005.

[152] Soares CN, Poitras JR, Prouty J, et al. Efficacy of citalopram as a monotherapy or as an adjunctive treatment to estrogen therapy for perimenopausal and postmenopausal women with depression and vasomotor symptoms. J Clin Psychiatry 2003;64: 473–9.

[153] Stearns V, Beebe KL, Iyengar M, et al. Paroxetine controlled release in the treatment of menopausal hot flashes: a randomized controlled trial. JAMA 2003;289:2827–34.

[154] Joffe H, Groninger H, Soares CN, et al. An open trial of mirtazapine in menopausal women with depression unresponsive to estrogen replacement therapy. J Womens Health Gend Based Med 2001;10:999–1004.

[155] Bateson AN. The benzodiazepine site of the GABAA receptor: an old target with new potential? Sleep Med 2004;5(Suppl 1):S9–15.

[156] Wagner J, Wagner ML. Non-benzodiazepines for the treatment of insomnia. Sleep Med Rev 2000;4:551–81.

[157] Krystal AD, Walsh JK, Laska E, et al. Sustained efficacy of eszopiclone over 6 months of nightly treatment: results of a randomized, double-blind, placebo-controlled study in adults with chronic insomnia. Sleep 2003;26:793–9.

[158] Dorsey CM, Lee KA, Scharf MB. Effect of zolpidem on sleep in women with perimeno-pausal and postmenopausal insomnia: a 4-week, randomized, multicenter, double-blind, placebo-controlled study. Clin Ther 2004;26:1578–86.

[159] Roth T, Walsh JK, Krystal A, et al. An evaluation of the efficacy and safety of eszopiclone over 12 months in patients with chronic primary insomnia. Sleep Med 2005;6:487–95.

[160] Soares CN, Utian W, Rubens R, et al. Evaluation of eszopiclone 3 mg in the treatment of insomnia associated with the menopausal transition. Obstet Gynecol 2006;107:24S.

Sleep and Psychiatric Disorders: Future Directions

Andrew D. Krystal, MD, MS[a,b,c,d,*]

[a]Department of Psychiatry and Behavioral Sciences, Duke University School of Medicine, Durham, NC, USA
[b]Insomnia and Sleep Research Program, Duke University School of Medicine, Durham, NC, USA
[c]Treatment-Resistant Depression Research Program, Duke University School of Medicine, Durham, NC, USA
[d]Quantitative EEG Laboratory, Duke University School of Medicine, Durham, NC, USA

T he view of the relationship between sleep and psychiatric disorders has undergone a radical change in the past 5 to 10 years. The longstanding perspective had been that sleep problems invariably are symptoms of psychiatric disorders. The emerging perspective includes the possibility that there may be complex, bidirectional relationships. This change has opened doors to important new directions in research and led to changes in guidelines for clinical practice. This article discusses promising future directions for building on this foundation. Although several important studies have been performed, they represent the beginnings of lines of research that will require a great deal of additional work to develop fully. For example, a few studies suggest that targeting treatment specifically to insomnia along with usual psychiatric treatment may result in improvements not only in sleep but also in the response of the non-sleep aspects of a psychiatric disorder. It will be important to map out which of the psychiatric disorders have this special relationship with the associated insomnia and which insomnia therapies are associated with this synergistic effect. Another example is that it is not yet known if treatment for insomnia mitigates the insomnia-associated increase in risk for psychiatric disorders that recently has been identified. In addition to developing current research directions, it also will be important to understand better the mechanisms that mediate the relationships between sleep and psychiatric disorders. Although little currently is known about these mechanisms, there are some alterations in physiology that

Consulting, advisory, or research grant support: Cephalon, Glaxo-Smith-Kline, Johnson and Johnson, King, Merck, National Institutes of Health, Neurocrine, Neurogen, Organon, Pfizer, Research Triangle Institute, Respironics, Sanofi-Synthelabo, Sepracor, Somaxon, and Transoral.

*Duke Insomnia and Sleep Research Program, Department of Psychiatry and Behavioral Sciences, Box 3309, Duke University Medical Center, Durham, NC 27710. E-mail address: kryst001@mc.duke.edu

are common to some sleep and psychiatric disorders, which are of particular interest. These include an interconnected set of changes in the hypothalamic-pituitary-adrenal (HPA) axis, central serotonergic function, and immune system inflammatory signaling peptides, referred to as cytokines. Understanding these mechanisms promises to lead to novel treatments that not only may ameliorate acute symptoms but also address the risks for the future development of sleep, psychiatric, and medical disorders.

INTRODUCTION

Sleep disturbances are extremely common in those who have psychiatric disorders. In fact, sleep disruption is among the diagnostic criteria for several psychiatric illnesses, including major depression, mania, generalized anxiety disorder (GAD), and posttraumatic stress disorder (PTSD) [1]. The longstanding view of the relationship of co-occurring sleep and psychiatric disorders had been one of unidirectional causality: psychiatric disorders cause sleep disorders (eg, depression or anxiety cause insomnia). In recent years, a growing body of research has emerged that contradicts that point of view. The emerging perspective includes the possibility that there may be complex, bidirectional relationships. This article briefly reviews the evolution of the understanding of this relationship and recent work that forms the foundation of the emerging new perspective. Important future directions for research and clinical practice are discussed, including (1) pursuing further current lines of research on the relationship between sleep and psychiatric disorders to fully develop their potential to improve clinical practice; (2) carrying out studies aimed at understanding the mechanisms that mediate the relationships between sleep and psychiatric disorders; and (3) developing novel treatments that target the mechanisms discovered.

THE TRADITIONAL MODEL: SLEEP PROBLEMS ARE SYMPTOMS OF AN UNDERLYING PSYCHIATRIC DISORDER

Sleep disturbances occurring in those who have psychiatric disorders long have been viewed as secondary symptoms of the associated psychiatric conditions [2]. As the sleep problems are seen as symptoms, they are expected to remit along with the other symptoms of the psychiatric disorder with effective psychiatric treatment. As a result, this model focuses treatment on the underlying psychiatric disorder while discouraging treatment of the sleep difficulties present. This model superficially seems to account for the high rate of sleep disturbances in several psychiatric conditions, which are reviewed briefly in this section, and the tendency for sleep problems to improve with treatments targeted at these psychiatric conditions.

Major Depression

Insomnia or daytime sleepiness is reported by up to 90% of patients who have major depression and is among the set of diagnostic criteria for this disorder [1,3]. Sleep-related findings in patients who are depressed include difficulty falling asleep, difficulty staying asleep, early morning awakening, nonrestorative sleep, fatigue, daytime sedation, increased awakenings, short rapid eye movement (REM) latency, increased percentage of the night spent in REM sleep, and diminished amount of slow wave sleep [4–6].

Consistent with the traditional model, nonsedating antidepressant treatment of patients who have insomnia co-occurring with depression resolves the sleep difficulty in the majority of cases [7–9].

Mania

More than 80% of manic patients experience a decrease in their ability to sleep [1,10]. Unlike depressed patients, who tend to report a lack of restoration from sleep, in mania there seems to be a decrease in the ability and need for sleep. Contrary to the tendency to think of insomnia as somehow opposite of depression, the sleep of manic patients also is marked by a loss of slow wave sleep, shortened REM latency, and relative increase in percentage of REM [10]. Therapies for mania tend to be sedating, and sleep generally increases with treatment [11–12].

Anxiety Disorders

The anxiety disorders associated most commonly with sleep disturbance are GAD and PTSD. More than half of patients who have GAD report problems initiating or maintaining sleep, which are among the diagnostic criteria for this disorder [1,13]. Although there are few studies of the response of sleep difficulties to GAD therapies, there is some evidence that selective serotonin reuptake inhibitors (SSRIs) often result in improvement of sleep problems [14]. Sleep problems also are among the diagnostic criteria for PTSD, though in this case the sleep difficulties include distressing dreams along with difficulties falling or staying asleep [1]. Although complaints of sleep difficulties are ubiquitous among those who have PTSD, accompanying polysomnographic alterations are reported inconsistently [15–17]. Several placebo-controlled studies of the treatment of PTSD with nonsedating agents are reported, which might reflect on whether or not treatment of the supposed primary condition might improve associated insomnia or nightmares [18]. The results are inconsistent, although one study of treatment with fluvoxamine reports a clear improvement in sleep compared with placebo [19].

Schizophrenia

Sleep disturbances are not among the diagnostic criteria for schizophrenia; however, difficulties with initiation, maintenance, and quality of sleep are frequent in this group [20–21]. As in mood disorders, short REM latency and a decrease in slow wave sleep also are observed commonly [22]. Further, many individuals who have schizophrenia experience a shift in circadian rhythm marked by a greater tendency to sleep during the day and remain awake at night [23,24]. Like antimanic agents, essentially all of the primary schizophrenia treatments generally enhance sleep, but there are no data on the effects of treatments on sleep problems in this population.

Alcoholism

Problems falling and staying asleep are noted in 36% to 72% of those who have alcoholism [25,26]. Despite alcohol's sedating effects, sleep problems arise because the sedation wears off over time and there tends to be a sleep-disrupting rebound effect in the middle of the night [27,28]. Regular daytime alcohol consumption also tends to promote daytime sleep and erosion of the usual circadian rhythm [27]. Alcoholism presents a challenge to the traditional symptom model in that there are no standard treatments for this condition that constitute effective therapy of the underlying condition. Cessation of alcohol use is problematic in this regard as it represents the resolution of one key phase of the disorder and at the same time involves the discontinuation of a sedating substance. It also is not possible to identify a change that might occur with treatment instituted during the abstinence phase that can claim to herald a successful therapeutic response.

THE EMERGING MODEL: A COMPLEX BIDIRECTIONAL RELATIONSHIP

The accumulated research on sleep problems occurring in those who have psychiatric disorders does not support the model in which sleep difficulties are seen only as symptoms. Instead, these data speak to a complex bidirectional relationship between sleep and some psychiatric disorders. Some of the most notable findings that have led to this change in viewpoint are reviewed briefly.

By far, the greatest evidence for the failure of the symptom model has been obtained related to sleep problems co-occurring with major depression. This evidence suggests that insomnia not only is a symptom but also that it has independent importance in terms of clinically relevant outcomes and the course of the disorder. Sleep disturbance seems to be associated with an independent increase in the risk of suicidal ideation and completed suicide [29–30]. Insomnia also seems to predict a greater future risk of depression (and anxiety disorders and alcoholism) [31–33]. Further, residual insomnia after otherwise successful antidepressant therapy is associated with an increased risk of depression relapse [34]. Data on the treatment of insomnia co-occurring with depression are the strongest blow to the symptom model. Initiating antidepressant treatment with a hypnotic agent in addition to an antidepressant medication leads not only to greater improvement in sleep but also a faster and more complete antidepressant response [35,36]. Preliminary suggestive data were obtained with lormetazepam [36]. A placebo-controlled study of 545 patients identifed that the addition of eszpiclone (3 mg) to fluoxetine had a significant therapeutic effect not only on sleep but also on nonsleep features of depression [35]. In addition, treatment of residual insomnia after otherwise successful SSRI therapy with zolpidem (10 mg) resulted in significant improvement in sleep and ratings of daytime function [37]. If sleep merely were a symptom, targeting treatment to sleep difficulties with hypnotic therapy would not be expected to improve antidepressant outcome over the administration of a therapeutic antidepressant regimen.

Compelling evidence of the independent importance of sleep problems also is observed related to alcoholism. Although alcoholism is associated with disrupted sleep, insomnia leads some individuals to drink as a means of addressing sleep difficulty [38]. As a result, insomnia may be a predisposing or perpetuating factor for alcohol consumption. Compared with the general population, alcoholics have a greater tendency to choose alcohol over other means of alleviating sleep problems [38,39]. Over a period of time of regular alcohol consumption, there also is evidence that alcohol is necessary to prevent significant sleep-onset difficulty [40]. Of particular importance, discontinuation of alcohol generally is accompanied by sleep difficulty, which may be extremely persistent and is correlated with an increased risk of relapsing to drinking [38,41,42].

These observations contradict the view that sleep difficulties invariably are symptoms of associated psychiatric disorders and have opened the door to the possibility that a complex-bidirectional relationship may exist between sleep difficulties and at least some psychiatric disorders. Some promising directions for future work that have the potential to build on this foundation are discussed.

FUTURE DIRECTIONS

Two areas for future work that seem to have potential to lead to improvements in the clinical treatment of patients who have comorbid sleep and psychiatric disorders are discussed. These are (1) to develop the fledgling lines of research that recently have been initiated in this area and (2) to carry out studies of the pathophysiologic mechanisms linking sleep and psychiatric disorders.

Developing Current Lines of Clinical Research

The studies that form the foundation for the emerging perspective of sleep and psychiatric disorders, although compelling, have important limitations. They are few enough in number and scope to at best represent seeds for several important lines of research. These research directions will require a great deal of additional work to develop fully their potential for leading to improvements in clinical treatment. Examination of the needed work reveals an intimidating matrix of important future studies.

Although the greatest amount of work has been performed with insomnia co-occurring with depression, this work leaves several key issues unaddressed that are needed before optimal treatment of insomnia comorbid with major depression can be achieved. Controlled studies of initial cotherapy so far have been performed only with flunitrazepam, lormetazepam, and eszopiclone, whereas only zolpidem and trazodone are the subjects of placebo-controlled studies of add-on therapy for residual insomnia [35–37,43]. Tthe dose-response characteristics of the effects of these insomnia agents used in this setting are not yet known nor is there data on the other insomnia therapies, which include other medications and nonpharmacologic therapies. The fact that one study reports a beneficial effect of insomnia cotherapy with lormetazepam but not flunitrazepam confirms the expected: that insomnia agents vary in the degree to which they are effective as cotherapies for depression [36]. This speaks to the need to map the risk-benefit profiles for each potential treatment as a function of dose in this setting to allow optimal choice of treatment for clinical practice.

Another important unresolved clinically relevant issue is the degree to which the therapeutic benefits of treating insomnia depend on the antidepressant therapy implemented. So far, the only large-scale placebo-controlled trial of initial cotherapy has been performed with fluoxetine [35]. Although unlikely, it must be established that the benefit of insomnia therapy observed in that study is not limited to treatment regimens that included fluoxetine as the antidepressant or some other subset of the antidepressant therapies. Considering that for each antidepressant treatment it may be necessary to carry out studies of cotherapy with severalf insomnia therapies, mapping the risk-benefit profile of the set of possible combinations of antidepressant and insomnia therapies is a daunting task.

It also will be of importance to determine whether or not the same beneficial effects noted with combination antidepressant and hypnotic therapy can be achieved with single-agent treatment with a sedating antidepressant, such as mirtazapine or a tricyclic antidepressant. This will require studies comparing nonsedating antidepressant therapy plus placebo versus nonsedating antidepressant plus insomnia therapy versus the sedating antidepressant plus placebo. The major potential advantages of single-agent therapy are the lower cost and ease of use, which are likely to translate into better adherence to therapy.

In addition, there is a need to determine the optimal time point in the course of depression treatment to institute insomnia therapy. It is not clear if adding insomnia treatment to the initial treatment regimen is a better strategy than waiting to see if there either is incomplete response to initial antidepressant or if individuals experience residual insomnia before initiating insomnia therapy. Although the former strategy seems advantageous in terms of speed of response, instituting treatment only after determining the response to initial therapy has the safety benefit of decreasing the number of patients exposed to treatment. Ideally, the means would be developed to predict before initial therapy who is most likely to benefit from insomnia cotherapy.

Studies assessing the effects of varying insomnia treatment duration also are likely to be of clinical usefulness. The convention is to identify two phases of treatment: the acute phase, which represents the period of the usual initial treatment response (approximately 1–3 months), and continuation, which constitutes the period after remission where the therapeutic challenge is preventing relapse [44]. The studies of initial insomnia cotherapy have examined acute treatment for 8 weeks and 4 weeks of continuation therapy [35–37]. There is no reason to assume that either of these treatment periods is optimal. In fact, approximately 11 months of treatment would seem natural to consider given that guidelines for the treatment of major depression recommend continuing therapy for up to 9 months after remission to prevent relapse [44,45]. Although longer insomnia treatment duration might be expected to decrease the risk of relapse, this has not yet been established and the evidence that residual insomnia is predictive of relapse suggests that it may be possible to maintain remission via a relatively short-term course of treatment if it eliminates residual insomnia [34]. Besides testing the hypothesis that short-term treatment that resolves residual insomnia might decrease relapse, the obvious advantages in cost, adherence, and safety also recommend this approach. The only data that suggest the possibility that a therapeutic advantage might persist beyond discontinuation of adjunctive insomnia treatment derive from the study of eszopiclone/fluoxetine cotherapy [35,46]. In that study, eszopiclone treatment led to significantly greater improvement in sleep and nonsleep features of depression than placebo not only during the 8 weeks of double-blind treatment but also during the subsequent 2-week discontinuation phase when all subjects received single-blind placebo and fluoxetine [46].

All of the studies that have been performed with major depression (and those enumerated previously) that represent important future directions also are needed in patients who have other psychiatric disorders. The most promising disorders seem to be GAD, PTSD, schizophrenia, and alcoholism, where there is some indication of an important relationship with disordered sleep. It will be important for work on alcoholism and schizophrenia to include not only studies of insomnia treatment, however, but also of treatment for circadian rhythm derangements, which are common in these disorders [23,24,27]. Similarly, for PTSD, it will be important to take into account nightmares [1].

Among the most promising areas of work for building on the current empiric base are explorations of the long-term course of individuals who have sleep disorders.

Longitudinal studies, although expensive and difficult to carry out, are the only means to address some key questions for the field. This includes determining whether or not effective treatment of insomnia eliminates the increased risk for the subsequent development of psychiatric disorders that has been associated with episodes of disturbed sleep [31,33].

The Mechanisms that Link Sleep and Psychiatric Disorders

Another promising direction for future work is to study the mechanisms that link sleep and psychiatric disorders. Although there have been few investigations addressing this issue, prior studies provide intriguing possibilities that have the potential to result in the development of more effective therapeutic approaches. Among these are several neurobiologic aberrations that are shared by some sleep and psychiatric disorders, including HPA system activation, alterations in serotonin system function, and elevated production of some immune system peptides that are part of the inflammatory response referred to as cytokines. Although cognitive-behavioral and other neurobiologic mechanisms also are of high potential importance, the focus of this discussion is on a set of neurobiologic mechanisms common to some of the disorders in the two domains that seem to be strongly interconnected and which also are implicated in the genesis of several medical disorders. These mechanisms may represent a web of processes that not only may link sleep and psychiatric disorders with each other but may also explain why both types of difficulties may be connected with risks for the development of a wide-range of psychiatric and medical disorders. This discussion also is restricted to the relationship of insomnia and major depression, because of the evidence of their complex bidirectionality and to limit the scope to one that is compatible with a review of this length.

Hypothalamic-pituitary-adrenal system activation

Elevated HPA axis activity is a hallmark of insomnia and depression. Conditions of corticosteroid level elevation, such as exogenous administration and Cushing's syndrome, often are accompanied by depression and insomnia [47,48]. In addition, elevated 24-hour urine cortisol is reported to accompany both conditions [49–51]. In patients who are depressed, there is some evidence of a relationship of HPA axis activation and the clinical treatment course [48]. Antidepressant response generally is preceded by a decrease in cortisol levels and sustained elevation is associated with a greater risk of relapse [48].

It is unlikely, however, that there is a simple relationship between HPA activation and the link between depression and insomnia, where each one can lead to cortisol elevation, which then causes an episode of the other. This is because significant hypercortisolemia occurs only in a subset of individuals who have these disorders and never rises to the level observed in individuals who have Cushing's syndrome or where exogenous administration results in symptom development [52,53]. A clear illustration of this point is that the typical sequelae of hypercortisolemia (buffalo hump, moon face, and so forth) are not characteristic of either insomnia or major depression [53]. There is some reason to believe, however, that a subset of individuals are prone to developing either depression or insomnia in response to relatively low-level HPA activation, which may, at least in part, account for why some individuals have associations between insomnia and depression [54].

Serotonin dysregulation

Of all of the neurotransmitter systems, major depression is associated most strongly with serotonin. Nearly all of the effective antidepressant medications are believed to mediate their effects via serotonin effects, including inhibition of reuptake, inhibition of the degradation of serotonin, and antagonism of serotonin type 2 receptors, which is believed to increase the binding to the serotonin1 receptors. On this basis, it long has been hypothesized that decreased serotonin activity is a fundamental mechanism that leads to major depression [55].

Serotonin also plays an important role in sleep. Neurons originating in the brainstem raphe nuclei form part of the activating system that promotes arousal and wakefulness [55]. From the point of view of pharmacotherapy, serotonin 2 antagonism enhances sleep and, in particular, increases the amount of slow wave sleep [56]. At the same time, activation of serotonin 1 receptors leads to an inhibition of REM sleep. Reuptake of serotonin suppresses REM and may be experienced either as sedating or disruptive of sleep [57].

Recent studies also link sleep and depression via a possible serotonin system genetic vulnerability to stress. A polymorphism in the gene for the serotonin transporter that affects the process of serotoninT reuptake is associated with a greater risk of developing insomnia [58] and depression [59–63] in response to stressful life events. A functional MRI study identified changes in perigenual cingulated/amygdala circuits in those who have the risk-associated serotonin transporter polymorphism, which is interpreted as a defect in negative feedback, resulting in an impaired ability to extinguish negative affective responses to stimuli [64].

This genetic serotonin-related polymorphism may explain why some individuals might be prone to experiencing depression and sleep disturbance in response to stressors. In addition, it may provide a mechanism whereby depression may lead to insomnia or insomnia may lead to depression. A period of either difficulty sleeping or depression symptoms may, in itself, be stressful enough life events to lead to the other type of disorder (depression may lead to insomnia and insomnia may lead to depression) in vulnerable individuals.

Inflammatory cytokines
Cytokines are immune-system peptides that play a signaling role in the inflammatory response [65]. More than 100 such molecules are identified and include interleukins (ILs), interferons (IFNs), and classical hormones, such as prolactin and growth hormone. Many can cross the blood-brain barrier and affect central nervous system function, and, although some are proinflammatory, other cytokines have anti-inflammatory effects [65,66].

A series of studies speaks to relationships of cytokines with insomnia and major depression. Studies in animals with various cytokines have identified dose-dependent sleep disruption and sedative effects [67,68]. Specific findings include IL-1 and tumor necrosis factor (TNF) enhancing slow wave sleep, whereas IL-10 and IL-6 tend to disrupt non-REM sleep [67]. In humans, as in the animal studies, IL-6 is found to diminish non-REM sleep, whereas elevated serum IL-6 levels are associated with worse sleep in the general population and among those exposed to caregiver stress [69–71]. IFN-α administration is noted to disrupt sleep in normal controls [72]. In addition, chronic insomnia patients are reported to have significant dysfunction in the usual circadian cycle of IL-6 and TNF production, such that IL-6 is greater than usual at night and TNF elevated during the day [73,74]. This is hypothesized to relate to the difficulty sleeping insomnia patients experience at night and as their daytime fatigue. Although there is evidence that sleep deprivation also leads to elevations in serum levels of IL-6 and TNF-α [75,76], sleep deprivation is a different phenomenon from insomnia. Unlike deprivation, insomnia is characterized by the inability to sleep when given the opportunity to do so.

Similar alterations in cytokines are associated with major depression. Studies of knockout mice lacking TNF receptors suggest that TNF-α leads to depression-like behaviors [77]. In humans, increased serum levels of IL-1β, IL-6, IL-8, IFN-γ, TNF-α, and prostaglandin E2 were found in depressed patients compared with normal controls [78,79]. In one study, however, although elevations in IL-6 were found in depressed subjects compared with controls, IL-6 levels correlated better with sleep-onset latency than the presence or severity of depression [80]. It is hypothesized that major depression is associated with an increase in IL-6 production that is responsible for the sleep disturbance that characterizes this disorder [81].

Overall, there is a limited number of studies of the relationship of cytokines to insomnia and depression. They draw particular attention to a few cytokines, including IL-6 and TNF-α. It may be the interactions of cytokines with the other mechanisms (HPA and serotonin systems), however, that are the most interesting for understanding the relationship between insomnia and major depression.

Hypothalamic-pituitary-adrenal system, serotonin, and cytokine interactions and the relationship of insomnia and depression

These three systems are highly interconnected in a manner that seems to link insomnia and depression and amplify the tendency for a disturbance in any of these systems to trigger both of the disorders.IL-1, IL-6, and TNF-αmodulate corticotrophin-releasing factor, resulting in elevations in serum cortisol and corticotropin [82–84]. Elevated IL-6 seems to be associated with significantly lower plasma tryptophan, which is known to predispose individuals to major depression [79]. Proinflammatory cytokines IL-2β and TNF-α also re reported to diminish peripheral tryptophan by enhancing the activity of the enzyme that is responsible for its degradation [83,84]. In addition, serum levels of IL-1β, IL-6, and TNF-αare found to correlate with synthesis of the serotonin transporter, such that higher levels of these cytokines would be expected to lead to more effective serotonin reuptake and are hypothesized to be a predisposing factor for major depression [78].

These observations provide several possible mechanisms that might account for the relationship between insomnia and depression. Assessment of their validity will be a valuable area for future research. The increased IL-6 that seems to accompany chronic insomnia may promote HPA activation and predispose individuals to major depression by decreasing central serotonin neurotransmission via decreasing tryptophan availability and increasing the effectiveness of serotonin reuptake. At the same time, major depression is suggested to lead to increases in IL-6, particularly at night, which may lead to sleep loss, which itself is associated with increases in IL-6 and daytime TNF-αproduction. The latter is associated with depression-like symptoms, daytime sleepiness, and fatigue. Both of these changes would be expected to increase HPA activation and decrease central serotonin neurotransmission further enhancing the likelihood of major depression. Although the etiologic role of HPA activation is not clear, cytokines seem to predispose toward increased activity in this system for insomnia and major depression. One group reports that cortisol enhances the serotonin reuptake mechanism and suggested a link between cortisol elevations and an increase in depression risk resulting from a decrease in central serotonin binding [85].

This complex interconnected system of processes not only would be expected to amplify factors that predispose individuals to insomnia and depression but also provide for multiple pathways that can lead to these disorders. Any factors that might lead to activation of some of the key cytokines or diminish central sertoninergic activity have the potential to initiate the chain of events that couple insomnia and depression and promote the development of both disorders. The degree to which these or related mechanisms are relevant to other sleep and psychiatric disorders remains unknown and provides another potentially fruitful future direction to pursue.

Developing treatment strategies based on understanding of mechanism
If it is possible to understand the mechanisms linking sleep and psychiatric disorders, this will provide valuable opportunities to improve clinical treatment. Treatments that specifically target these mechanisms have the potential to not only treat the presenting problem but also may mitigate the future risks of both types of disorders. This understanding also might allow identifying vulnerable subgroups of the population, such as individuals who have the serotonin transporter polymorphism that could be targeted for preventative treatment of the specific processes that mediate the risk. Another possible opportunity might be the availability of physiologic markers that could be monitored in clinical practice to ensure that treatment has effectively addressed the processes that increase risks. In terms of the mechanisms discussed previously, the antidepressant bupropion has been found to lead to a decrease in TNF production [86]. The effects of other depression and insomnia treatments on the serum markers of interest are not known.

Lastly, developing treatments that address the mechanisms that link sleep and psychiatric disorders also have the potential to provide the capacity to address long-term health risks that are associated with these disorders, including hypertension, diabetes, and coronary artery disease [87–90]. As an example, IL-6 and TNF-αare identified as mediators of long-term risks for coronary artery disease and diabetes [91–93].

SUMMARY AND CONCLUSIONS
As recent work has opened the door to a more complex view of the potential relationships between sleep and psychiatric disorders, it also has provided a springboard to many areas of potential future work. This includes continuing the research directions that recently have been initiated and studying the mechanisms that link sleep and psychiatric disorders. Understanding these mechanisms has the potential to change the way we think about sleep and psychiatric disorders and lead to novel treatments that not only may ameliorate acute symptoms but also address the risk for future development of associated sleep, psychiatric, and medical disorders. Hypnotics are not indicated by the Food and Drug Administration (FDA) for the treatment of depression; antidepressants are not indicated by the FDA for the treatment of insomnia.

References

[1] American Psychiatric Association. Diagnostic and statistical manual of mental disorders. 4th edition, text revision. Washington (DC): American Psychiatric Press; 2004.

[2] NIH Consensus Conference. Drugs and insomnia. JAMA 1984;251:2410–4.

[3] Thase ME. Antidepressant treatment of the depressed patient with insomnia. J Clin Psychiatry 1999;60(Suppl 17):28–31.

[4] Kupfer DJ, Frank E, Ehlers CL. EEG sleep in young depressives: first and second night effects. Biol Psychiatry 1989;25:87–97.

[5] Benca RM, Obermeyer WH, Thisted RA, et al. Sleep and psychiatric disorders: a meta-analysis. Arch Gen Psychiatry 1992;49:651–68.

[6] Gillin JC, Duncan WC, Pettigrew KD, et al. Successful separation of depressed, normal and insomniac subjects by EEG sleep data. Arch Gen Psychiatry 1979;36:85–90.

[7] Hirschfeld RM, Mallinckrodt C, Lee TC, et al. Time course of depression-symptom improvement during treatment with duloxetine. Depress Anxiety 2005;21:170–7.

[8] Nelson JC, Wohlreich MM, Mallinckrodt CH, et al. Duloxetine for the treatment of major depressive disorder in older patients. Am J Geriatr Psychiatry 2005 Mar;13:227–35.

[9] Nierenberg AA, Keefe BR, Leslie VC, et al. Residual symptoms in depressed patients who respond acutely to fluoxetine. J Clin Psychiatry 1999;60:221–5.

[10] Hudson JI, Lipinski JF, Keck PE Jr, et al. Polysomnographic characteristics of young manic patients. Comparison with unipolar depressed patients and normal control subjects. Arch Gen Psychiatry 1992;49:378–83.

[11] Wehr TA, Goodwin FK, Wirz-Justice A, et al. 48-hour sleep-wake cycles in manic-depressive illness: naturalistic observations and sleep deprivation experiments. Arch Gen Psychiatry 1982 May;39:559–65.

[12] Zimanova J, Vojtechovsky M. Sleep deprivation as a potentiation of antidepressive pharmacotherapy? Act Nerv Super (Praha) 1974;16:188–9.

[13] Monti JM, Monti D. Sleep disturbance in generalized anxiety disorder and its treatment. Sleep Med Rev 2000;4:263–76.

[14] Rosenthal M. Tiagabine for the treatment of generalized anxiety disorder: a randomized, open-label, clinical trial with paroxetine as a positive control. J Clin Psychiatry 2003;64:1245–9.

[15] Ross RJ, Ball WA, Sullivan KA, et al. Sleep disturbance as the hallmark of posttraumatic stress disorder. Am J Psychiatry 1989;146:697–707.

[16] Mellman TA, Kumar A, Kulick-Bell R, et al. Nocturnal/daytime urine noradrenergic measures and sleep in combat-related PTSD. Biol Psychiatry 1995;174–9.

[17] Hurwitz TD, Mahowald MW, Kuskowski M, et al. Polysomnographic sleep is not clinically impaired in Vietnam combat veterans with chronic posttraumatic stress disorder. Biol Psychiatry 1998;44:1066–73.

[18] Van Liempt S, Vermetten E, Geuze E, et al. Pharmacotherapeutic treatment of nightmares and insomnia in posttraumatic stress disorder: an overview of the literature. Ann N Y Acad Sci 2006;1071:502–7.

[19] Neylan TC, Metzler TJ, Schoenfeld FB, et al. Fluvoxamine and sleep disturbances in posttraumatic stress disorder. J Trauma Stress 2001;14:461–7.

[20] Chouinard S, Poulin J, Stip E, et al. Sleep in untreated patients with schizophrenia: a meta-analysis. Schizophr Bull 2004;30:957–67.

[21] Doi Y, Minowa M, Uchiyama M, et al. Psychometric assessment of subjective sleep quality using the Japanese version of the Pittsburgh Sleep Quality Index (PSQI-J) in psychiatric disordered and control subjects. Psychiatry Res 2000;97:165–72.

[22] Poulin J, Daoust AM, Forest G, et al. Sleep architecture and its clinical correlates in first episode and neuroleptic-naive patients with schizophrenia. Schizophr Res 2003;62:147–53.

[23] Martin JL, Jeste DV, Ancoli-Israel S. Older schizophrenia patients have more disrupted sleep and circadian rhythms than age-matched comparison subjects. J Psychiatr Res 2005;39: 251–9.

[24] Hofstetter JR, Mayeda AR, Happel CG, et al. Sleep and daily activity preferences in schizophrenia: associations with neurocognition and symptoms. J Nerv Ment Dis 2003;191: 408–10.

[25] Baekeland F, Lundwall L, Shanahan TJ, et al. Clinical correlates of reported sleep disturbance in alcoholics. Q J Stud Alchol 1974;35:1230–41.

[26] Brower KJ, Aldrich MS, Robinson EAR, et al. Insomnia, self-medication, and relapse to alcoholism. Am J Psychiatry 2001;158:399–404.

[27] Gillin JC, Drummond SPA. Medication and substance abuse. In: Kryger MH, Roth T, Dement WC, editors. Principles and practice of sleep medicine. 3rd edition. Philadelphia (PA): W.B. Saunders; 2000. p. 1176–95.

[28] Lobo LL, Tufik S. Effects of alcohol on sleep parameters of sleep-deprived healthy volunteers. Sleep 1997;20:52–9.

[29] Turvey CL, Conwell Y, Jones MP, et al. Risk factors for late-life suicide: a prospective, community-based study. Am J Geriatr Psychiatry 2002;10:398–406.

[30] Agargun MY, Kara H, Solmaz M. Sleep disturbances and suicidal behavior in patients with major depression. J Clin Psychiatry 1997;58:249–51.

[31] Ford DE, Kamerow DB. Epidemiologic study of sleep disturbance and psychiatric disorders: an opportunity for prevention? JAMA 1989;262:1479–84.

[32] Breslau N, Roth T, Rosenthal L, et al. Sleep disturbance and psychiatric disorders: a longitudinal epidemiologic study of young adults. Biol Psychiatry 1996;39:411–8.

[33] Chang PP, Ford DE, Mead LA, et al. Insomnia in young men and subsequent depression. Am J Epidemiol 1997;146:105–14.

[34] Reynolds CF III, Frank E, Houck PR, et al. Which elderly patients with remitted depression remain well with continued interpersonal psychotherapy after discontinuation of antidepressant medication? Am J Psychiatry 1997;154:958–62.

[35] Fava M, McCall WV, Krystal AD, et al. Eszopiclone co-administered with fluoxetine in patients with insomnia co-existing with major depressive disorder. Biol Psychiatry 2006;59: 1052–60.

[36] Nolen WA, Haffmans PM, Bouvy PF, et al. Related Hypnotics as concurrent medication in depression. A placebo-controlled, double-blind comparison of flunitrazepam and lormetazepam in patients with major depression, treated with a (tri)cyclic antidepressant. J Affect Disord 1993;28:179–88.

[37] Asnis GM, Chakraburtty A, DuBoff EA, et al. Zolpidem for persistent insomnia in SSRI-treated depressed patients. J Clin Psychiatry 1999;60:668–76.

[38] Brower KJ. Alcohol's effects on sleep in alcoholics. Alcohol Res Health 2001;25:110–25.

[39] Roehrs T, Papineau K, Rosenthal L, et al. Ethanol as a hypnotic in insomniacs: self administration and effects on sleep and mood. Neuropsychopharmacology 1999;20:279–86.

[40] Skoloda TE, Alterman AI, Gottheil E. Sleep quality reported by drinking and non-drinking alcoholics. In: Gottheil EL, editor. Addiction research and treatment. Elmsford (NY): Pergamon Press; 1979. p. 102–12.

[41] Foster JH, Peters T. Impaired sleep in alcohol misusers and dependent alcoholics and the impact upon outcome. Alcohol Clin Exp Res 1999;23:1044–51.

[42] Drummond SPA, Gillin JC, Smith TL, et al. The sleep of abstinent pure primary alcoholic patients: natural course and relationsip to relapse. Alcohol Clin Exp Res 1988;22: 1796–802.

[43] Nierenberg AA, Adler LA, Peselow E, et al. Trazodone for antidepressant-associated insomnia. Am J Psychiatry 1994;151:1069–72.

[44] American Psychiatric Association. Practice guidelines for major depressive disorder in adults. Am J Psychiatry 1993;150:1–26.

[45] Bauer M, Whybrow PC, Angst J, et al. World federation of societies biological psychiatry task force on treatment guidelines for unipolar depressive disorders. World federation of societies of biological psychiatry (WFSBP) guidelines for biological treatment of unipolar depressive disorders. part 1: acute and continuation treatment of major depressive disorder. World J Biol Psychiatry 2002;3:5–43.

[46] Krystal AD, Fava M, Rubens R, et al. Evaluation of eszopiclone discontinuation after co-therapy with fluoxetine for insomnia with co-existing depression. J Clin Sleep Med, in press.

[47] Starman MN, Schtingart DE. Neuropsychiatric manifestations of patients with Cushing's syndrome. Relationship to cortisol and aderenocorticotropic hormone levels. Arch Intern Med 1981;141:215–9.

[48] Wolkowitz OM, Reus VI. Treatment of depression with antiglucocorticoticoid drugs. Psychosom Med 1999;61:698–711.

[49] Carroll BJ, Curtis GC, Mendels J. Neuroendocrine regulation in depression. Arch Gen Psychiatry 1976;33:1039–58.

[50] Vgontzas AN, Tsigos C, Bixler EO, et al. Chronic insomnia and activity of the stress system: a preliminary study. J Psychosom Res 1998;45(1 Spec No):21–31.

[51] Vgontzas AN, Bixler EO, Lin H-M, et al. Chronic insomnia is associated with nyctohemeral activation of the hypothalamic-pituitary-adrenal axis: clinical implications. J Clin Endocrinol Metab 2001;86:3787–94.

[52] Vgontzas AN, Chrousos GP. Sleep, the hypothalamic pituitary-adrenal axis, and cytokins: multiple interactions and disturbances in sleep disorders. Endo Metab Clin North Am 2002;31:15–36.

[53] Brown ES, Varghese FP, McEwen BS. Association of depression with meeical illness: does cortisol play a role? Biol Psychiatry 2004;55:1–9.

[54] Rodenbeck A, Hajak G. Neuroendocrine dysregulation in primary insomnia. Rev Neurol (Paris) 2001;157:S57–61.

[55] Adrien J. Neurobiological bases for the relation between sleep and depression. Sleep Med Rev 2002;6:341–51.

[56] Landolt HP, Meier V, Burgess HJ, et al. Serotonin-2 receptors and human sleep: effect of a selective antagonist on EEG power spectra. Neuropsychopharmacology 1999;21:455–66.

[57] Oberndorfer S, Saletu-Zyhlarz G, Saletu B. Effects of selective serotonin reuptake inhibitors on objective and subjective sleep quality. Neuropsychobiology 2000;42:69–81.

[58] Brummett BH, Krystal AD, Kuhn C, et al. Sleep quality varies as a function of 5-HTTLPR genotype and stress. Psychosomatic Med, in press.

[59] Collier DA, Stober G, Li T, et al. A novel functional polymorphism within the promoter of the serotonin transporter gene: possible role in susceptibility to affective disorders. Mol Psychiatry 1996;1:453–60.

[60] Caspi A, Sugden K, Moffitt TE, et al. Influence of life stress on depression: moderation by a polymorphism in the 5-HTT gene. Science 2003;301:386–9.

[61] Eley TC, Sugden K, Corsico A, et al. Gene-environment interaction analysis of serotonin system markers with adolescent depression. Mol Psychiatry 2004;9:908–15.

[62] Lenze EJ, Munin MC, Ferrell RE, et al. Association of the serotonin transporter gene-linked polymorphic region (5-HTTLPR) genotype with depression in elderly persons after hip fracture. Am J Geriatr Psychiatry 2005;13:428–32.

[63] Kendler KS, Kuhn JW, Vittum J, et al. The interaction of stressful life events and a serotonin transporter polymorphism in the prediction of episodes of major depression: a replication. Arch Gen Psychiatry 2005;62:529–35.

[64] Pezawas L, Meyer-Lindenberg A, Drabant EM, et al. 5-HTTLPR polymorphism impacts human cingulate-amygdala interactions: a genetic susceptibility mechanism for depression. Nat Neurosci 2005;8:828–34.

[65] Majde JA, Krueger JM. Links between the innate immune system and sleep. J Allergy Clin Immunol 2005;116:1188–98.

[66] Wilson CJ, Finch CE, Cohen HJ. Cytokines and cognition—the case for a head-to-toe inflammatory paradigm. J Am Geriatr Soc 2002;50:2041–56.

[67] Krueger JM, Toth LA. Cytokines as regulators of sleep. Ann N Y Acad Sci 1994;31:299–310.

[68] Benca RM, Quintas J. Sleep and host defenses: a review. Sleep 1997;20:1027–37.

[69] Spath-Schwalbe E, Hansen K, Schmidt F, et al. Acute effects of recombinant human interleukin-6 on endocrine and central nervous sleep functions in healthy men. J Clin Endocrinol Metab 1998;83:1573–9.

[70] von Kanel R, Dimsdale JE, Ancoli-Israel S, et al. Poor sleep is associated with higher plasma proinflammatory cytokine interleukin-6 and procoagulant marker fibrin D-dimer in older caregivers of people with Alzheimer's disease. J Am Geriatr Soc 2006;54:431–7.

[71] Hong S, Mills PJ, Loredo JS, et al. The association between interleukin-6, sleep, and demographic characteristics. Brain Behav Immun 2005;19:165–72.

[72] Spath-Schwalbe E, Lange T, Perras B, et al. Interferon-alpha acutely impairs sleep in healthy humans. Cytokine 2000;12:518–21.

[73] Vgontzas AN, Zoumakis M, Papanicolaou DA, et al. Chronic insomnia is associated with a shift of interleukin-6 and tumor necrosis factor secretion from nighttime to daytime. Metabolism 2002;51:887–92.

[74] Burgos I, Richter L, Klein T, et al. Increased nocturnal interleukin-6 excretion in patients with primary insomnia: a pilot study. Brain Behav Immun 2006;20:246–53.

[75] Vgontzas AN, Zoumakis E, Bixler EO, et al. Adverse effects of modest sleep restriction on sleepiness, performance, and inflammatory cytokines. J Clin Endocrinol Metab 2004;89:2119–26.

[76] Shearer WT, Reuben JM, Mullington JM, et al. Soluble TNF-alpha receptor 1 and IL-6 plasma levels in humans subjected to the sleep deprivation model of spaceflight. J All Clin Immunol 2001;107:165–70.

[77] Simen BB, Duman CH, Simen AA, et al. TNF-alpha signaling in depression and anxiety: behavioral consequences of individual receptor targeting. Biol Psychiatry 2006;59:775–85.

[78] Tsao CW, Lin YS, Chen CC, et al. Cytokines and serotonin transporter in patients with major depression. Prog Neuropsychopharmacol Biol Psychiatry 2006;30:899–905.

[79] Song C, Lin A, Bonaccorso S, et al. The inflammatory response system and the availability of plasma tryptophan in patients with primary sleep disorders and major depression. J Affect Disord 1998;49:211–9.

[80] Motivala SJ, Sarfatti A, Olmos L, et al. Inflammatory markers and sleep disturbance in major depression. Psychosom Med 2005;67:187–94.

[81] Maes M. A review on the acute phase response in major depression. Rev Neurosci 1993;4:407–16.

[82] O'Brien SM, Scott LV, Dinan TG. Cytokines: abnormalities in major depression and implications for pharmacological treatment. Hum Psychopharmacol 2004;19:397–403.

[83] Wichers M, Maes M. The psychoneuroimmuno-pathophysiology of cytokine-induced depression in humans. Int J Neuropsychopharmacol 2002;5:375–88.

[84] Wang J, Dunn AJ. Mouse interleukin-6 stimulates the HPA axis and increases brain tryptophan and serotonin metabolism. Neurochem Int 1998;33:143–54.

[85] Tafet GE, Toister-Achituv M, Shinitzky M. Enhancement of serotonin uptake by cortisol: a possible link between stress and depression. Cogn Affect Behav Neurosci 2001;1:96–104.

[86] Brustolim D, Ribeiro-dos-Santos R, Kast RE, et al. A new chapter opens in anti-inflammatory treatments: the antidepressant bupropion lowers production of tumor necrosis factor-alpha and interferon-gamma in mice. Int Immunopharmacol 2006;6:903–7.

[87] Ayas NT, White DP, Manson JE, et al. A prospective study of sleep duration and coronary heart disease in women. Arch Intern Med 2003;163:205–98.

[88] Elwood P, Hack M, Pickering J, et al. Sleep disturbance, stroke, and heart disease events: evidence from Caerphilly cohort. J Epidemiol Community Health 2006;60:69–73.

[89] Taggi HK, Araujo AB, McKinlay JB. Sleep duration as a risk factor for the development of Type 2 diabetes. Diabetes Care 2006;29:657–61.

[90] Gagnon LM, Patten SB. Major depression and its association with long-term medical conditions. Can J Psychiatry 2002;47:149–52.

[91] Pickup JC. Inflammation and activated innate immunity in the pathogenesis of type 2 diabetes. Diabetes Care 2004;27:813–23.

[92] Cesari M, Penninx BW, Newman AB, et al. Inflammatory markers and onset of cardiovascular events: results from the Health ABC study. Circulation 2003;108:2317–22.

[93] Haddy N, Sass C, Droesch S, et al. IL-6, TNF-alpha and atherosclerosis risk indicators in a healthy family population: the STANISLAS cohort. Atherosclerosis 2003;170:277–83.

INDEX

A

Acetylcholine, in sleep and wakefulness, 848–849

Actigraphy, in children, 1068
in excessive sleepiness syndrome, 923

Adenosine, in sleep and wakefulness, 847–848

Adolescents, delayed sleep phase syndrome in, 1062–1063
sleep and sleep disorders in, **1059–1076**
sleep in, 1059

Advanced sleep phase syndrome (ASPS), chronotherapy for, 994
description of, 993
light therapy for, 994
in older adults, 994
pathophysiology of, 993–994
prevalence of, 993

Age, changes in, depression-related, 1012
sleep and, 844–845, 1075–1076

Alcohol, for insomnia, 882–883

Amino acid neurotransmitters, in depression, 1017

Amphetamine, for narcolepsy, 959–960

Anticonvulsants, for restless legs syndrome, 965

Antidepressants. See also *Tricyclic antidepressants.*
effect on sleep quality, 1021
for insomnia, in anxiety disorder, 1052
off-label use of, 879
past use of, 872
recent use of, 872–873
in women, 1102
sedating, in coexistent insomnia, 881–882
efficacy of, 880–881
hypnotic use of, 879–882
safety of, 881
side effects of, 881

Anxiety, in adolescents, sleep disorders in, 1071
in children, sleep problems in, 1070–1071

Anxiety disorders, sleep and, **1047–1058**
sleep disturbances in, 1115
antidepressants for, novel, 1052
benzodiazepine receptor agonist medications for, 1052
cognitive behavioral treatment of, 1051
relaxation techniques for, 1051

Arousal disorders, 973–974
in children, 1065

Arousal system, in sleep, 896

Attention-deficit/hyperactivity disorder (ADHD), in children, sleep and, 1069–1070

Autism spectrum disorders (ASDs), in children, sleep problems in, 1070
sleep disorders in, 1070

Autonomic nervous system, during sleep, 843

B

Barbiturates, for insomnia, past use of, 871

Behavioral insomnia of childhood, limit-setting type, 1060–1061
sleep-onset association type, 1060

Benzodiazepine receptor agonists (BzRAs), for insomnia, 887, 1052
adverse reactions, 877
dosing of, 887–888
effectiveness of, 875
effects of, 887
efficacy of, 874–875
FDA approved, 873–874
intermittent administration of, 875
rebound insomnia from, 877
safety of, 876–877
side effects of, 887

Benzodiazepines, for insomnia, past use of, 871
in women, 1102–1103

Bipolar affective disorder, genetic factors in, 1019
sleep architecture in, 1011–1012
sleep loss in, 1022

0193-953X/06/$ – see front matter
doi:10.1016/S0193-953X(06)00094-3

Moving?

Make sure your subscription moves with you!

To notify us of your new address, find your **Clinics Account Number** (located on your mailing label above your name), and contact customer service at:

E-mail: elspcs@elsevier.com

800-654-2452 (subscribers in the U.S. & Canada)
407-345-4000 (subscribers outside of the U.S. & Canada)

Fax number: 407-363-9661

Elsevier Periodicals Customer Service
6277 Sea Harbor Drive
Orlando, FL 32887-4800

*To ensure uninterrupted delivery of your subscription, please notify us at least 4 weeks in advance of move.

United States Postal Service
Statement of Ownership, Management, and Circulation

1. Publication Title	2. Publication Number								3. Filing Date
Psychiatric Clinics of North America	0	0	0	—	7	0	0	3	9/15/06

4. Issue Frequency	5. Number of Issues Published Annually	6. Annual Subscription Price
Mar, Jun, Sep, Dec	4	$180.00

7. Complete Mailing Address of Known Office of Publication *(Not printer) (Street, city, county, state, and ZIP+4)*

Elsevier Inc.
360 Park Avenue South
New York, NY 10010-1710

Contact Person
Sarah Carmichael
Telephone
(215) 239-3681

8. Complete Mailing Address of Headquarters or General Business Office of Publisher *(Not printer)*

Elsevier Inc., 360 Park Avenue South, New York, NY 10010-1710

9. Full Names and Complete Mailing Addresses of Publisher, Editor, and Managing Editor *(Do not leave blank)*

Publisher *(Name and complete mailing address)*

John Schrefer, Elsevier Inc., 1600 John F. Kennedy Blvd., Suite 1800, Philadelphia, PA 19103-2899

Editor *(Name and complete mailing address)*

Sarah Barth, Elsevier Inc., 1600 John F. Kennedy Blvd., Suite 1800, Philadelphia, PA 19103-2899

Managing Editor *(Name and complete mailing address)*

Catherine Bewick, Elsevier Inc., 1600 John F. Kennedy Blvd., Suite 1800, Philadelphia, PA 19103-2899

10. Owner *(Do not leave blank. If the publication is owned by a corporation, give the name and address of the corporation immediately followed by the names and addresses of all stockholders owning or holding 1 percent or more of the total amount of stock. If not owned by a corporation, give the names and addresses of the individual owners. If owned by a partnership or other unincorporated firm, give its name and address as well as those of each individual owner. If the publication is published by a nonprofit organization, give its name and address.)*

Full Name	Complete Mailing Address
Wholly owned subsidiary of	4520 East-West Highway
Reed/Elsevier Inc., US holdings	Bethesda, MD 20814

11. Known Bondholders, Mortgagees, and Other Security Holders Owning or Holding 1 Percent or More of Total Amount of Bonds, Mortgages, or Other Securities. If none, check box ➤ None

Full Name	Complete Mailing Address
N/A	

12. Tax Status *(For completion by nonprofit organizations authorized to mail at nonprofit rates) (Check one)*
The purpose, function, and nonprofit status of this organization and the exempt status for federal income tax purposes:
Has Not Changed During Preceding 12 Months
Has Changed During Preceding 12 Months *(Publisher must submit explanation of change with this statement)*
(See Instructions on Reverse)

PS Form 3526, October 1999

---

13. Publication Title		14. Issue Date for Circulation Data Below
Psychiatric Clinics of North America		September, 2006

15.	Extent and Nature of Circulation		Average No. Copies Each Issue During Preceding 12 Months	No. Copies of Single Issue Published Nearest to Filing Date
a.	Total Number of Copies *(Net press run)*		2,675	2,500
b. Paid and/or Requested Circulation	(1)	Paid/Requested Outside-County Mail Subscriptions Stated on Form 3541. *(Include advertiser's proof and exchange copies)*	1,405	1,299
	(2)	Paid In-County Subscriptions Stated on Form 3541 *(Include advertiser's proof and exchange copies)*		
	(3)	Sales Through Dealers and Carriers, Street Vendors, Counter Sales, and Other Non-USPS Paid Distribution	394	406
	(4)	Other Classes Mailed Through the USPS		
c.	Total Paid and/or Requested Circulation *(Sum of 15b. (1), (2), (3), and (4))* ➤		1,799	1,705
d. Free Distribution by Mail *(Samples, complimentary, and other free)*	(1)	Outside-County as Stated on Form 3541	113	114
	(2)	In-County as Stated on Form 3541		
	(3)	Other Classes Mailed Through the USPS		
e.	Free Distribution Outside the Mail *(Carriers or other means)* ➤		113	114
f.	Total Free Distribution *(Sum of 15d. and 15e.)* ➤			
g.	Total Distribution *(Sum of 15c. and 15f)* ➤		1,912	1,819
h.	Copies not Distributed		763	681
i.	Total *(Sum of 15g. and h.)* ➤		2,675	2,500
j.	Percent Paid and/or Requested Circulation *(15c. divided by 15g. times 100)*		94.09%	93.73%

16. Publication of Statement of Ownership
Publication required. Will be printed in the **December 2006** issue of this publication. ☐ Publication not required

17. Signature and Title of Editor, Publisher, Business Manager, or Owner   Date

[signature]
John Tanucci – Executive Director of Subscription Services   9/15/06

I certify that all information furnished on this form is true and complete. I understand that anyone who furnishes false or misleading information on this form or who omits material or information requested on the form may be subject to criminal sanctions (including fines and imprisonment) and/or civil sanctions (including civil penalties).

Instructions to Publishers

1. Complete and file one copy of this form with your postmaster annually on or before October 1. Keep a copy of the completed form for your records.
2. In cases where the stockholder or security holder is a trustee, include in items 10 and 11 the name of the person or corporation for whom the trustee is acting. Also include the names and addresses of individuals who are stockholders who own or hold 1 percent or more of the total amount of bonds, mortgages, or other securities of the publishing corporation. In item 11, if none, check the box. Use blank sheets if more space is required.
3. Be sure to furnish all circulation information called for in item 15. Free circulation must be shown in items 15d, e, and f.
4. Item 15h., Copies not Distributed, must include (1) newsstand copies originally stated on Form 3541, and returned to the publisher, (2) estimated returns from news agents, and (3), copies for office use, leftovers, spoiled, and all other copies not distributed.
5. If the publication had Periodicals authorization as a general or requester publication, this Statement of Ownership, Management, and Circulation must be published; it must be printed in any issue in October or, if the publication is not published during October, the first issue printed after October.
6. In item 16, indicate the date of the issue in which this Statement of Ownership will be published.
7. Item 17 must be signed.
Failure to file or publish a statement of ownership may lead to suspension of Periodicals authorization.

PS Form **3526**, October 1999 *(Reverse)*